Hct	Hematocrit	**NTG**	Nitroglycerin
HDL	High-density lipid	**PAC**	Premature atrial contraction
Hgb	Hemoglobin	**PAP**	Pulmonary artery pressure
HR	Heart rate	**PCWP**	Pulmonary capillary wedge pressure
HTN	Hypertension	**PND**	Paroxysmal nocturnal dyspnea
IABP	Intra-aortic balloon pump	**PT**	Prothrombin time
ICS	Intercostal space	**PTT**	Partial thromboplastin time
IE	Infective endocarditis	**PTCA**	Percutaneous transluminal coronary angioplasty
JVD	Jugular venous distention	**PVC**	Premature ventricular contraction
JVP	Jugular venous pulse	**PVR**	Pulmonary vascular resistance
LA	Left atrium; left atrial	**RA**	Right atrium; right atrial
LAD	Left anterior descending	**RAP**	Right atrial pressure
LBBB	Left bundle branch block	**RBBB**	Right bundle branch block
LDH	Lactate dehydrogenase	**RCA**	Right coronary artery
LDL	Low-density lipid	**RV**	Right ventricle; right ventricular
LOC	Level of consciousness (loss of consciousness)	**RVH**	Right ventricular hypertrophy
LSB	Left sternal border	**SA**	Sinoatrial
LV	Left ventricle; left ventricular	**SBE**	Subacute bacterial endocarditis
LVEDP	Left ventricular end-diastolic pressure	**SOB**	Shortness of breath
LVH	Left ventricular hypertrophy	**SVR**	Systemic vascular resistance
MAP	Mean arterial pressure	**t-PA**	Tissue-plasminogen activator
MCL	Modified chest lead	**VAD**	Ventricular assist device
MI	Myocardial infarction	**VHD**	Valvular heart disease
MRI	Magnetic resonance imaging	**VLDL**	Very low density lipid
MVo$_2$	Myocardial oxygen consumption	**VSD**	Ventricular septal defect
MVP	Mitral valve prolapse	**WBC**	White blood cell

CARDIOVASCULAR DISORDERS

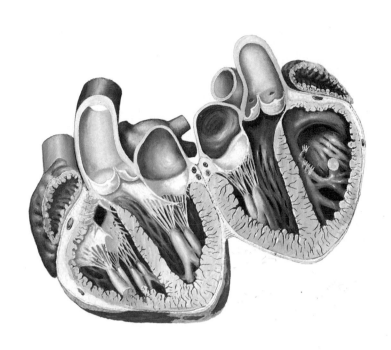

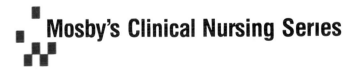

Mosby's Clinical Nursing Series

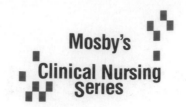

Mosby's Clinical Nursing Series

Cardiovascular Disorders
by Mary Canobbio

Respiratory Disorders
by Susan Wilson and June Thompson

Infectious Diseases
by Deanna Grimes

Immunologic Disorders
by Christine Mudge-Grout

Neurologic Disorders
by Victor Campbell

Musculoskeletal Disorders
by Leona Mourad

Gastrointestinal Disorders
by Debra Broadwell

Renal and Genitourinary Disorders
by Dorothy Brundage and Mikel Gray

Neoplastic and Hematologic Disorders
by Anne Belcher

Eye, Ear, Nose, and Throat Disorders
by Jane Hirsch

CARDIOVASCULAR DISORDERS

MARY M. CANOBBIO, RN, MN

Cardiovascular Clinical Specialist
Assistant Clinical Professor
School of Nursing
University of California, Los Angeles
Los Angeles, California

THE C. V. MOSBY COMPANY

SAINT LOUIS ▪ BALTIMORE ▪ PHILADELPHIA ▪ TORONTO 1990

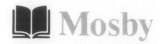

Editor: *William Grayson Brottmiller*
Senior developmental editor: *Sally Adkisson*
Developmental writer: *Daphna Gregg*
Project Manager: *Mark Spann*
Designer: *Liz Fett*

Printed in the United States of America

The C.V. Mosby Company
11830 Westline Industrial Drive, St. Louis, Missouri 63146

C/C/VH 9 8 7 6 5 4 3 2 1

Contributors

Mary Liz Bilodeau, RN, MS, CCRN, CS
Clinical Nurse Specialist
Intensive Care Nursing Service
Massachusetts General Hospital
Boston, Massachusetts

Adrienne Greco, RN, MSN
Cardiovascular Clinical Nurse Specialist
Coordinator, Acute Myocardial Infarction Program
The Heart Institute
The Hospital of the Good Samaritan
Los Angeles, California

Kenneth T. Kokubun, Pharm. D.
Director of Inpatient Pharmacy Services
Kaiser Foundation Hospital
Harbor City, California

Preface

Cardiovascular Disorders is the first volume in *Mosby's Clinical Nursing Series*, a new kind of resource for practicing nurses.

The *Series* is the result of the most elaborate market research ever undertaken by The C.V. Mosby Company. We first surveyed hundreds of working nurses to determine what kind of resources practicing nurses want in order to meet their advanced information needs. We then approached clinical specialists—proven authors and experts in 10 practice areas, from cardiovascular to ENT—and asked them to develop a common format that would meet the needs of nurses in practice, as specified by the survey respondents. This plan was then presented to nine focus groups composed of working nurses over a period of 18 months. The plan was refined between each group, and in the later stages we published a 32-page full-color sample of this book so that detailed changes could be made to improve the physical layout and appearance of the book, section by section and page by page.

The result is a new genre of professional books for nursing professionals.

Cardiovascular Nursing begins with an innovative Color Atlas of Structure and Function. This is not a mere review of anatomy and physiology taught in undergraduate curriculums; it is actually a collection of highly detailed full-color drawings designed to explain how cardiovascular problems develop. Every effort was made to explain cardiovascular structure and function in a way that rationalizes nursing interventions.

Chapter 2 is a pictorial guide to the nurse's assessment of the cardiovascular system. Clear, full-color photographs show proper position and technique in sharp detail, aided by concise instructions, rationales, and tips.

Chapter 3 presents the latest in diagnostic tests, again using full-color photographs of equipment, techniques, monitors, and output. A consistent format for each diagnostic procedure gives nurses information about the purpose of the test, indications and contraindications, and nursing care associated with each test, including patient teaching.

Chapters 4, 5, and 6 present the nursing care of patients experiencing specific cardiac disorders, vascular disorders, and major medical interventions, respectively. Nurses in our focus groups specifically requested information on vascular disorders, which is hard to obtain elsewhere.

Each disease is presented in a format that you invented to meet your advanced practice needs. Information on pathophysiology answers questions nurses often have. A unique box alerting nurses to possible complications provides this information to the health professionals in the best position to observe, respond to, and report dangerous changes in patient conditions.

Definitive diagnostic tests and the physician's treatment plan are briefly reviewed to promote collaborative care among members of the health care team.

The heart of the book is the nursing care, presented according to the nursing process. These pages are bordered in red to make them easy to find and use on the unit. The nursing care is structured to integrate the five steps of the nursing process, centered around appropriate nursing diagnoses accepted by the North American Nursing Diagnosis Association (NANDA). The material can be used to develop individualized care plans quickly and accurately, and it meets the standards of nursing care required by the Joint Commission on the Accreditation of Hospitals (JCAH). By facilitating the development of individualized and authoritative care plans, this book can actually save you time to spend on direct patient care.

In response to requests from scores of nurses participating in our research, a distinctive feature of this book is its use in patient teaching. Background information on diseases and medical interventions enables nurses to answer with authority questions patients often ask. The illustrations in the book, particularly those in the Color Atlas and diagnostic tests chapters, are specifically designed to support patient teaching. Chapter 7 consists of 16 Patient Teaching Guides written at a ninth-grade level so they can be copied, distributed to patients and their families, and used for self-care after discharge. Patient teaching sections in each care plan provide nurses with checklists of concepts to teach, promoting this increasingly vital aspect of nursing care.

The book concludes with a concise guide to cardiovascular drugs and, inside the back cover, a "yellow pages" directory to organizations and other resources on cardiovascular health for nurses and patients.

This book is intended for medical-surgical nurses, who invariably care for patients with acute cardiovascular disorders. Critical care nurses in our survey and focus groups also expressed a need for the book. We expect that students will find the book an indispensable help in developing clinical skills and judgment in caring for patients with cardiovascular disorders, as it will also be for nurses returning to practice after a hiatus, nurses seeking advanced certification, and nurses transferring to medical-surgical or critical-care settings.

We hope that this book contributes to the advancement of professional nursing by serving as a first step toward a body of professional literature for nurses to call their own.

Contents

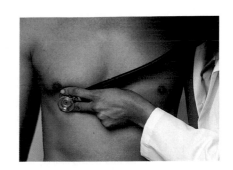
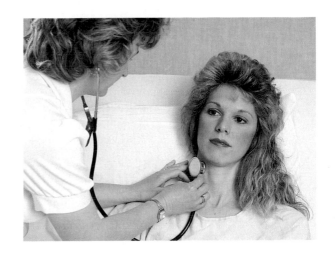
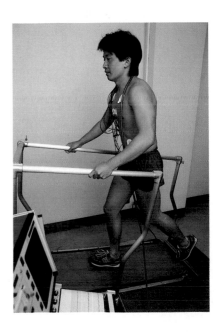

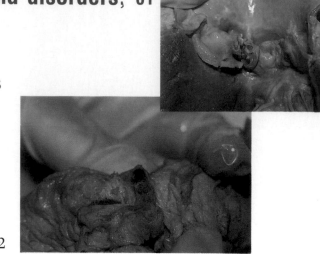
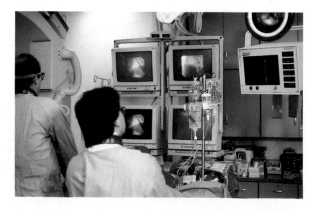

7 Patient teaching guides, 262

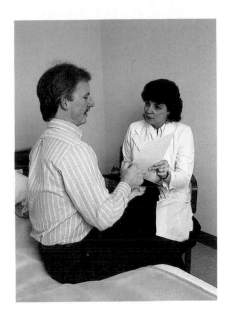

8 Cardiovascular drugs, 283

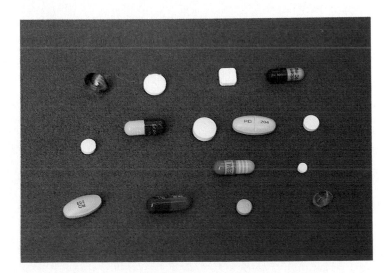

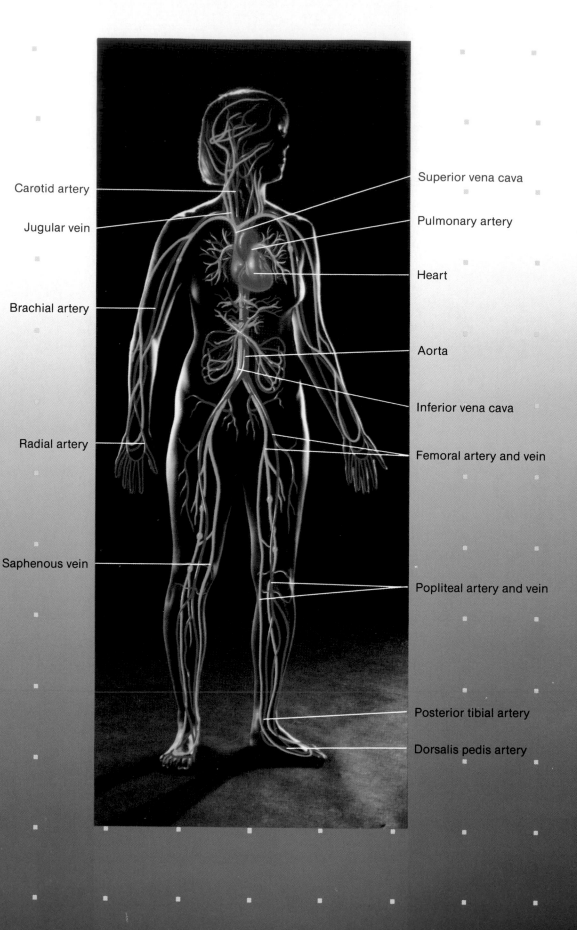

Carotid artery

Jugular vein

Brachial artery

Radial artery

Saphenous vein

Superior vena cava

Pulmonary artery

Heart

Aorta

Inferior vena cava

Femoral artery and vein

Popliteal artery and vein

Posterior tibial artery

Dorsalis pedis artery

CHAPTER 1

Color Atlas of Cardiovascular Structure and Function

The primary purpose of the cardiovascular system is to supply enough blood to peripheral tissues to meet their metabolic demands at all times. Through the arterial system, it supplies organs and tissues throughout the body with oxygen, nutrients, hormones, and immunologic substances. Through venous return it removes wastes from tissues, routing deoxygenated blood through the lungs for excretion of metabolic wastes.

Although relatively small, the heart carries an impressive workload over a lifetime. It beats 60 to 100 times per minute without resting. The heart and circulatory system must be able to adjust to changes in the body's metabolic demands, often in a matter of seconds. For example, vigorous exercise can increase metabolic requirements of muscles as much as 20 times over their needs during rest. The heart responds by accelerating its rate to increase cardiac output. Vessels undergo local changes to redistribute blood flow, shunting a greater proportion of blood to muscle tissues and away from internal organs.

To meet the demands placed on it, the heart possesses several unique properties. As a pump, it expands and contracts without placing stress on the cardiac muscle. It can withstand continual activity without developing muscle fatigue. It also has the inherent capability to generate electrical impulses that maintain proper rhythm regardless of other factors, such as heart rate, and ignores inappropriate electrical signals that would overstimulate the cardiac muscle.

A healthy cardiovascular system seldom calls attention to itself, even though it performs a remarkable number of complex activities every minute throughout a lifetime.

The heart weighs only 250 to 350 g and is about the size of a fist. With each beat the heart pumps an average of 148 ml, totalling more than 6,813 liters per day.

FIGURE 1-1
Location of heart in
chest cavity.

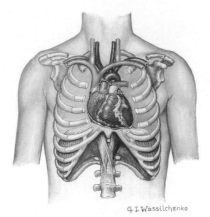

G. J. Wassilchenko

FIGURE 1-2
Cross section of left
ventricular heart mus-
cle.

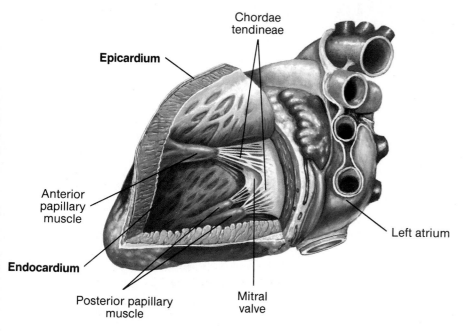

Chordae
tendineae

Epicardium

Anterior
papillary
muscle

Endocardium

Posterior papillary
muscle

Mitral
valve

Left atrium

FIGURE 1-3
Cross section of cardiac muscle.

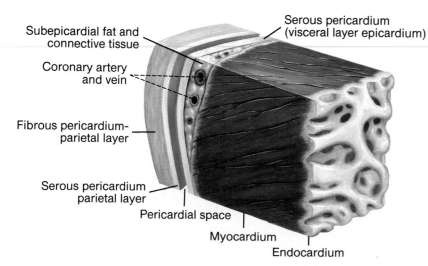

Subepicardial fat and
connective tissue

Coronary artery
and vein

Fibrous pericardium-
parietal layer

Serous pericardium
parietal layer

Pericardial space

Myocardium

Endocardium

Serous pericardium
(visceral layer epicardium)

LOCATION OF THE HEART

The heart is a hollow, muscular organ situated in the middle of the thoracic cavity, cradled in a cage of bone, cartilage, and muscle (Figure 1-1). It lies just left of the midline of the mediastinum and just above the diaphragm. The heart is protected anteriorly by the sternum and posteriorly by the vertebral column. The lungs are located on either side. The entire heart is enclosed in the fluid-filled pericardial sac (Figures 1-4 and 1-5). The pericardium helps to shield the heart against infection and trauma and aids cardiac function by helping with the free pumping motion of the heart.

CARDIAC MUSCLE

The cardiac muscle is arranged in three layers (Figures 1-2 and 1-3):
 The epicardium—the outermost layer
 The myocardium—the contractile muscle layer
 The endocardium—the inner layer
The **epicardium** covers the surface of the heart and extends to the great vessels. It is a visceral layer of serous pericardium.

The **myocardium,** the center layer of thick muscular tissue, is responsible for the major pumping action of the ventricles. Myocardial cells are composed of striated muscle fibrils consisting of contractile elements known as myofibrils (described on page 9).

The **endocardium** is made up of a thin layer of endothelium and a thin layer of underlying connective tissue. It lines the inner chambers of the heart, valves, chordae tendineae, and papillary muscles.

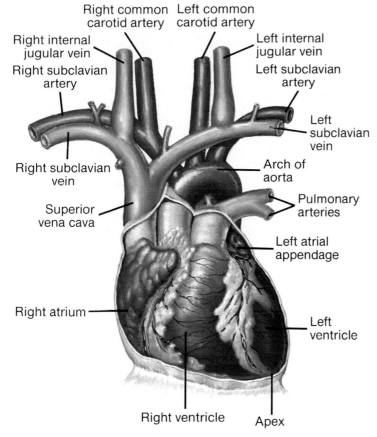

FIGURE 1-4
Heart within the pericardium.

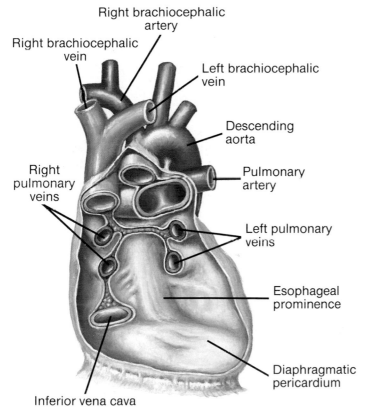

FIGURE 1-5
Pericardial sac with heart removed (frontal view).

PERICARDIUM

The heart is encased in the **pericardium,** a loose, double-walled sac of elastic connective tissue that shields the heart from trauma and infection (Figures 1-4 and 1-5). The outer layer, the fibrous pericardium, is a strong, loosely fitting sac that surrounds the heart. The inner layer, the serous pericardium, is made up of the parietal layer and the visceral layer. The parietal layer lines the inside of the fibrous pericardium. The visceral layer (also known as the epicardium) adheres to the outside of the heart. This layer forms the inner layer of the heart muscle (Figure 1-3).

The space between the visceral and parietal layers, known as the **pericardial space,** contains a clear, lymphlike fluid that is secreted by the serous membrane. This fluid lubricates the surface of the heart, allowing easy movement during contraction and expansion of the heart. The pericardial space, which normally contains 10 to 30 ml of fluid, can hold up to 300 ml without interfering with cardiac function. In certain chronic disease states, the pericardial space can hold up to a liter of fluid. However, with sudden rapid filling, as little as 100 ml can compromise cardiac function and cause cardiac tamponade.

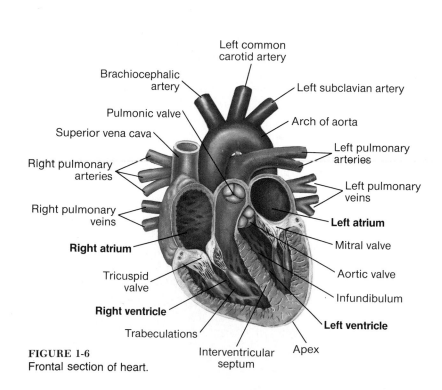

CARDIAC CHAMBERS

The heart has four chambers, but it functions as a two-sided pump. The atria serve as reservoirs, and the ventricles provide the pumping action (Figure 1-6). The right side is a low-pressure system that pumps venous (deoxygenated) blood to the lungs. The left side is a high-pressure system that propels arterial (oxygenated) blood into the systemic circulation. As a result of this difference in pressure, the walls of the left ventricle are thicker than those of the right.

Right Atrium

The **right atrium** (RA) receives systemic venous blood from the **superior vena cava** (SVC), which drains the upper portion of the body, and from the **inferior vena cava** (IVC), which drains blood from the lower extremities. The **coronary sinus** (Figure 1-21) also empties into the RA just above the tricuspid valve. The pressure exerted during normal filling of the RA varies with respira-

tion. Because fluid moves more rapidly from high pressure areas to low pressure areas, right atrial filling occurs primarily during inspiration, when pressure inside the right atrium drops below that of the veins outside the chest cavity.

Right Ventricle

The **right ventricle** (RV) is normally the most anterior chamber of the heart and lies directly beneath the sternum. Functionally the RV can be divided into an inflow and an outflow tract. The inflow tract includes the tricuspid area and the criss cross muscular bands called trabeculations, which make up the inner surface of the ventricle. The outflow tract is commonly referred to as the infundibulum and extends to the pulmonary artery.

Left Atrium

The **left atrium** (LA), the most posterior cardiac structure, receives oxygenated blood from the lungs via the right and left pulmonary veins. The wall of the LA is slightly thicker than that of the RA. Filling pressures vary little with respiration.

Left Ventricle

The **left ventricle** (LV) lies posterior to and to the left of the RV. It is ellipsoid, with a wall composed of thick muscular tissue measuring 8 to 16 mm, two to three times thicker than that of the RV (3 to 5 mm). This increased muscle mass is necessary to generate sufficient pressure to propel blood into the systemic circulation. The inflow tract is formed by the mitral annulus, the two mitral leaflets, and the chordae tendineae. The outflow tract is surrounded by the anterior mitral leaflet, the interventricular septum, and the left ventricular free wall. During systole, blood is propelled superiorly and to the right across the aortic valve.

Normal oxygen saturations

RA 75%	LA 95%
RV 75%	LV 95%

RA 0-7 mm Hg	LA 5-10 mm Hg
RV 20-25 mm Hg (peak-systolic) 0-5 mm Hg (end-diastolic)	LV 100-120 mm Hg (peak-systolic) 0-10 mm Hg (end-diastolic)

FIGURE 1-6
Frontal section of heart.

Left common carotid artery
Brachiocephalic artery
Pulmonic valve
Superior vena cava
Right pulmonary arteries
Right pulmonary veins
Right atrium
Tricuspid valve
Right ventricle
Trabeculations
Interventricular septum
Apex
Left subclavian artery
Arch of aorta
Left pulmonary arteries
Left pulmonary veins
Left atrium
Mitral valve
Aortic valve
Infundibulum
Left ventricle

CARDIAC VALVES

The heart's efficiency as a pump depends on the four cardiac valves, whose sole function is to ensure one-way blood flow and prevent backflow (Figures 1-6 and 1-7).

Atrioventricular Valves

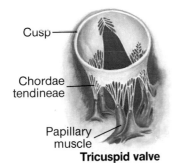

Cusp

Chordae tendineae

Papillary muscle

Tricuspid valve

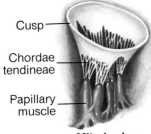

Cusp

Chordae tendineae

Papillary muscle

Mitral valve

The two **atrioventricular (AV) valves** are functionally similar but differ in several anatomic details. They are positioned between the atria and the ventricles, with the tricuspid valve on the right and the mitral valve on the left. The anatomic elements that make up the tricuspid and mitral valves include the **annulus fibrosus** (a tough, fibrous ring), the valvular tissue (leaflets) to which the **chordae tendineae** are attached, and the **papillary muscles** connecting the chordae to the floor of the ventricular wall. This arrangement allows the leaflets to balloon upward during ventricular systole but prevents eversion of the cusps into the atria. These components should be considered as a single unit, since disruption of any one element can result in serious hemodynamic dysfunction.

The **tricuspid valve** is larger in diameter and thinner than the mitral valve and has three separate leaflets: anterior, posterior, and septal. Competence of the leaflets depends on RV lateral wall function. The septal leaflet attaches to portions of the interventricular septum and sits close to the AV node.

The **mitral valve** has two leaflets. The anterior leaflet descends deep into the LV during diastole, snapping quickly back during systole to meet the posterior leaflet. The posterior leaflet is smaller and more restricted in its motion. The orifice is normally 4 to 6 cm^2 in diameter in adults.

Atrial contraction forces the AV valves open and propels blood into the ventricles. Ventricular contraction creates pressure against the leaflets, which balloon upward toward the atria. The chordae tendineae restrain the leaflets from opening into the atria.

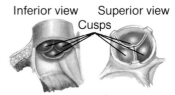

Inferior view   Superior view

Cusps

Semilunar valves

The two **semilunar valves** are the pulmonic and aortic valves. They are smaller than the AV valves. Each is composed of three pocket-like valve leaflets and is surrounded by an annulus. The normal valve orifice is 2.6 to 3.6 cm^2. The names of the valves describe their locations—the **pulmonic valve** lies between the right ventricle and the pulmonary artery, and the **aortic valve** leads from the left ventricle into the aorta.

Pressure inside the ventricles during contraction forces the valves open, and loss of pressure at the end of diastole allows them to close.

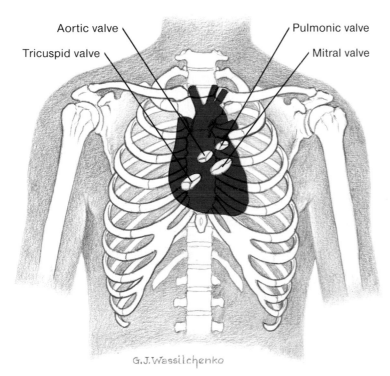

Aortic valve

Tricuspid valve

Pulmonic valve

Mitral valve

G.J. Wassilchenko

FIGURE 1-7
Anatomic location of cardiac valves.

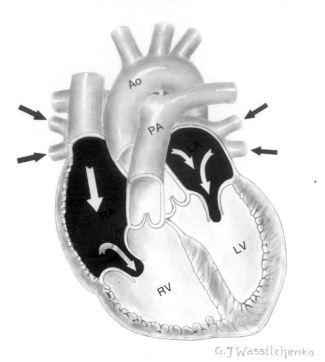

FIGURE 1-8
Blood flow during diastole.

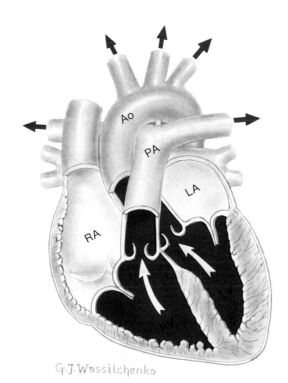

FIGURE 1-9
Blood flow during systole.

CARDIAC CYCLE

The cardiac cycle is divided into two phases—diastole and systole. During **diastole** the ventricles relax and fill with blood from the atria. During **systole** blood is ejected from the ventricles.

Diastole

Diastole has two distinct phases. In the first phase, the atria contract and force the AV valves open, propelling about 70% of the blood from the atria into the relaxed ventricles (Figures 1-8 and 1-10). In the second phase, the flow of blood slows until atrial contraction accelerates, forcing the remainder of the blood into the ventricles. This added atrial thrust compels diastolic filling of the ventricles and is reflected as the "a" wave on the atrial pressure tracing (Figure 1-12). Blood remaining in the ventricles at the end of diastole is the **end-diastolic volume.**

Systole

Once the ventricles are filled, systole, or ejection, begins. Systolic pressure rises during the initial phase, forcing the AV valves to snap shut and preventing backflow into the atria, and the ventricles begin contracting (Figures 1-9 and 1-11). Closure of the AV valves is the source of the first heart sound (S_1). Once ventricular pressure exceeds aortic pressure, the semilunar valves open, and blood is ejected into the pulmonary artery and aorta.

As the ejection phase ends, the ventricular muscle relaxes, decreasing intraventricular pressures and causing reversal of blood flow in the aorta, which forces the semilunar valves to close. The onset of ventricular relaxation with the closure of the semilunar valves is the source of the second heart sound (S_2), reflected by a dicrotic notch on the pressure waveform of the aorta.

After the semilunar valves close, ventricular pressure falls rapidly. On the atrial pressure tracing the "v" wave reflects this period in which the ventricles are relaxing and blood is entering the atrium (Figure 1-12). The down sloping following the "v" wave is the signal that ventricular relaxation is complete.

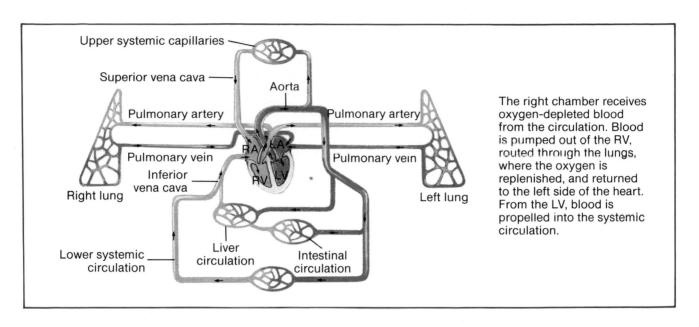

Upper systemic capillaries

Superior vena cava

Aorta

Pulmonary artery

Pulmonary artery

Pulmonary vein

Pulmonary vein

Inferior vena cava

RA LA

RV LV

Right lung

Left lung

Lower systemic circulation

Liver circulation

Intestinal circulation

The right chamber receives oxygen-depleted blood from the circulation. Blood is pumped out of the RV, routed through the lungs, where the oxygen is replenished, and returned to the left side of the heart. From the LV, blood is propelled into the systemic circulation.

FIGURE 1-10
Cardiac valves during diastole (superior view).

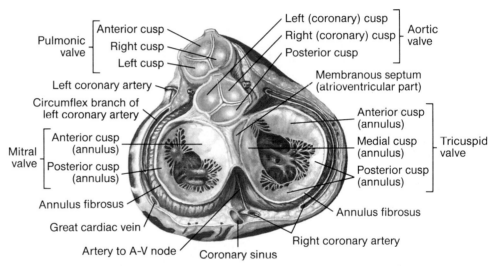

Pulmonic valve — Anterior cusp
Right cusp
Left cusp

Left (coronary) cusp
Right (coronary) cusp — Aortic valve
Posterior cusp

Left coronary artery

Circumflex branch of left coronary artery

Membranous septum (atrioventricular part)

Mitral valve — Anterior cusp (annulus)
Posterior cusp (annulus)

Anterior cusp (annulus)
Medial cusp (annulus) — Tricuspid valve
Posterior cusp (annulus)

Annulus fibrosus

Annulus fibrosus

Great cardiac vein

Artery to A-V node

Coronary sinus

Right coronary artery

FIGURE 1-11
Cardiac valves during systole (superior view).

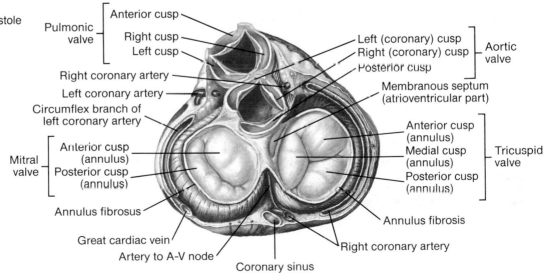

Pulmonic valve — Anterior cusp
Right cusp
Left cusp

Right coronary artery

Left coronary artery

Circumflex branch of left coronary artery

Left (coronary) cusp
Right (coronary) cusp — Aortic valve
Posterior cusp

Membranous septum (atrioventricular part)

Mitral valve — Anterior cusp (annulus)
Posterior cusp (annulus)

Anterior cusp (annulus)
Medial cusp (annulus) — Tricuspid valve
Posterior cusp (annulus)

Annulus fibrosus

Annulus fibrosis

Great cardiac vein

Artery to A-V node

Coronary sinus

Right coronary artery

CARDIAC FUNCTION

Cardiac function is based on the adequacy of the cardiac output (CO), which is the amount of blood pumped from the left ventricle per minute. (See box on Cardiac Output.) The circulating volume of blood to the heart varies according to the needs of tissue cells. Any increase in the work of the cells causes an increase in blood flow and a subsequent increase in the work of the heart and myocardial oxygen consumption (MVo_2).

The primary factors affecting CO include the following:
Preload—filling of the heart during diastole
Afterload—the resistance against which the heart must pump
Contractility of heart muscle
Heart rate

CARDIAC OUTPUT

Cardiac output (CO) is calculated by multiplying the amount of blood ejected from one ventricle with one heart beat (stroke volume, or SV) by the heart rate (HR, the number of times the heart beats per minute [bpm]).

$$CO = SV \times HR$$

For a normal 150 pound (70 kg) adult at rest, the CO is 5 L/minute.

Preload

Preload is the degree of fiber stretch that occurs as a result of load or tension placed on the muscle before contraction. The term *load* refers to the quantity of blood; the term *tension* refers to the pressure it exerts in the left ventricle at the end of diastole (filling) just before systole (ejection). This is commonly referred to as **left ventricular end-diastolic pressure** (LVEDP) (Figure 1-12).

The intrinsic ability of the muscle fibers to stretch in response to increasing loads of incoming blood (venous return) is related to the Frank-Starling principle (see box).

FRANK-STARLING PRINCIPLE

The greater the fiber stretch before systole, the stronger the ventricular contraction. In other words, the more blood that enters the ventricle during diastole, the greater the quantity of blood that will be pumped during systole.

Afterload

Afterload is the resistance to blood flow as it leaves the ventricles. Afterload is a function of both arterial pressure and left ventricular size. Any increase in vascular resistance (pressure against which the heart is forced to pump) causes increased ventricular contractility in order to maintain stroke volume and cardiac output. For example, as arterial pressure increases, more energy is required to generate enough pressure to eject blood. As more energy is required for ventricular systole, the myocardial oxygen demand increases. Conditions that increase afterload include those causing obstruction to ventricular outflow, such as aortic stenosis, and those causing high peripheral vascular resistance, such as hypertension.

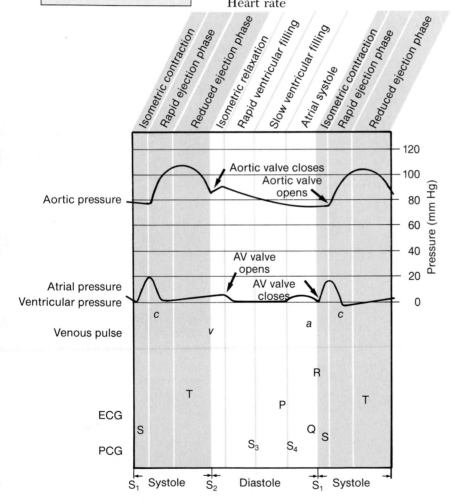

FIGURE 1-12
Events of cardiac cycle. Shows ventricular pressures in systole and diastole, ECG, heart sounds (phonocardiogram, or PCG), and venous pressure.

Contractility of Heart Muscle

The myocardium is a unique muscle with intrinsic properties that contribute to its effective pumping action. The ability of cardiac cells to contract in an organized manner rests in the unique structure of myocardial cells. Thin membranes (intercalated discs) loosely join the myocardial cells. Within each myocardial cell are numerous striated muscle cells that contain fibers called myofibrils (Figure 1-13).

The **myofibrils** are composed of repeating structures called **sarcomeres,** the basic protein units responsible for contraction. Sarcomeres are longitudinally arranged, with dark Z lines dividing the myofibrils. The area between two Z lines is composed of overlapping thick (myosin) and thin (actin) myofilaments. These myofilaments are the contractile elements of the heart. The actin filaments are referred to as the I bands, and the myosin filaments are referred to as the A bands. When heart muscle is stimulated, the length of the A band remains constant, but the I band shortens, pulling actin filament toward the center of the sarcomere (H zone). The myofibrils slide together and overlap, producing a contraction of the cell. During relaxation, the filaments pull away from each other and return to their former positions.

Heart Rate

Cardiac output can be decreased or increased directly by changes in heart rate. The normal heart rate is 60 to 100 bpm. With a heart rate of less than 40 bpm, the cardiac output often falls. This leads to an increased tendency for dysrhythmias, because inherent automaticity contributes to uncoordinated myocardial contraction, which further depresses contractility. Increased heart rates reduce the time that the heart is in diastole. As a result, left ventricular filling decreases, as does coronary blood flow to the myocardium.

Inotropic Force: Force of Contraction
Chronotropic Force: Rate of Contraction

FACTORS AFFECTING THE HEART'S CONTRACTILITY

Decreased contractility is generally caused by loss of contractile muscle mass due to injury, disease, dysrhythmias, or drugs

Increased contractility can be caused by sympathetic nerve stimulation or inotropic drugs, such as isoproterenol, epinephrine, and dopamine

---

Key
Myosin = black fibers
Actin = red fibers

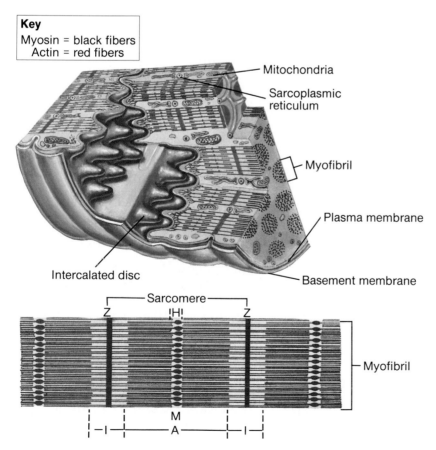

Mitochondria
Sarcoplasmic reticulum
Myofibril
Plasma membrane
Basement membrane
Intercalated disc
Sarcomere
Z   !H!   Z
Myofibril
M
I   A   I

FIGURE 1-13
Magnification of cardiac muscle cell.

ARTERIAL PRESSURE AND PERIPHERAL RESISTANCE

Arterial blood pressure is a measure of the pressure blood exerts within the blood vessels. It depends on cardiac output, blood volume, peripheral resistance and the elasticity of arterial walls.

Peripheral resistance is the resistance to blood flow imposed by the force created by the aorta and arterial system. The amount of pressure exerted on the blood is highest in the aorta and becomes progressively lower in the arteries, arterioles, capillaries, and veins (Figure 1-14). Because blood flows naturally from high pressure to low pressure areas, this pressure gradient is one determinant of blood flow.

Two other factors are the diameter of the vessels and the blood viscosity. The diameter of the vessels is controlled by vascular tone, which allows them to constrict or dilate, thus changing the resistance to blood flow. *Viscosity* refers to the thickness of the blood. Greater pressure is required to propel viscous fluid.

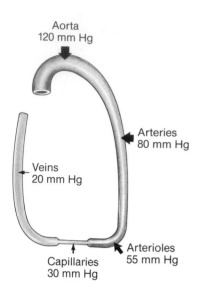

FIGURE 1-14
Decreasing pressures in vascular system.

Aorta
120 mm Hg

Arteries
80 mm Hg

Veins
20 mm Hg

Arterioles
55 mm Hg

Capillaries
30 mm Hg

FORMULA FOR SYSTEMIC VASCULAR RESISTANCE

Systemic vascular resistance (SVR) is calculated to be the resistance to blood flow imposed by the force of friction between the blood and walls of the blood vessels.

$$SVR = \frac{Mean\ arterial\ BP\ -\ Right\ atrial\ pressure}{Cardiac\ output\ \times\ 80}$$

Normal value: 800 to 1200 dynes/sec/cm^{-5}

FACTORS INFLUENCING CIRCULATION

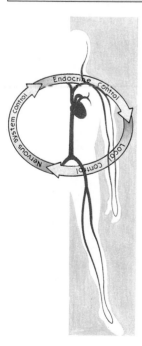

An elaborate system of control mechanisms is needed to orchestrate circulatory changes to supply the body's changing needs. Although these mechanisms fall into three categories—neural, endocrine, and local control—they interact closely in a continuous feedback cycle.

Autonomic Nervous System Control

Although the heart has the ability to initiate its own impulse through the SA node, physical activity, pain, temperature, emotions, and drugs can activate the autonomic nervous system. Sympa-

thetic and parasympathetic fibers combine to form the cardiac plexuses located near the aortic arch. Nerve fibers from the plexuses innervate the SA node, the AV node, and the atrial myocardium.

Sympathetic nerves accelerate the heart rate by releasing epinephrine. The parasympathetic system releases acetylcholine, which slows the heart rate.

Arteries, arterioles, and capillaries are also under sympathetic nervous system control. The muscle layer in the arterial wall is supplied by **vasoconstrictors,** which cause the arterial walls to contract, and **vasodilators,** which relax them. This permits blood distribution to change in response to the body's changing needs. For example, eating prompts vasodilation of arteries in the digestive tract and vasoconstriction of arteries supplying skeletal muscles.

Baroreceptor cells in the carotid sinus and aortic arch respond to stretch and pressure. Stimulation of the cells inhibits the vasomotor center and stimulates parasympathetic fibers. As a result, the heart beat slows and blood vessels dilate.

Vasomotor chemoreceptors in the aortic arch and carotid bodies are sensitive to decreases in arterial oxygen pressure and pH and increases in arterial carbon dioxide pressure. When stimulated, impulses are sent to the vasoconstrictor centers in the medulla, and the arterioles constrict.

Endocrine Control

Several hormones contribute to the regulation of the circulation and the heart. For example, in response to physical activity and stress, catecholamines are released, influencing heart rate, myocardial contractility, and peripheral vascular resistance. Other hormones that play a major role in the regulation of circulation include angiotensin, ACTH, vasopressin, bradykinin, and prostaglandins.

Local Control

Local tissue pH and concentrations of oxygen, carbon dioxide, and metabolic products affect vascular tone. Local vascular tone regulates blood flow in the area to meet tissue needs.

In the normal adult, 5 liters of blood circulate through about 60,000 miles (96,560.6 kilometers) of blood vessels. The distribution of blood volume is about 20% in the arterial system and 60% to 70% in the venous system.

VASCULAR SYSTEM

The vascular system is a network of three types of blood vessels—arteries, capillaries, and veins.

Arteries

The arterial tree, which carries oxygenated blood to all body tissues, comprises arteries, arterioles, and capillaries (Figure 1-17). **Arteries** are thick, high-pressure vessels. The walls include a tough, elastic layer that allows the arteries to distend to accommodate the blood pumped from the heart (Figure 1-16). **Arterioles,** the smaller branches, contain less elastic tissue and more smooth muscle. Constriction or dilation of the arterioles is the primary mechanism of blood pressure control.

Arteries and arterioles respond to autonomic nervous system control, to chemical stimulation, and temperature. Chemical substances can change the size of a blood vessel by acting directly on the vessel or by stimulating sensory receptors.

Capillaries

Capillaries are microscopic endothelial vessels that connect the arterioles and venules. They are permeable to the molecules that are exchanged between blood cells and tissue cells (Figure 1-15). It is in the capillary bed that the exchange of oxygen, nutrients, and metabolic waste products takes place. Oxygen is extracted from the blood, and waste products are collected from the cells.

Blood flow through the capillaries is regulated by cellular oxygen demand, with assistance of the precapillary sphincter. As oxygen demand increases, the precapillary sphincter dilates and the capillaries open up, increasing blood flow to the tissue.

The capillaries are also responsive to ANS control. However, local capillary response is due primarily to humoral factors, that is, chemical substances resulting from tissue metabolism or the presence of chemical substances in the blood. Such substances include histamine (a powerful capillary dilator) and hormones such as epinephrine, which have a constricting effect. Oxygen and pH can also influence local blood flow.

Veins

The venous system, comprising venules and veins, is responsible for returning blood to the heart (Figure 1-18). **Venules** are small, thin tubules that collect blood from the capillary bed. The venules converge to form **veins,** which then carry the deoxygenated blood back to the heart. The walls of the veins are thinner and more distensible than arterial walls. This allows the veins to accommodate larger amounts of blood and to serve as a reservoir, ready to supply tissue needs. Veins contain valves at varying intervals to maintain forward blood flow to the heart (venous return) (Figure 1-19).

Venous blood flow is influenced by a variety of factors, including arterial flow, skeletal muscle contractions, changes in thoracic and abdominal pressure, and pressure in the right atrium.

Lymphatic System

Lymph vessels, ending in lymphatic capillaries, are part of the capillary bed. Fluid and protein move from the circulatory system capillaries into the interstitial space, where they are collected by lymphatic capillaries. Similarly, the lymph system transfers components of the immune system, such as antibodies and lymphocytes, into the circulatory system.

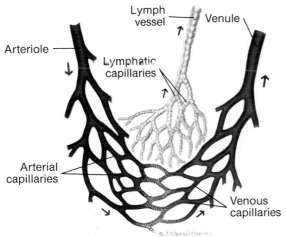

FIGURE 1-15
Microcirculation involving blood, interstitial fluid, oxygen, and nutrients.

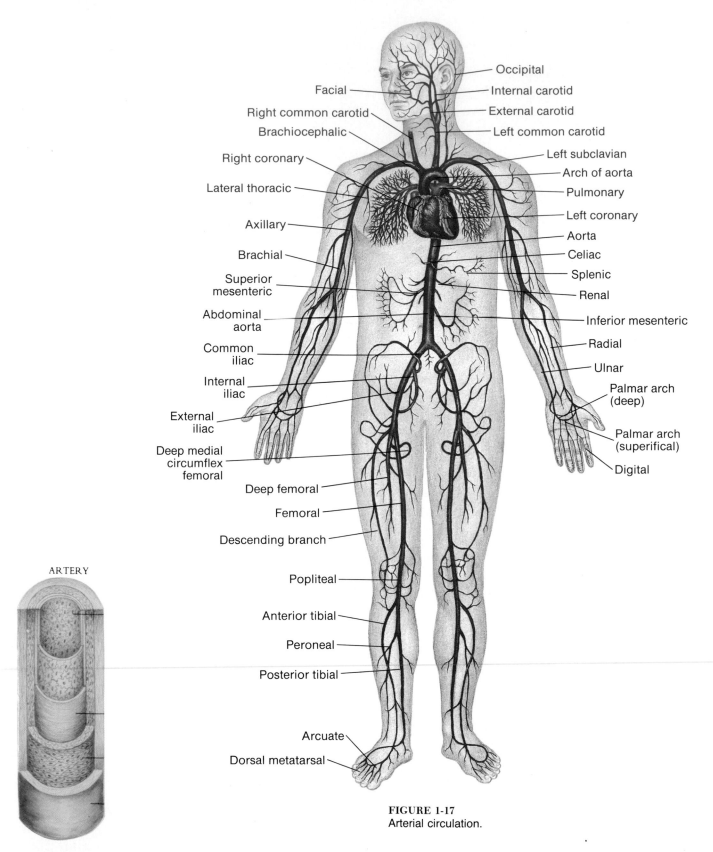

Facial

Right common carotid

Brachiocephalic

Right coronary

Lateral thoracic

Axillary

Brachial

Superior
mesenteric

Abdominal
aorta

Common
iliac

Internal
iliac

External
iliac

Deep medial
circumflex
femoral

Deep femoral

Femoral

Descending branch

Popliteal

Anterior tibial

Peroneal

Posterior tibial

Arcuate

Dorsal metatarsal

Occipital

Internal carotid

External carotid

Left common carotid

Left subclavian

Arch of aorta

Pulmonary

Left coronary

Aorta

Celiac

Splenic

Renal

Inferior mesenteric

Radial

Ulnar

Palmar arch
(deep)

Palmar arch
(superifical)

Digital

FIGURE 1-17
Arterial circulation.

ARTERY

FIGURE 1-16
Cross section of artery.

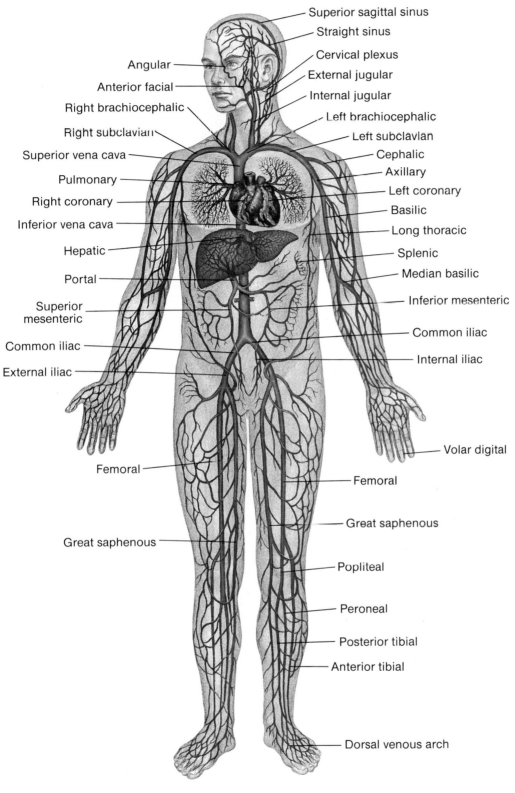

Superior sagittal sinus
Straight sinus
Angular
Cervical plexus
Anterior facial
External jugular
Internal jugular
Right brachiocephalic
Left brachiocephalic
Right subclavian
Left subclavian
Superior vena cava
Cephalic
Pulmonary
Axillary
Right coronary
Left coronary
Inferior vena cava
Basilic
Hepatic
Long thoracic
Portal
Splenic
Superior mesenteric
Median basilic
Inferior mesenteric
Common iliac
Common iliac
External iliac
Internal iliac
Volar digital
Femoral
Femoral
Great saphenous
Great saphenous
Popliteal
Peroneal
Posterior tibial
Anterior tibial
Dorsal venous arch

FIGURE 1-18
Venous circulation.

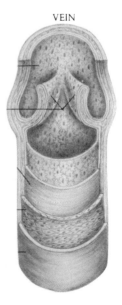

VEIN

FIGURE 1-19
Cross section of vein.

CORONARY ARTERIES

Right coronary artery

Supplies: Right atrium, anterior right ventricle

Posterior aspect of septum (90% of population)

Posterior and papillary muscle

Sinus and AV nodes (80-90% of population)

Inferior aspect of left ventricle

Left coronary arteries
Left anterior descending (LAD)

Supplies: Anterior left ventricular wall

Anterior interventricular septum
  Septal branches supply conduction system, bundle of His, and bundle branches

Anterior papillary muscle

Left ventricular apex

Circumflex

Supplies: Left atrium

Posterior surfaces of left ventricle

Posterior aspect of septum

CORONARY CIRCULATION
Coronary Arteries

The myocardium receives blood from the right and left coronary arteries (Figures 1-20 to 1-22). They arise from the aorta just above and behind the aortic valve (see Figures 1-10 and 1-11). Although exact courses of the coronary arteries may vary, the most abundant blood supply feeds the left ventricular myocardium. This is because the left ventricle does most of the work of the heart (see page 4).

Although coronary blood flow continues throughout the cardiac cycle, blood flow to the myocardium is depressed during systole but then increased during diastole.

The flow of blood through the myocardium is influenced by the myocardial oxygen demand. In normal resting situations, the heart extracts 60% to 70% of oxygen present in coronary artery blood flow. However, a variety of factors, such as exercise, can increase myocardial oxygen demand, which in turn increases coronary blood flow. When oxygen demands exceed the coronary circulation's capacity, myocardial ischemia results.

Cardiac Veins

The heart is drained by the cardiac veins. Veins draining the left ventricle empty into the coronary sinus and then enter into the right atrium. Several veins that drain blood from the right ventricle empty directly into the right atrium and ventricle.

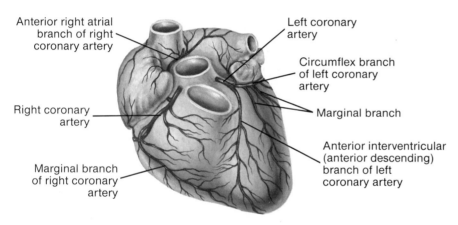

Anterior right atrial branch of right coronary artery

Left coronary artery

Circumflex branch of left coronary artery

Right coronary artery

Marginal branch

Anterior interventricular (anterior descending) branch of left coronary artery

Marginal branch of right coronary artery

FIGURE 1-20
Coronary circulation—anterior view.

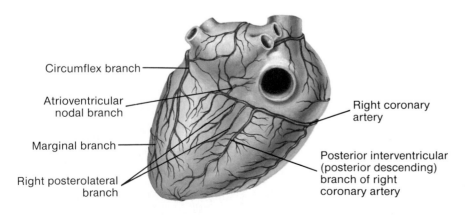

Circumflex branch

Atrioventricular nodal branch

Marginal branch

Right posterolateral branch

Right coronary artery

Posterior interventricular (posterior descending) branch of right coronary artery

FIGURE 1-21
Coronary circulation—posterior view.

ELECTRICAL ACTIVITY OF THE HEART

Conduction System

Specialized areas of the myocardium exert electrical control over the cardiac cycle. Although not anatomically distinct, these areas exhibit physiologic differences from the rest of the myocardium, forming a pathway for electrical impulses.

The sinoatrial (SA), or sinus node, which initiates a self-generating impulse, is the primary pacemaker and sets the pace for the heart at about 60 to 100 bpm. It is located at the border (junction) of the superior vena cava and right atrium (Figure 1-22). Once generated, this electrical impulse sets the rhythm of contractions and travels through both atria over a specialized conduction network to the atrioventricular (AV) node. The AV node located in the floor of the right atrium receives the impulse and transmits it to the bundle of His. The bundle of His then divides into a right-bundle branch and two left-bundle branches. These terminate in a complex network called Purkinje fibers, which spread throughout the ventricle. When the impulse reaches the ventricle, stimulation of the myocardium causes depolar-

ization of the cells, and contraction occurs. The AV node serves as a gate to delay electrical conduction and in this way to prevent an excessive number of atrial impulses from entering the ventricle.

Both the SA and AV nodes are supplied with sympathetic and parasympathetic fibers. This permits nearly instantaneous changes in the heart rate in response to physiologic changes in oxygen demand.

Electrophysiology

Transmission of an electrical impulse and response of the myocardium occurs as a result of a series of sequential ionic changes across the cell membrane. At the cellular level, electrical charges are regulated primarily by two electrolytes—potassium (the primary intracellular ion) and sodium (the primary extracellular ion) (Figure 1-23, *1*). The ionic gradient—that is, the difference in concentrations of these ions across the cell—determine the cell's electrical charge. Any stimulus that increases the permeability of the membrane will generate an electrical potential and is referred to as an action potential. The action potential of myocardial muscle cell consists of 5 phases (labeled 0 to 4) (Figure 1-24). A polarized or resting state during which no electrical activity occurs is called the resting membrane potential. It has a net charge of −90 mV.

Once an electrical impulse is generated, sodium moves rapidly into the cell and potassium begins to exit, converting the electrical forces within the cell to a positive charge (Figure 1-23, *2*). The cell is then depolarized, resulting in shortening of the cardiac cell. This is depicted by the upstroke of the action potential curve (Figure 1-24) and is referred to as Phase 0.

Phase 1 is the brief rapid change toward the repolarization process, during which the membrane potential returns to 0 mV.

Phase 2 is a plateau, or stabilization period, caused by the slow influx of sodium and the slow exit of potassium. During this period, calcium ions enter

> **If the SA node falters,** a hierarchy of pacemakers can take over. Atrial, AV node, and ventricular escape pacemakers can function as subsidiary pacemakers, although they generate impulses at much slower rates; for example:
> AV—40 to 60 bpm
> Purkinje fibers—20 to 40 bpm

FIGURE 1-22
Cardiac conduction.

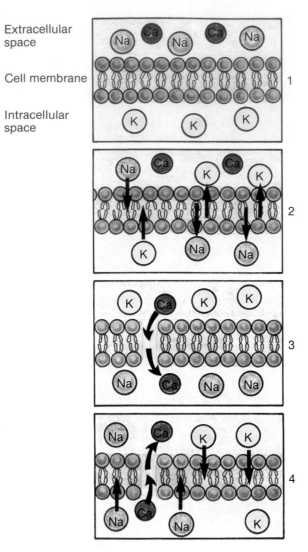

Extracellular space

Cell membrane

Intracellular space

FIGURE 1-23
Ionic exchanges across the cell membrane.

the cell through slow calcium channels, triggering the release of large quantities of calcium. Calcium functions in the process of cellular contraction (Figure 1-23, 3).

Phase 3 represents sudden acceleration in repolarization as potassium leaves rapidly, causing the inside of the cell to move toward a more negative state.

Phase 4 represents the return to the resting phase during which the intracellular charge is once again electronegative (Figure 1-23, 4), and the process is ready to be repeated (Phase 0). It is also at this time that any excess sodium is eliminated from the cell and exit of potassium speeds up.

Throughout these phases the cardiac cell goes through a series of refractory periods during which the cell is incapable of accepting another electrical stimulus and responding with a full action potential. An absolute refractory period occurs during depolarization and at the beginning of repolarization (phases 0, 1, and 2). During this period, excitation of the cardiac cell will not result in another impulse, no matter how strong the stimulus. The relative refractory period represents the time when the cell is once again electronegative. A stronger than threshold stimulus can initiate another impulse. A vulnerable, or supernormal, period occurs as phase 4 begins and the cell is returning to its resting potential. During this time a weaker than threshold stimulus can initiate an action potential.

The resting membrane potential is associated with potassium concentrations of about 150 mEq/L intracellularly and 3.5 to 5 mEq/L extracellularly. Sodium concentrations are about 132-142 mEq/L in extracellular fluid and 10 mEq/L in intracellular concentrations.

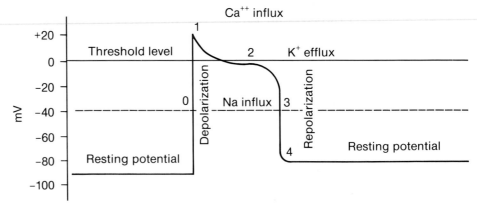

FIGURE 1-24
Cardiac action potentials.

CHAPTER 2

Assessment

Cardiovascular nursing assessment involves careful, systematic evaluation of a patient's medical, family, social, cultural, psychologic, and occupational history and examination of the heart and vascular system.

The patient and examiner should be relaxed to help ensure a more comprehensive assessment. Avoid technical terms, and use language that is age-appropriate and matched to the patient's experience. Be sensitive to intellectual, socioeconomic, cultural, and language barriers that can influence the patient's response. The assessment process serves to: (1) determine the patient's chief complaint, (2) discover elements in the patient's history that relate to the present problem, and (3) allow the examiner to observe the patient for clues to the patient's health and emotional status. The interview is an opportunity to establish rapport with the patient. By demonstrating interest and concern, the nurse can elicit valuable information that will help in the evaluation of symptoms.

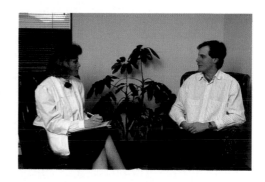

Awareness of nonverbal communication during the interview increases the nurse's understanding of the patient. Facial expression, body position, and tone of voice can provide important diagnostic clues. The patient's chief complaint is best elicited by asking the patient "What has brought you here?" or "What is bothering you?" The response is recorded in the patient's own words. The examiner determines when the patient first began having symptoms. The nature of the complaint will direct the line of questioning. Complete information should be requested by specific questions to determine the location, radiation quality, and quantity (severity, duration); precipitating or aggravating factors; relieving factors; associated findings; and treatment sought.

A person's response to stress and coping methods are sometimes difficult to assess directly on the initial interview, but this information is important to obtain. Direct questioning about recent stresses and major life changes can often elicit pertinent information on the patient's coping abilities and symptoms. However, the examiner should never assume a major life change was stressful for the patient simply because it sounds stressful. Similarly, an event that seems minor may be interpreted by the patient as extremely stressful.

HISTORY

Chief Complaint: Guidelines for the Interview

Chest pain (myocardial ischemia)
 Location
  Substernal or precordial
  Diffuse or localized
  Radiates from chest to jaw, arm, or neck
 Character
  Dull, aching, pressure, burning, tightness, crushing, indigestion
  Variable or continuous
 Intensity
  Mild, moderate, or severe
 Onset and duration
  Sudden or gradual
  Brief (1 to 10 minutes) or continuous
 Precipitating factors
  Exertion, emotion, eating, elimination, exposure (the 5 Es)
 Relieving factors
  Stopping aggravating activity, rest, warmth, walking
  Sublingual nitroglycerin
  Not relieved
 Accompanying symptoms
  Anxiety, apprehensiveness, restlessness
  Dyspnea
  Lightheadedness or dizziness
  Diaphoresis
  Nausea or vomiting
Limb pain (peripheral ischemia)
 Intermittent claudication
 Location
  Calves, thighs, buttocks
  Can occur in other sites
  Localized or radiates from calf to thigh
 Character
  Cramplike pain occurs after walking a distance
 Precipitating factors
  Physical activity, walking, climbing stairs
 Relieving factors
  Relieved by rest or stopping activity
 Pain at rest
 Location
  Distal forefoot
 Character
  Burning, numbness, tingling
 Onset
  Occurs at night, when legs elevated
 Relieving factors
  Relieved by assuming upright position with feet in dependent position
Palpitation (or consciousness of rapid and/or irregular heart action)

 Rapid and/or irregular heart beat
 Skipped beats
 Palpitations
 Thumping in the chest
Dyspnea, difficulty breathing
 Shortness of breath (SOB)
 Dyspnea on exertion (DOE)
  Type of activities that bring on DOE
 Orthopnea
  Number of pillows required to alleviate symptoms
  Relieved by changing position
 Paroxysmal nocturnal dyspnea (PND)
Cough
 Dry
 Precipitated or worsened by lying down
 Paroxysmal with exertion
 Occurs at night
Fatigue
 Inability to perform activities of daily living
 Progressive decrease in activity tolerance
Syncope or transient loss of consciousness (LOC)
 Stokes-Adams syncope (associated with marked bradycardia or dysrhythmia)
 Effort syncope—LOC occurs shortly after heavy activity (associated with hypotension, aortic stenosis, or cyanotic congenital heart disease)
 Carotid sinus syncope—precipitated by suddenly turning the neck, shaving the neck, or tight collar (associated with atherosclerosis of the carotid artery)

Patient History: Factors Relating to Cardiovascular Disorders

Concurrent disorders
 Atherosclerosis, hyperlipoproteinemia, hypertension, diabetes or other systemic diseases, chronic pulmonary disorders, obesity
Medical history
 Infancy and childhood
  Cyanosis at birth, congenital heart disease or murmurs, rheumatic fever, scarlet fever, Kawasaki disease, streptococcal infections
 Previous disorders
  Angina, myocardial infarction, endocarditis, peripheral vascular disease, stroke, heart failure, pulmonary or renal problems
 Injuries
  Recent accidents, chest trauma
 Hospitalizations and surgeries
  Heart surgery, vascular surgery, obstetric surgery, any recent invasive procedure
 Cardiovascular risk profile (see box on page 19)
 Gynecologic history
  Pregnancies, outcome, complications

Past and present contraceptive methods
Dental care
  Recent surgery or treatment for gum disease
  Recent routine procedures, including cleaning

Medication History

Prescription drugs
  Past or current use of antihypertensives, antiarrhythmics, anticoagulants, diuretics, digitalis, nitroglycerin, oral contraceptives
  Peripheral vascular vasodilators, antiinflammatory steroids
Nonprescription drugs
  Recent use of aspirin, cold and flu preparations, sleeping agents, antacids, herbal remedies, vitamin or mineral supplements; illicit drug use (cocaine, IV drug use)
Family history
  Family members with hypertension, coronary heart disease, hyperlipidemia, cerebrovascular disease, diabetes
  Age, sex, and health of grandparents, parents, siblings, and children
  Age and cause of death of deceased family members
Diet and nutrition
  Weight
    Actual and ideal
    Recent loss or gain; deliberate or unintentional
  Dietary or fluid restriction
    Prescribed by physician or self-prescribed
    How well tolerated
  Usual diet
  Food intolerances or allergies

Sociocultural history
  Educational level
  Occupation
    Sedentary or physically active
    Usual occupation, hours worked per week
  Exercise and usual activity level
    Recent changes due to increased symptoms
    Distance able to walk before becoming symptomatic
  Tobacco use (cigarettes, pipe, cigar, chewing tobacco, snuff)
    Number of pack years (number of years smoked multiplied by the packs smoked per day)
  Alcohol and caffeine intake
  Sleep patterns
  Cultural and spiritual values
  Economic resources
Psychosocial history
  Recent stress or major life change
  Support systems
    Marital status, number of children
    Significant other
  Perception of illness
  Understanding of past and present illness
  Response to pain
  Coping pattern

CARDIOVASCULAR RISK FACTORS

Family history of heart disease	Overweight/obesity
Age >60 years	Elevated serum cholesterol and triglycerides
Sex	Diabetes mellitus
Men (35 to 55 years)	Physical inactivity; sedentary life-style
Women (postmenopausal)	Stress
Hypertension	Women <40 years
Smoking	Smoking, birth control pills

THE ENVIRONMENT AND EQUIPMENT

Before starting the physical examination, it is important to ensure that the examining room is well-lit, quiet, and private. Natural lighting is necessary to assess subtleties of color and changes in contour, and a minimal noise level is necessary for the examiner to detect low-pitched sounds during auscultation. Every effort should be made to ensure patient privacy with no interruptions. This encourages the patient to relax and increases the patient's confidence and the examiner's concentration.

The basic equipment for cardiovascular assessment should be at hand. This includes a stethoscope, sphygmomanometer with the appropriate-size cuff, centimeter ruler, and penlight or flashlight. The stethoscope must have both bell and diaphragm to detect high and low pitched sounds. Its tubing should be flexible and no longer than 12 to 15 inches, since longer tubing diminishes sound conduction (Figure 2-1).

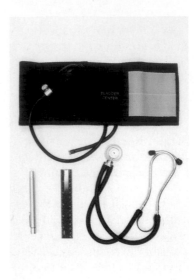

FIGURE 2-1
Equipment for cardiovascular assessment.

GENERAL EXAMINATION

The physical examination actually begins with the initial interview by observing the patient's general state of health and degree of distress. Signs of retarded growth, malnutrition, or physical abnormalities should be noted. Evaluate the patient's general health status and correlate this with his chronologic age and emotional status.

The examiner should make every effort to reassure the patient, explaining briefly what is transpiring at each step ("Now I am going to listen to your heart") and giving clear directions when needed ("Take a deep breath and hold it"). A calm, matter-of-fact manner can often allay anxiety, even for patients who are in distress.

The cardiovascular assessment should be conducted in an organized manner. It begins with an overall evaluation of the patient, assessing the skin, nails, and extremities for general signs of circulatory compromise. It proceeds to a more direct evaluation of cardiovascular integrity, consisting of palpating the pulses, evaluating the major arteries and veins, measuring the blood pressure, and assessing the heart by palpation and auscultation.

Skin

The skin should be evaluated for color, turgor, temperature, and moisture. The general condition of the skin reflects the patient's age and frequently the general state of health. Chronic cardiovascular disease that interferes with the patient's ability to perform activities of daily living, for example, may be reflected in poor hygiene.

Color

The range of normal skin varies from pink to deep or light brown. Normal skin color varies widely, reflecting differences in ethnic tone, age, and exposure to sun and wind. The presence of generalized or local pallor or cyanosis is easily detected in light-skinned persons and suggests some compromise in circulation. In dark-skinned persons, however, changes in color can be more difficult to determine. In such cases, skin color changes are best evaluated in the conjunctiva, tongue, buccal mucosa, and palms. Normal variations include a bluish hue of the lips, gums, and nailbeds.

Pallor. Pallor reflects decreased oxyhemoglobin concentration. A generalized pallor may be caused by a number of conditions, some of which are nonpathological, such as vasoconstriction of superficial vessels from anxiety or cold. More ominous causes include anemia, hypovolemia, low cardiac output states, infective endocarditis, and malignant hypertension.

In peripheral vascular disorders, a marbled appearance and pallor will develop after 30 seconds of elevation of the legs. This reflects absence of adequate collateral veins. Placing the extremity in a dependent position results in a rubious (red) color that develops after 1 minute. In severe ischemia, the skin takes longer to become red.

Cyanosis. The bluish hue of cyanosis is caused by an increased amount of deoxygenated hemoglobin (at least 5 gm/100 ml). It is best observed at the nailbeds and lips, and inside the mouth. The distribution of cyanosis often provides a clue to the cause. Cyanosis may be either generalized (central cyanosis) or localized (peripheral) (Figure 2-2).

Central cyanosis reflects decreased arterial oxygenation of blood. If present from birth it is usually due to congenital heart disease with a right-to-left shunt but if it develops in late adolescence, cyanosis suggests reversal of a left-to-right shunt. Cyanosis with acute myocardial infarction reflects right-to-left shunt from ventricular septum rupture. In older adults, it can develop from chronic obstructive pulmonary disease or pulmonary hypertension.

Peripheral cyanosis can result from diminished peripheral perfusion from low cardiac output or vasoconstriction of the arteries.

Turgor

Turgor reflects skin elasticity and the water content of the skin and subcutaneous tissues. It is assessed by lifting a fold of skin and observing how quickly it returns to normal position (Figure 2-3). Loss of normal turgor occurs with dehydration, but it is also a normal process of aging.

Temperature and moisture

The skin should be warm and dry, unless environmental temperatures are extreme. Lower body temperatures can occur with a decreased systemic blood flow, as is seen in shock states. An extremity that is cooler and drier than other body surfaces suggests arterial insufficiency. A generalized or local elevation in temperature occurs with inflammatory processes.

Increased skin moisture can occur in shock states as a result of sympathetic nerve stimulation. Abnormally dry skin may reflect dehydration.

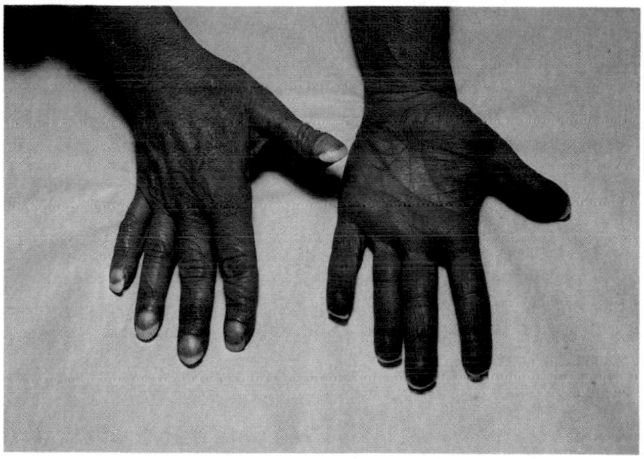

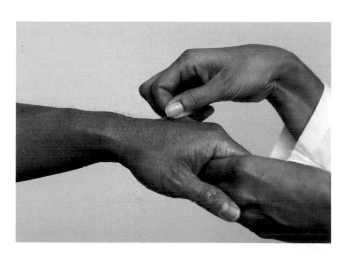

FIGURE 2-2
Cyanosis of hands and fingers. (Also note severe clubbing.)

FIGURE 2-3
Examination of skin turgor.

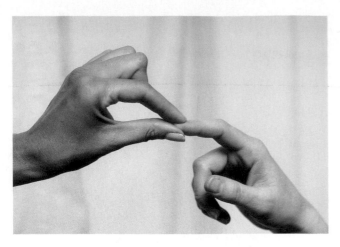

FIGURE 2-4
Testing nail bed adherence.

Nails

Nails should be assessed for color, shape, thickness, symmetry, and nail adherence. Normal nail color is some variation of pink, although in dark-skinned persons the nail may have a bluish hue, as well as pigmented deposits or bands. The shape and texture of nails can vary widely. Nail thickness generally is 0.3 to 0.65 mm, but may be thicker in men. The nail should be smooth, flat or gently curved, and adhere to the nail bed (Figure 2-4). The nail base lies at about a 160-degree angle to the finger.

Nail abnormalities

Peripheral vascular disease can produce nail depression, pitting, longitudinal striations, thinning, and brittleness. However, these findings are not diagnostic of circulatory disorders, because a number of other events such as trauma, dietary factors, and age can also produce such nail abnormalities. Koilonychia, or spoon-shaped nail, is associated with several conditions, including Raynaud's disease (Figure 2-5).

Clubbing

Clubbing of the fingers accompanies longstanding cyanosis and is associated with decreased oxygen. The distal tips of the fingers become bulbous. The nails are thickened, hard, and curved at the tip, and the nailbed feels boggy when squeezed. Separation from the nail bed produces a white, yellowish, or greenish color on the nonadherent portion of the nail. Early in the clubbing process, the normal angle of the nail is lost, leaving the nail flat. In advanced cases, the base of the nail becomes elevated and may feel boggy or spongy (Figure 2-6).

Spoon nail (koilonychia)

FIGURE 2-5
Koilonychia (spoon-shaped nail).

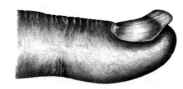

Clubbing—early

FIGURE 2-6
Clubbing of fingers.

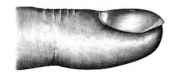

Clubbing—middle

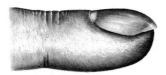

Clubbing—severe

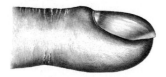

Extremities

The upper and lower extremities should be evaluated for signs and symptoms of acute and chronic changes due to arterial or venous disorders.

Chronic arterial insufficiency can over time lead to trophic changes such as uneven hair distribution or hair loss and atrophy of the skin, which becomes smooth, shiny, and thin. The nails thicken, demonstrating irregular growth and shape and opacification.

Severe ischemia of the lower extremity results in varying degrees of tissue loss, including ulceration or gangrene. Ulcerations, due to arterial insufficiency, have well-defined margins and tend to occur between the toes, on the tips of toes, and around pressure points.

The presence of gangrene indicates complete occlusion of the arterial circulation to a portion of the extremity that has been ongoing for several days. It is demonstrated when the skin is black, dry, and hard. Pre-gangrene signs can be recognized by a deep cyanosis or purple-black color that is not affected by pressure or changes in position.

Venous incompetence can lead to a number of chronic problems. Varicose veins appear as dilated, often tortuous veins when the legs are in a dependent position. The Trendelenburg test is used to evaluate venous incompetence. With the patient supine, lift the leg above the level of the heart until the veins empty and then lower the leg quickly. Venous incompetency is distinguished by rapid filling of the veins.

Stasis dermatitis, chronic inflammation of the lower legs and ankles, also is caused by venous incompetence. Occurring primarily in older patients, it is characterized by pruritis, erythema, mild scaling, hair loss, and brown discolorations. Edema and varicose veins may be present. If left unattended, complications such as ulcers can develop.

PITTING EDEMA SCALE

Scale	Degree	Response
1+ Trace	Slight	Rapid
2+ Mild	0-0.6 cm (0-¼ in)	10-15 seconds
3+ Moderate	0.6-1.3 cm (¼-½ in)	1-2 minutes
4+ Severe	1.3-2.5 cm (½-1 in)	2-5 minutes

Venous ulcers, which occur on the anteromedial malleolus and pretibial areas, are shallow with ragged edges and contain granulation tissue. Edema and swelling are usually present.

Redness, thickening, and tenderness along a superficial vein suggest thrombophlebitis. Deep vein thrombosis (DVT) cannot be confirmed on physical examination alone, but it should be suspected if swelling, pain, and tenderness appear over a vein. Homan's sign, which is used to test for DVT, involves having the patient quickly dorsiflex the foot while the knee is slightly flexed. Calf pain is a positive sign and usually indicates a thrombosis.

The lower extremities should be evaluated for edema. Edema is a sign of increased interstitial fluid. Bilateral edema of the lower extremities can be a sign of heart failure or venous insufficiency. To check for edema, press the bony prominence over the tibia or medial malleolus for several seconds and lift the finger. If the depression does not fill almost immediately, pitting edema is present.

Edema observed in only one extremity may be caused by deep venous thrombosis. Nonpitting edema caused by circulatory disorders must be distinguished from lymphedema, which causes the same symptoms.

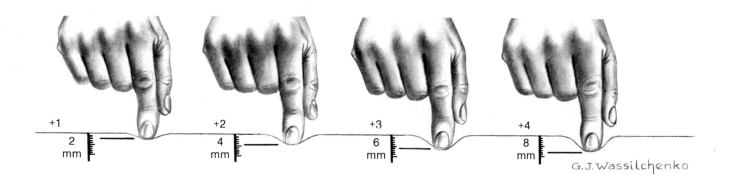

+1	+2	+3	+4
2 mm	4 mm	6 mm	8 mm

G.J. Wassilchenko

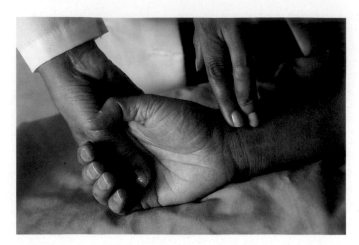

FIGURE 2-7
Radial pulse. Use gentle pressure over the medial inner wrist.

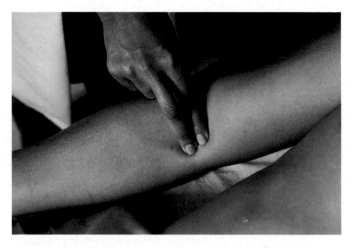

FIGURE 2-8
Brachial pulse. Palpate just medial to the biceps tendon.

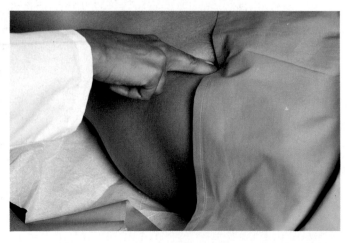

FIGURE 2-9
Femoral pulse. Exert firm pressure just below the inguinal ligament.

EXAMINATION OF ARTERIAL PULSES

Careful examination of the arterial pulses provides valuable information about the cardiovascular system, including the overall function of the ventricles, the quality of the arterial blood vessels, and the condition of the aortic valve. The arterial pulses include the carotid, radial, brachial, femoral, popliteal, dorsalis pedis, and posterior tibial. Because the carotid artery is usually given special consideration in the examination, it is discussed separately on page 28.

HOW TO PALPATE ARTERIAL PULSES

Examine the arterial pulses with the distal pads of the second and third fingers. Do not use your thumb, because your own pulse may be more readily felt than the patient's. Palpate firmly but not so hard that the artery is occluded. If pulses are difficult to locate, vary the amount of pressure and feel carefully throughout the area (Figures 2-7 to 2-12).

- Palpate each pulse individually to analyze rate, rhythm, amplitude, and contour.
- Palpate each pulse separately as well as simultaneously to detect changes in timing or amplitude.
- Palpate upper and lower extremity pulses on the same side (for example, left femoral and brachial pulses) to detect variations.
- Compare pulses on left and right extremities to detect variations. (Asymmetrical pulses suggest arterial occlusion.)

The **femoral artery,** located behind the inguinal ligament, is easily palpable in most persons (Figure 2-9). However, it may be difficult to locate in obese patients. In these cases, the femoral pulse can be palpated (exerting greater pressure than when palpating other areas) midway between the anterior superior iliac spine and the pubic tubercle. The right and left femoral pulses should be of equal intensity. A femoral pulse that is delayed, absent, or weaker when compared with the radial pulses suggests coarctation of the aorta. Absence of the femoral pulse or a bruit suggests occlusive disease of the aortoiliac artery.

The vigor of blood flow diminishes with distance from the heart, so amplitude is normally somewhat decreased in the lower extremities. The **popliteal artery** is difficult to palpate in most persons (Figure 2-10). Occlusive disease in the superficial femoral artery can result in a diminished or absent popliteal pulse.

The dorsalis pedis and posterior tibial arteries are the most distal pulses. The **dorsalis pedis pulse** has a variable location over the dorsum of the foot and is absent in approximately 15% of normal individuals[111] (Figure 2-11). The **posterior tibial pulse** is more readily palpated. A decreased or absent pulse is therefore reflective of occlusive vascular disease[71] (Figure 2-12). The posterior tibial pulse can be obscured by obesity or edema.

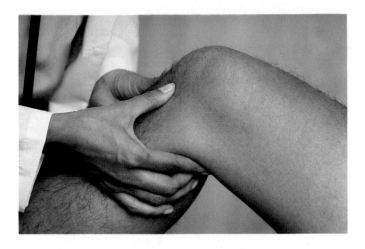

FIGURE 2-10
Popliteal pulse. Use firm pressure behind the knee at the popliteal fossae. The patient may be positioned supine **(A)** or prone **(B).**

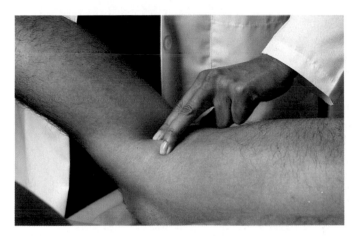

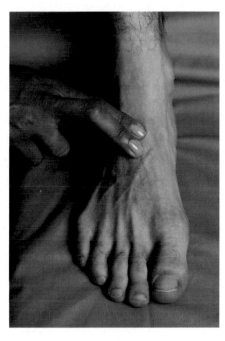

FIGURE 2-11
Dorsalis pedis pulse. Slightly dorsiflex the patient's foot and palpate the top medial portion of the foot above the great and second toe rays.

PULSE AMPLITUDE RATINGS	
4+	Full volume, bounding, hyperkinetic
3+	Full volume
2+	Normal
1+	Diminished, barely palpable
0+	Absent

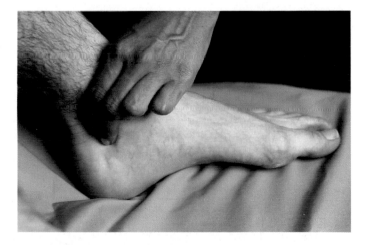

FIGURE 2-12
Posterior tibial pulse. Palpate behind and slightly below the medial malleolus of the ankle.

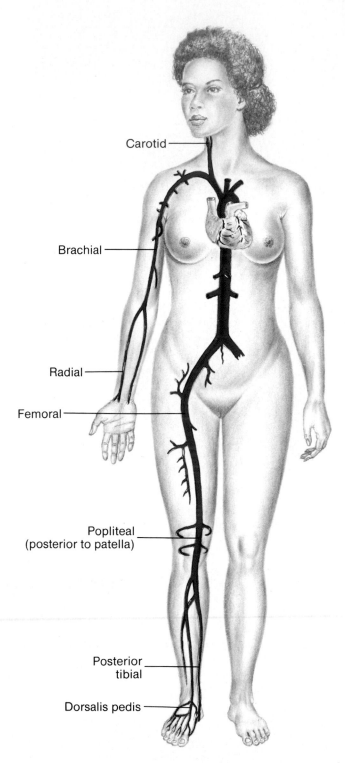

Carotid

Brachial

Radial

Femoral

Popliteal
(posterior to patella)

Posterior
tibial

Dorsalis pedis

Arteries for taking pulses

ARTERIAL PULSES—NORMAL AND ABNORMAL FINDINGS

Assessment	Findings
Resting heart rate	**Normal**
	60-90 bpm; rate may be lower in conditioned athletes
	Abnormal
	Tachycardia (>100 bpm) occurs with fever, anemia, and low cardiac output states
	Bradycardia (<50 bpm) may indicate parasympathetic nerve stimulation or atrioventricular node conduction disturbance
Rhythm	**Normal**
	Regular; normal cyclic variation can occur with respiration, increasing on inspiration, decreasing on expiration (more commonly seen in children)
	Abnormal
	Irregular rhythm usually is associated with dysrhythmias such as atrial fibrillation
	Regular pulses with pauses (dropped beats) or extra beats reflect premature atrial or ventricular contraction
Volume or amplitude	**Normal**
	Easily palpable, does not fade in and out; all pulses are full and symmetrical, with full, strong, brisk upstrokes
	Abnormal
	Diminished, weak, thready, or hypokinetic pulse is associated with left ventricular dysfunction, hypovolemia, or outflow obstruction (for example, aortic stenosis)
	Strong, brisk, or hyperkinetic pulse reflects rapid ejection from left ventricle generally caused by increased blood volume (for example, chronic aortic regurgitation)
Contour	**Normal**
	Pulse wave has a smooth and rounded or domed shape
	Abnormal
	Pulse wave has variation or irregularities

ARTERIAL PULSE ABNORMALITIES

Type	Description	Possible causes
Diminished, weak, hypokinetic	Pulse is difficult to feel, easily obliterated by the fingers, and may fade out Pulse is slow to rise, has a sustained summit, and falls slowly If both weak and variable in amplitude, pulse is termed "thready"	Hypovolemia Depressed left ventricular function (low ejection fraction) Aortic stenosis
Increased, strong, bounding, hyperkinetic	Pulse is readily palpable, not easily obliterated by fingers, and does not fade Pulse is felt as a brisk impact; can occur with or without increased pulse pressure	Exercise Fever Rigid arterial walls and systolic hypertension Hyperthyroidism (in combination with normal pulse pressure) Chronic severe mitral regurgitation
Water-hammer, collapsing	Pulse has greater amplitude than normal pulse Pulse marked by rapid rise to a narrow summit followed by a sudden descent	Chronic aortic regurgitation Patent ductus arteriosus
Pulsus bisferiens (double-peaked)	Best felt by palpating carotid artery Two systolic peaks can occur in disorders that cause rapid left ventricular ejection of large stroke volume with wide pulse pressure	Aortic regurgitation Large left-to-right shunt Patent ductus arteriosus Hypertrophic obstructive cardiomyopathy
Pulsus alternans	Pulses have large amplitude beats followed by pulses of small amplitude Rhythm remains normal	Depressed left ventricular function
Bigeminal pulse	Normal pulses are followed by premature contractions Amplitude of premature contraction is less than that of normal pulse Rhythm is irregular	Dysrhythmias Premature ventricular contraction
Pulsus paradoxus	Pattern is exaggerated (>10 mm Hg) during inspiration, and amplitude is increased during expiration Heart rate and rhythm are unchanged	Cardiac tamponade Constrictive pericarditis Pulmonary emphysema (non-cardiac)

Inspiration   Expiration   Inspiration

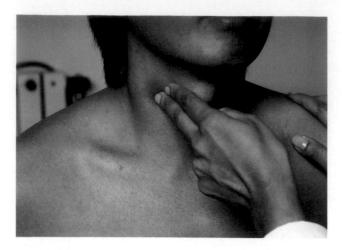

FIGURE 2-13
Palpation of carotid artery. Palpate just medial to and below the angle of the jaw. NEVER PALPATE BOTH SIDES SIMULTANEOUSLY.

CAROTID PULSE

Numerous vagus fibers of the parasympathetic system are grouped in the carotid sinus, located high in the neck near the angle of the jaw.

Palpation

The carotid artery should be palpated in the lower third of the neck to avoid excessive pressure on the carotid artery (Figure 2-13). Excessive pressure could result in slowing of the heart rate and hypotension. Palpation of the right and left carotid arteries should be done one side at a time to avoid reduction in cerebral blood flow.

Auscultation

Auscultation follows palpation. Instruct the patient to hold the breath while the stethoscope is placed over the carotid artery (again, one artery at a time) (Figure 2-14). The normal carotid artery pulse is seen on the ECG as a single, smooth rapid upstroke during ventricular systole and is best felt after the first heart sound. This is followed by a dicrotic notch, which signals the closure of the aortic valve (Figure 2-15). During examination, the dicrotic notch may not be felt. The pulse reaches a peak, or plateau (dome shape on an ECG), followed by a downstroke that is less steep than the upstroke. Carotid artery pulsations are not commonly visible on the ECG nor is a sound heard during auscultation.

B R U I T S

Bruits are low-pitched blowing sounds that are best heard with the bell of the stethoscope. Instruct the patient to hold the breath for several heartbeats during auscultation to facilitate your hearing abnormal sounds. Auscultate at several points along the length of the artery. Bruits occur during systole but may extend into diastole.

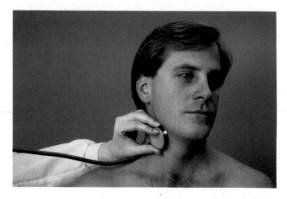

FIGURE 2-14
Auscultation of carotid artery for bruits.

Sites to routinely auscultate for bruits are the carotid, temporal, abdominal, aortic, renal, and femoral arteries. In addition, the finding of a diminished pulse in an extremity should be followed by auscultation for bruits (Figure 2-14).

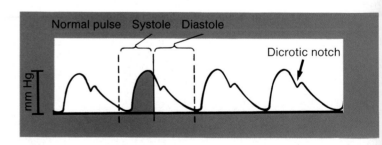

FIGURE 2-15
Normal pulse waveform.

CAROTID PULSE ABNORMALITIES

Finding	Cause	Associated conditions
Systolic bruit or blowing sound	Vessel narrowed by arteriosclerosis	Carotid artery disease
Prominent pulsations	Increased pulse pressure	Aortic regurgitation (Bisferiens pulse); hyperthyroidism
DeMusset's sign (rhythmic nodding of the head)	Marked pulsation of the carotid arteries	Severe aortic insufficiency
Hyperkinetic carotid pulse	Increased stroke volume and decreased peripheral resistance	Increased cardiac output, aortic regurgitation, complete heart block, anemia, hyperthyroidism
Hypokinetic carotid pulse	Diminished stroke volume of left ventricle; increased peripheral vascular resistance; narrowed pulse pressure; resistance to flow across the cardiac valves	Left ventricular failure from MI; constrictive pericarditis; aortic valve stenosis
Palpable thrill	Local atherosclerotic obstruction; fistula between the carotid artery and jugular vein; high cardiac output states	Anemia; thyrotoxicosis; aortic stenosis

EXAMINATION OF JUGULAR VEINS

Assessment of jugular veins provides information regarding the volume and pressure in the right side of the heart. The external jugular vein is visible above the clavicle, but the larger internal vein crosses under the sternocleidomastoid muscles (Figure 2-16).

Because palpation obliterates the jugular pulse, veins are assessed by visual inspection. They are usually not visible when the patient is sitting upright; examination of jugular venous pulse and pressure is best achieved with the patient reclining at a 30- to 45-degree angle. This position achieves maximum excursion of the internal vein, which pulsates in response to the phasic changes in right atrial pressure. The external vein, by comparison, is generally not pulsatile but can be used to estimate the mean right atrial pressure.

A 45-degree angle will cause the venous pulsation to rise to 1 to 3 cm above the level of the manubrium. The upper limit of normal for jugular venous pressure (JVP) is 3 cm H_2O above the sternal angle. Clinically this represents a JVP of 8 cm (since the sternal angle is equal to 5 cm above the right atrium).

Increases in JVP greater than 8 cm are most often the result of increased blood volume. It is usually seen in conditions that

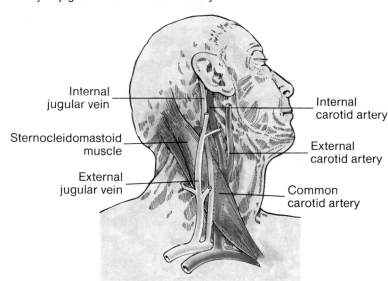

FIGURE 2-16
Anatomy of jugular veins and carotid artery.

cause RV failure such as tricuspid valve regurgitation and pulmonary hypertension.

Hepatojugular reflex

Increased venous pressure can be further demonstrated by compressing the upper right quadrant of the abdomen for 30 to 60 seconds. A slight rise in venous pulsation may be seen in normal persons, but in patients with right-sided failure, both venous pressure and pulsation are increased. This is recorded as a positive hepatojugular reflex.

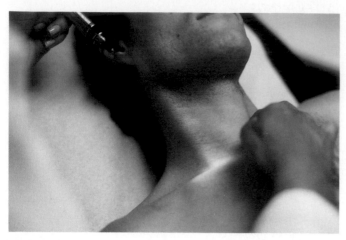

FIGURE 2-17
Use a tangential light source to illuminate the jugular veins and pulsations.

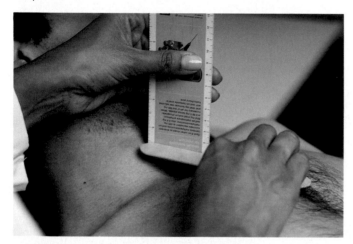

FIGURE 2-18
Measuring jugular venous pressure.

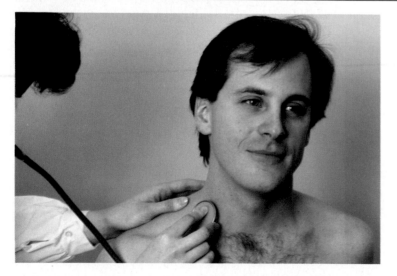

FIGURE 2-19
Auscultation for venous hum.

HOW TO MEASURE JUGULAR VENOUS PRESSURE

1. The head of the bed should be raised until the venous pulsation in the internal jugular vein is seen. A tangential light source aids in illuminating the veins and pulsations (Figure 2-17). The pulse represents the top of the oscillating column of blood and is usually seen between 30 degrees and 45 degrees. If the venous pressure is elevated, it may be necessary to elevate the head of bed to 90 degrees.

2. Using a centimeter ruler, measure the vertical distance above the manubriosternal joint (angle of Louis) and the highest level that jugular vein pulsations are visible (Figure 2-18). The height of the column of blood is established by drawing an imaginary horizontal line from the column to the sternal angle.

The internal jugular vein closely parallels the carotid artery; therefore the arterial pulse may be confused with jugular pulsations. It is easier to distinguish the two pulses if you palpate the carotid on one side of the neck while looking at the jugular vein on the other side.

VENOUS HUM

Venous hum is caused by turbulent blood flow in the internal jugular vein. Venous hum usually occurs on the right side and is best heard with the bell of the diaphragm over the supraclavicular space with the patient sitting upright with head turned to the left and tilted slightly (Figure 2-19). It is continuous, low in pitch, and loudest during diastole. Gentle pressure between the trachea and sternocleidomastoid muscle at the level of the thyroid cartilage stops the hum. Venous hum is common in children, probably resulting from vigorous myocardial contraction, and is usually benign.

JUGULAR VENOUS PULSE—NORMAL AND ABNORMAL FINDINGS

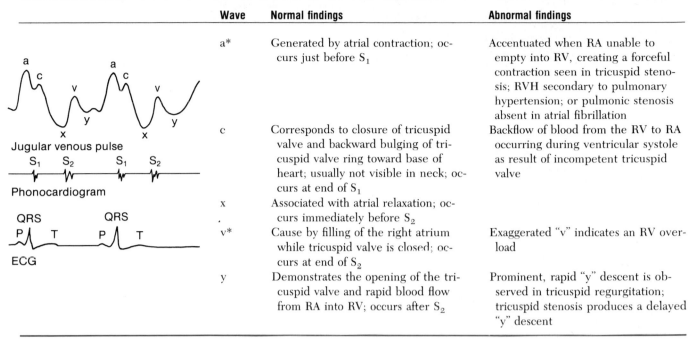

Jugular venous pulse

Phonocardiogram

ECG

Wave	Normal findings	Abnormal findings
a*	Generated by atrial contraction; occurs just before S_1	Accentuated when RA unable to empty into RV, creating a forceful contraction seen in tricuspid stenosis; RVH secondary to pulmonary hypertension; or pulmonic stenosis absent in atrial fibrillation
c	Corresponds to closure of tricuspid valve and backward bulging of tricuspid valve ring toward base of heart; usually not visible in neck; occurs at end of S_1	Backflow of blood from the RV to RA occurring during ventricular systole as result of incompetent tricuspid valve
x	Associated with atrial relaxation; occurs immediately before S_2	
v*	Cause by filling of the right atrium while tricuspid valve is closed; occurs at end of S_2	Exaggerated "v" indicates an RV overload
y	Demonstrates the opening of the tricuspid valve and rapid blood flow from RA into RV; occurs after S_2	Prominent, rapid "y" descent is observed in tricuspid regurgitation; tricuspid stenosis produces a delayed "y" descent

*Usually only the "a" and "v" waves are visible on physical examination.

BLOOD PRESSURE

Systolic blood pressure is the force exerted against the arterial wall as the ventricle contracts. Diastolic blood pressure is the force produced during ventricular relaxation and filling. Pulse pressure is the difference between systolic and diastolic pressures.

Blood pressure is determined by two factors: cardiac output and peripheral vascular resistance. Thus blood pressure measurements reflect blood volume and elasticity of the arterial walls.

In most cases, blood pressure measurements provide an accurate evaluation of cardiovascular status. Under some circumstances, however, blood pressure measurements are inaccurate, even with the most careful technique. Cardiac dysrhythmias may cause readings to vary widely. The sounds produced by aortic regurgitation can obscure the diastolic pressure. Pathologic venous congestion can cause the systolic pressure to be heard lower and the diastolic pressure higher than they actually are. Repeated slow inflations of the cuff can also cause venous congestion.

Assessment

Upper extremities

Although blood pressure is routinely measured in one arm, a complete cardiovascular examination requires that measurements are made in both arms. Pressure in the dominant arm is usually as much as 10 mm Hg higher, but a greater differential may indicate an obstruction. The higher reading should be accepted as the patient's blood pressure reading.

Lower extremities

Blood pressure measurements should be made in the legs if the diastolic pressure in the arms is above 90 mm Hg or if coarctation or insufficiency of the aorta is suspected. The patient should be prone, if possible. If the patient is supine, the leg is flexed as little as possible. Center the bladder over the posterior surface and wrap the cuff around the distal third of the femur to auscultate the popliteal artery. Leg pressures are usually higher than arm pressures, but they are lower in cases of aortic insufficiency or coarctation of the aorta.

NORMAL BLOOD PRESSURES

	Systolic	Diastolic
Infants	60-96 mm Hg	30-62 mm Hg
Age 2	78-112 mm Hg	48-78 mm Hg
Age 8	85-114 mm Hg	52-85 mm Hg
Age 12	95-135 mm Hg	58-88 mm Hg
Adult	100-140 mm Hg	60-90 mm Hg

Systolic pressure in the thigh can be higher by 10 to 40 mm Hg as compared with brachial artery pressure. Diastolic pressure remains the same.

SIZES OF BLOOD PRESSURE CUFF BLADDERS

	Width (cm)	Length (cm)
Newborn	2.5-4.0	5.0-10.0
Infant	6.0-8.0	12.0-13.5
Child	9.0-10.0	17.0-22.5
Adult, standard	12.0-13.0	22.0-23.5
Adult, large arm	15.5	30.0
Adult, thigh	18.0	36.0

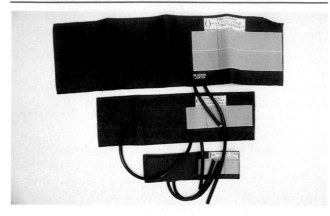

FIGURE 2-20
Three sizes of blood pressure cuffs: infant, child, and obese adult.

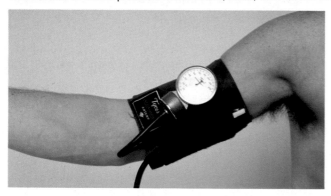

FIGURE 2-21
Proper placement of blood pressure cuff on arm.

How to Measure Blood Pressure

The correct-size cuff should be selected according to the diameter of the patient's limb (Figure 2-20). Too narrow a cuff produces an erroneously high reading, and too wide a cuff results in an erroneously low reading.

Wrap the cuff snugly around the upper arm so that the bottom edge is 2 to 5 cm (1 to 2 inches) above the antecubital space (Figure 2-21). While palpating the brachial artery, rapidly inflate the cuff to 20 to 30 mm Hg above the point at which the pulse disappears. Position the stethoscope bell over the pulse area. Deflate the cuff slowly (2 to 3 mm Hg per second), listening for the three Korotkoff sounds:

1. The first sound is the systolic pressure. Occasionally the sound disappears, reappearing 10 to 15 mm Hg later. This period of silence, called the auscultatory gap, has no significance.
2. The first diastolic sound is marked by muffling of the Korotkoff sound and is the closest approximation to the diastolic arterial pressure.
3. The second diastolic sound is the point at which all sounds disappear.

The American Heart Association recommends recording all three values for the blood pressure—the systolic and both diastolic measures (for example, 118/76/58). If only two values are recorded, the systolic pressure and the second diastolic pressure are recorded (120/58) (Figure 2-22).

	Systolic	Auscultatory gap		First diastolic	Second diastolic	
mm Hg 120		110	100	90	80	mm Hg
			Muffling			
	Sharp "thud"	Blowing or swishing sound	Softer thud than phase 1, still crisp	Softer blowing sound that disappears	Silence	
	PHASE 1	PHASE 2	PHASE 3	PHASE 4	PHASE 5	

FIGURE 2-22
Phases of Korotkoff sounds.

Abnormal Findings

Hypertension is usually defined on the basis of the diastolic pressure, since this is generally more stable than systolic pressure, which responds to a wide variety of emotional and physical stimuli. A diagnosis of hypertension is made only after three consecutive diastolic pressures are 90 mm Hg or above. A diastolic pressure between 85 and 89 mm Hg is considered high normal and requires close monitoring.

Mild hypertension	Diastolic pressure 90 to 104 mm Hg
Moderate hypertension	Diastolic pressure 105 to 114 mm Hg
Severe hypertension	Diastolic pressure above 115 mm Hg

Systolic pressure over 160 mm Hg and diastolic pressures under 90 mm Hg are common in persons over 65 and generally considered a function of aging.

Hypotension is defined as persistent blood pressure less than 95/60 mm Hg. In the absence of other signs and symptoms, hypotension is usually benign.

Postural hypotension is a common cause of dizziness and syncope, especially in older patients. It is easily diagnosed by first measuring the blood pressure while the patient is supine, then repeating the measurement with the patient standing. A slight or no drop in systolic pressure and a slight rise in diastolic pressure is expected. If postural hypotension is present, systolic pressure decreases 15 mm Hg or more, and diastolic pressure drops. Severe hypotension may be caused by hypovolemia, severe injury that produces shock, or endotoxin shock.

Patients who are taking antihypertensive drugs or are over 50 should be assessed for postural hypotension.

Pulse Pressure

Pulse pressure, which is normally 30 to 40 mm Hg, is influenced by heart rate. Bradycardia lowers diastolic pressure without affecting systolic pressure, causing the pulse pressure to widen. High output states and increased peripheral vascular resistance may also cause increased pulse pressure, whereas decreased stroke volume narrows the pulse pressure.

EXAMINATION OF THE PRECORDIUM

Thorough assessment of cardiac function should begin with inspection, then palpation, and finally auscultation of the precordium (chest). The room should be quiet without distractions, and the patient should be warm and comfortable.

The patient's age, size of the chest, and state of health influence the precordial examination. Obesity, large breasts, and muscularity can make the precordial examination more difficult.

Inspection

The chest should be inspected with the patient in the supine position, with the head slightly elevated to 30 degrees. A pocket flashlight can be used as a tangential light source to highlight any exaggerated precordial movement such as visible pulsations, lifts, heaves, or retractions.

The apical impulse, which provides information on LV function, is visible in the fifth left intercostal space 5 to 7 cm from the midsternal line (midclavicular line) in about half of normal adults. Fig. 2-23.

A slight retraction medial to the midclavicular line at the fifth intercostal space is a normal finding, but a marked retraction can reflect pericardial disease. Turning the patient to the left lateral decubitus position or sitting upright may aid in identification. A stronger impulse, characterized as a lift or heave, along the left sternal border occurs with increased right ventricular force.

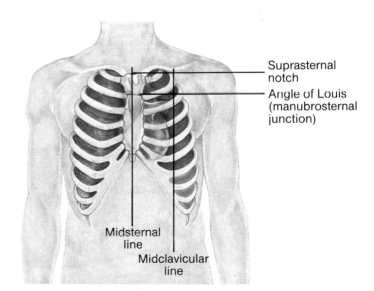

FIGURE 2-23
Landmarks of anterior chest.

Suprasternal notch

Angle of Louis (manubrosternal junction)

Midsternal line

Midclavicular line

FIGURE 2-24
Simultaneous palpation of the carotid artery and apical impulse to time systolic events.

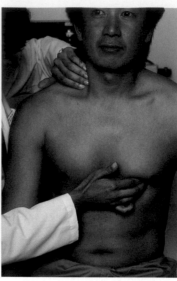

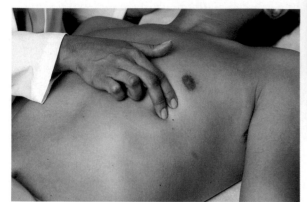

A

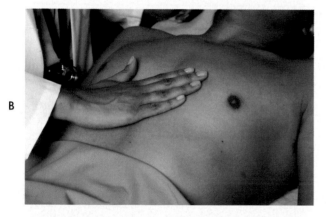

B

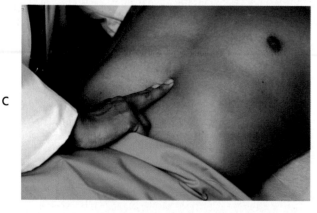

C

Palpation

A gentle touch is necessary in palpating the precordium, allowing movements of the chest to lift the hand. Heavy pressure obscures the pulsations. Palpation of the precordium can often be conducted with the patient supine, but it may be necessary to have the patient sit upright in order to feel the impulses. By simultaneously palpating the precordium and the carotid artery, systolic events can be timed. Be aware of any lifts or thrills (Figure 2-24).

The apical impulse may be difficult to feel with the patient supine; thus, having the patient assume the left lateral decubitus position or sit upright will help to identify it. The apical impulse is normally felt as a gentle, unsustained tap in an area about the size of a nickel (a radius of 2 to 3 cm) (Figure 2-25, A).

A slow lifting or sustained and forceful apical impulse that pushes upward into the examiner's hand indicates LV enlargement. Displacement of the apical impulse can be caused by dextrocardia, diaphragmatic hernia, abdominal distention, or pulmonary abnormality.

Palpation of the left sternal border provides information on right ventricular (RV) function. Using the heel of the hand and keeping the fingers elevated, the RV is best felt between the third, fourth, and fifth in-

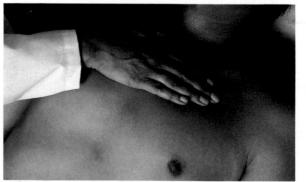

D

FIGURE 2-25
Palpation of precordium. A, The apical impulse is usually felt over the fifth intercostal space 5 to 7 cm from the left sternal border. B, Right ventricular impulses are detected at the left sternal border along the third, fourth, and fifth intercostal

spaces. C, Palpation of right ventricular impulse just below the sternum. D, The base of the heart is palpated at the right and left second intercostal spaces along the sternal border.

tercostal spaces (Figure 2-25, *B*). The RV impulse can also be palpated by gently placing the finger just below the sternum (Figure 2-25, *C*). Sustained and diffuse systolic lifts suggest RV hypertrophy that may be associated with pulmonary valvular disease, pulmonary hypertension, or chronic lung disease. A systolic thrill or parasternal lift suggests presence of a ventricular septal defect.

Palpation of the base of the heart, which is the area to the right and left of the second intercostal space, reflects events involving the pulmonic and aortic valves (Figure 2-25, *D*). This area should feel quiet, although in persons with thin chest walls, slight pulsation may be felt over the second and third interspaces near the sternum. Increased cardiac output caused by anemia, fever, exertion, or pregnancy may accentuate this, but the pulsation should be brief.

A thrill at the first and third interspaces is associated with aortic stenosis. (A thrill is a palpable vibration over the precordium or an artery.) The accentuated vibration of aortic valve closure during S_2 may be palpated in hypertensive patients. On the left side, pulmonic valve stenosis is associated with a thrill at the second and third left interspaces near the sternum. Marked pulsations can occur in the same area in patients with pulmonary hypertension or atrial septal defect.

AUSCULTATION

Normal heart sounds are relatively low in pitch, making them somewhat difficult to hear. Consequently, a quiet environment is essential when auscultating the heart. The patient should also be warm and relaxed, since tense muscles, movement, and shivering increase ambient sounds.

The sequence for auscultating the heart usually begins with the patient sitting up, although the patient's condition may require altering the procedure. There are three basic positions for auscultating heart sounds (Figure 2-26). A systematic approach to examination should be used, for example, beginning at the apex, then moving to the lower sternal border, and then ascending gradually along the left sternal border up to the right and left base. At each auscultation site, listen to one event at a time. All sites should be auscultated first with the diaphragm using firm pressure, and then with the bell using light pressure. Instruct the patient to breathe normally and then hold the breath in expiration. This permits the listener to better hear the sound.

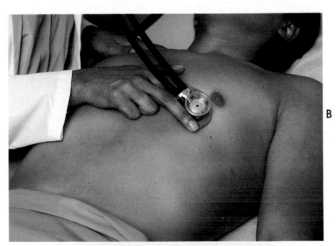

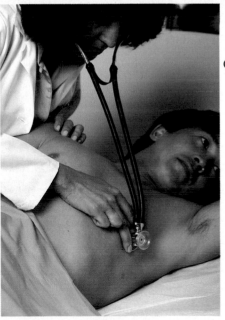

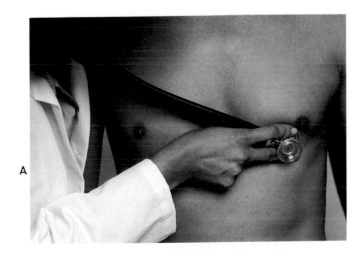

FIGURE 2-26
A, Have the patient sit up and lean slightly forward. B, Position the patient in a recumbent position with the thorax and chest elevated about 30 degrees. The head is comfortably supported with a pillow so the neck is relaxed. C, Position the patient in the left lateral recumbent position.

TIPS FOR IMPROVING AUSCULTATION OF HEART SOUNDS

Heart sounds are produced by sudden deceleration of a column of blood when the valves close. AV valve closure generates the "lubb" sounds (S_1). The "dubb" sound (S_2)—which may be heard as two sounds (split S_2)—is the closing of the aortic valve followed by the closing of the pulmonic valve.

1. Use a systematic approach, beginning at the mitral area, and proceed upward to the base.
2. Listen at each point for S_1, S_2, and extra cardiac sounds or murmurs.
3. Use the diaphragm first, then the bell. Low-pitched sounds are best heard with the stethoscope bell. High-pitched sounds are best heard with the diaphragm.
4. Heart sounds can be accentuated by positioning the patient in the left lateral decubitus position with the hips and knees flexed.
5. Systolic ejection clicks can be increased or decreased by postural changes such as standing and squatting.

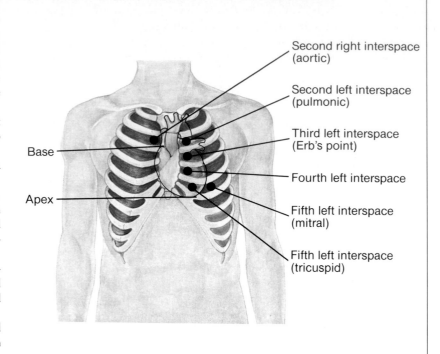

Second right interspace (aortic)

Second left interspace (pulmonic)

Third left interspace (Erb's point)

Fourth left interspace

Fifth left interspace (mitral)

Fifth left interspace (tricuspid)

Base

Apex

There are five auscultatory sites (see box above). At each of the sites, listen to one event at a time, identifying the first heart sound (S_1), then the second (S_2). Consider the following points as you examine each auscultatory site:

1. Overall rate and rhythm of the heart
2. Intensity, pitch, duration, and timing in the cardiac cycle
   a. Intensity (or loudness) is the degree to which a heart sound can be heard. This varies widely.
   b. Pitch is the frequency of the heart sound. Heart sounds are of relatively low intensity; however, extra sounds, such as diastolic murmur of mitral stenosis and S_3, are of lower frequencies. The diastolic murmur of aortic regurgitation or a normal S_2 are higher frequency sounds.
   c. Duration refers to how long the heart sound lasts. Heart sounds are brief, lasting much less than 1 second. The silent periods between S_1 and S_2, which reflect systole, and S_2 and S_1, which reflect diastole, are longer.
   d. Timing describes the heart sounds as they occur during the cardiac cycle. For example, systole begins with S_1 and extends to S_2. Diastole, which is a longer interval, begins with S_2 and extends to the next S_1. Simultaneously palpating the carotid artery while auscultating the heart aids in identifying systole.
3. Extra sounds: Listen for extra sounds, such as systolic clicks or ejection sounds, diastolic opening snaps, gallops, and murmurs.
4. Physiologic splitting: Listen for physiologic splitting associated with respiration.

NORMAL HEART SOUNDS

S_1

The first heart sound is produced by closure of the tricuspid (T_1) and mitral (M_1) valves and marks the beginning of systole (Figure 2-27). It is best heard at the apex and the fourth intercostal space–left sternal border. It corresponds with the upswing of the carotid pulse. Although the tricuspid valve closes slightly before the mitral valve, S_1 is normally heard as a single sound.

S_1 becomes more intense in high output states and with mitral valve stenosis. A decreased intensity occurs in systemic or pulmonary hypertension and valve fibrosis or calcification. Obesity, emphysema, and excess pericardial fluid can also obscure S_1. A varying intensity of S_1 suggests severe dysrhythmia or complete heart block.

S_2

The second heart sound is produced by closure of the pulmonic (P_2) and aortic (A_2) valves and marks the beginning of diastole (Figure 2-27). It is higher in pitch and of shorter duration than S_1. The relative intensity of S_1 and S_2 vary from the base to the apex. Instruct the patient to breathe normally while you listen for two distinct components of S_2 (split S_2). Instruct the patient to exhale and hold the breath, then inhale and hold the breath. Normally, S_2 tends to merge on expiration, becoming a single sound. Aortic valve closure (A_2) is best heard at the second right intercostal space, and pulmonic valve closure (P_2) is best heard at the second left intercostal space. Physiologic S_2 splitting typically is accentuated in older persons. In young children, S_2 is accentuated.

Systemic hypertension may cause S_2 to ring or boom. A_2 is accentuated in cases of systemic hypertension, syphilis of the aortic valve, and during exercise and excitement. P_2 is intensified in pulmonary hypertension, mitral stenosis, and congestive heart failure. A decreased intensity of S_2 occurs in severe arterial hypotension and in immobile, thickened, calcified, or stenosed valves. Overlying tissue, fat, or fluid also mutes S_2.

Split S_2 Abnormalities

Wide splitting of S_2 occurs when contraction or emptying of the right ventricle is delayed, resulting in delayed pulmonic clo-

HEART SOUNDS	AREA BEST HEARD
A — S_1 S_2 — Intense first sound	Apex
B — S_1 (M T) S_2 — Split first sound	Tricuspid
C — S_1 S_2 — Intense second sound	Base
D — S_1 S_2 — Physiological splitting—S_2 Expiration; S_1 S_2 (A P) — Inspiration	Base
E — S_1 S_2 S_3 — Third sound (ventricular gallop)	Apex
F — S_4 S_1 S_2 — Fourth sound (atrial gallop)	Apex
G — S_1 S_2 S_{3-4} — Summation gallop	Apex

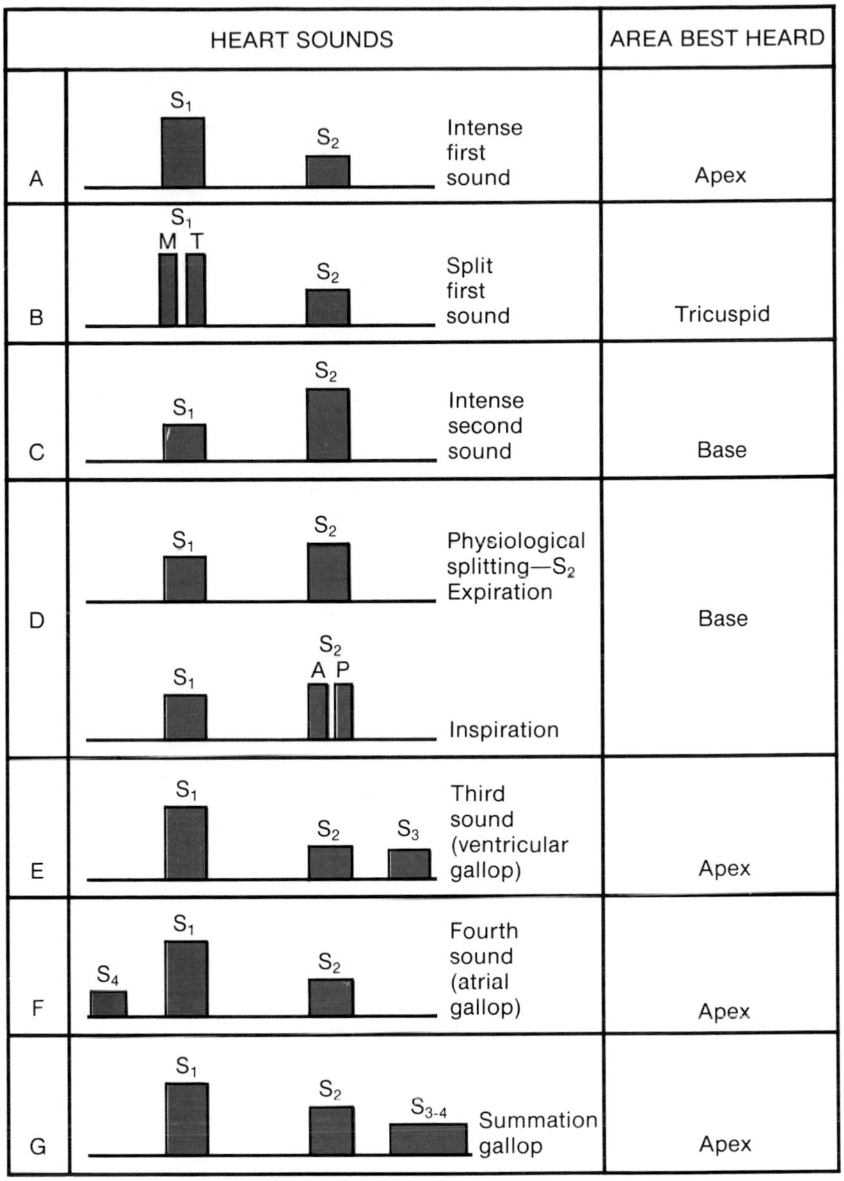

FIGURE 2-27
Normal heart sounds.

sure. This occurs in right bundle branch block and is accompanied by a split S_1. Other conditions causing wide splitting include pulmonic valve stenosis and mitral regurgitation that induces premature aortic valve closure.

Fixed splitting is unaffected by respirations. It is caused by delayed closure of the pulmonic valve when right ventricle output is greater than the left, as occurs with large septal defects and right ventricular failure.

Paradoxical splitting occurs with delayed aortic valve closure so that P_2 occurs first. The splitting disappears with inspiration. Paradoxical splitting is associated with left bundle branch block.

S₃

Vibration of the ventricular walls during rapid passive filling in early diastole produces the third heart sound—S_3 (also referred to as ventricular gallop). It occurs after closure of the semilunar valves. Best heard with the stethoscope bell at the apex while the patient is supine or in the left lateral decubitus position, S_3 is a soft, low-pitched sound.

An accentuated S_3 sound can result from conditions that cause more rapid filling, including exercise and elevation of the legs, or any factors that increase the heart rate. S_3 is commonly heard in children and young adults and is considered normal (physiologic S_3). In older persons, S_3 gallop signals heart failure.

S₄

S_4 (atrial gallop) is normally a soft, low-pitched sound caused by vibration of the valves, supporting structure, and ventricular walls during the second phase of rapid ventricular filling in late diastole. S_4 is related to augmentation of ventricular filling by a forceful atrial ejection into a distended ventricle. It is best heard with the bell of the apex and, because it occurs just before S_1, may be confused for a split S_1. Intensified S_4 or pre-systolic gallop may be heard in infants and children with thin chests but is rarely a normal finding in adults. S_4 gallop is caused by loss of ventricular wall compliance from hypertension or coronary artery disease or from increased stroke volume in high cardiac output states. A quadruple rhythm, resulting from rapid ventricular filling, produces an audible S_3 and S_4. At increased heart rates, diastole becomes shorter, and the two sounds may become fused. The result is a summation gallop with three cardiac sounds—S_1, S_2, and the summation sounds of S_3-S_4.

ABNORMAL HEART SOUNDS

Abnormal heart sounds can be classified into 3 categories: extracardiac, miscellaneous, and murmurs. **Extracardiac (extra heart) sounds,** which include opening snaps and ejection clicks, are generated from thickened, roughened valves or valves that have been damaged. They usually accompany a heart murmur. Opening of the mitral valve is generally a silent event; however, in the presence of stenosis, this becomes audible and is referred to as an **opening snap.** It occurs early in diastole and is best heard near the apex toward the left sternal border; it may radiate toward the base. The sound is high-pitched, brief, and has a snapping or clicking quality. It is generally associated with a loud S_1, and respiration does not alter the timing.

The **ejection click,** produced by opening of the semilunar valve, occurs early in systole. Aortic valve ejection click is heard at both the base and the apex and does not change with respiration. The less common pulmonic ejection click is best heard at the second left intercostal space. It increases with expiration and decreases with inspiration.

Pericardial friction rub produces grating, machine-like sounds heard throughout systole and diastole. They are heard widely but are more distinct at the apex and sternum. It is caused by roughened visceral and parietal surfaces of an inflamed pericardial sac rubbing together. A three-component friction rub, which is more grating in quality, indicates pericarditis. It is loud enough to obscure the heart sounds. A one- or two-component friction rub, which may not be as loud, is more indicative of a pleural friction rub.

MURMURS

Heart murmurs are a series of prolonged sounds heard during either systole or diastole. They are produced by vibrations that are created by disruption in the blood flow as it passes through the heart or great vessels. They can arise from structural changes or defects in the valves, the heart itself, or the great vessels. Like normal heart sounds, murmurs are best heard over the auscultatory areas, rather than directly over the defective structure.

Murmurs are classified by timing (systolic or diastolic), pitch, (high, medium, low), intensity, sound pattern, quality, location, radiation, and effects of respiration.

Murmurs occurring during the ventricular ejection phase of the cardiac cycle are referred to as systolic sounds. The majority of systolic murmurs are caused either by obstruction to the outflow tract (semilunar valves) or by incompetent atrioventricular valves. The vibratory sound may be heard through part or all of systole.

There are other causes of systolic murmurs, including structural deformities of the aorta or pulmonary arteries. A ventricular septal defect results in a murmur classified as pansystolic or holosystolic because it occupies all of systole.

Murmurs occurring during the filling phase of the cardiac cycle are referred to as diastolic murmurs. In-

GRADING OF CARDIAC MURMURS

Classification	Description
Grade I	Soft, barely audible in quiet room
Grade II	Quiet but clearly audible
Grade III	Moderately loud, without thrill
Grade IV	Loud, associated with thrill
Grade V	Very loud, thrill easily palpable
Grade VI	Very loud, audible with stethoscope off the chest, thrill palpable and visible

HEART MURMURS

Pattern	Types	Detection	Quality	Variables
Holosystolic murmur	Mitral regurgitation Tricuspid regurgitation Ventricular septal defect	Diaphragm at apex, radiates to left axilla or base	High pitch with harsh blowing quality	Thrill may be palpable at base; S_1 decreased; S_2 increased with P_2 often accentuated; S_3 often present. If mild, late systolic crescendo present; if severe, early systolic decrescendo and summation gallop present.
Systolic ejection murmur	Aortic stenosis	Heard over aortic valve area; ejection sound at second right intercostal border	Medium pitch, coarse, with crescendo-decrescendo pattern	May radiate as far as apex and to carotid with thrill; S_1 may be followed by ejection click; S_2 soft or absent; S_4 palpable.
	Pulmonic stenosis	Heard over pulmonic valve; radiates left to neck; thrill at second and third left intercostal spaces	Same as for aortic stenosis	S_1 usually followed by quick ejection click; S_2 often diminished with wide split; P_2 may be soft or absent; S_4 common if right ventricular hypertrophy present.
Diastolic murmur	Mitral stenosis	Bell at apex with patient in left lateral decubitus position	Low rumble more intense in early and late diastole	Thrill at apex in late diastole common; S_1 increased and often palpable at left sternal border; accentuated P_2 common followed closely by opening snap. Decreased arterial pulse amplitude.
	Tricuspid stenosis	Bell over tricuspid area	Similar to mitral stenosis but louder on inspiration	Thrill over right ventricle; S_2 may split during inspiration. Decreased arterial pulse amplitude. Jugular pulse prominent, especially a wave; v wave falls slowly.
Diastolic regurgitant murmur	Aortic regurgitation	Diaphragm, patient sitting and leaning forward Austin-Flint: bell, ejection click at second intercostal space	High pitch, blowing in early diastole Austin-Flint: low pitch rumbling at apex	Decrescendo midsystolic murmur common; early ejection click may be present; S_1 soft; S_2 split may have tambour-like quality; summation gallop common. Wide pulse pressure; bisferiens pulse common in carotid, brachial, and femoral arteries.
	Pulmonic regurgitation	Same as aortic regurgitation	Same as aortic regurgitation	Difficult to distinguish from aortic regurgitation on physical examination.

competent semilunar or stenotic AV valves create diastolic murmurs.

Diastolic murmurs almost always indicate heart disease. Early diastolic murmurs usually result from insufficiency of a semilunar valve or dilation of the valvular ring. Mid- and late-diastolic murmurs are generally caused by narrowed, stenosed mitral or tricuspid valves that obstruct blood flow.

A loud heart murmur that is accompanied by a thrill usually indicates a pathologic condition.

Innocent Murmurs

Murmurs are often a normal finding, particularly in children and adolescents. Innocent murmurs appear to result from vigorous myocardial contraction, resulting in stronger blood flow in early or midsystole, and are more easily heard through the thinner chest walls of the young. They also are seen in high output states, including pregnancy, anxiety, anemia, fever, and thyrotoxicosis.

Innocent murmurs are usually grade I or II, without radiation, of medium pitch, blowing, and brief. Typically they increase in intensity during held expiration and may change with the patient's position. They usually occupy only a portion of systole and are unaccompanied by a thrill. They are most easily heard with a bell placed lightly over the second intercostal space near the left sternal border with the patient recumbent. The murmur often disappears when the patient sits or stands.

TYPES OF INNOCENT MURMURS

Vibratory systolic murmur
Pulmonic ejection systolic murmur
Aortic midsystolic murmur
Supraclavicular systolic murmur
Systolic or continuous mammary soufflé
Venous hum

Diagnostic Procedures

ELECTROCARDIOGRAM

The electrocardiogram (ECG) produces a graphic recording of the heart's electrical activity. Each ECG waveform represents a single electrical impulse as it travels through the heart. The ECG is commonly used to detect abnormal transmission of impulses, but it also provides information on the electrical position of the heart (the axis) and the sizes of cardiac chambers.

ECG LEADS

The standard ECG records electrical activity of the heart from twelve locations, or leads: six on the chest and six on the limbs (Figures 3-1 and 3-2). The six precordial leads (V1 through V6) measure electrical activity of the anterior, posterior, and lateral cardiac walls and record cardiac forces on the horizontal plane. The limb

leads measure forces on the frontal plane. Leads I, II, and III are bipolar limb leads that record the difference in electrical force between two electrode sites. The augmented limb leads (aVR, aVL, and aVF) are unipolar leads used to compare the electrical potential at one site with the center of the heart (zero point).

Because the ECG leads record the electrical forces from different sites, the tracing of a single impulse looks different from each lead.

Continuous beat-to-beat monitoring is accomplished by connecting either one of the bipolar limb leads or a modified chest lead (MCL) to an oscilloscope. The modified chest lead is created by placing the positive electrode at the V1 position and the negative electrode

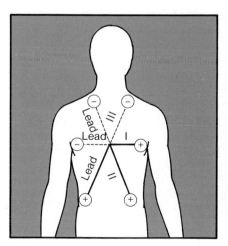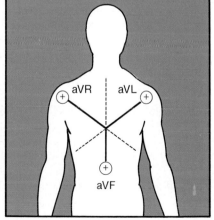

FIGURE 3-1
Positions for ECG leads. **A,** Standard bipolar limb leads I, II, and III (Einthoven triangle). **B,** Augmented unipolar limb leads aVR, aVL, and aVF. (From Thelan.)

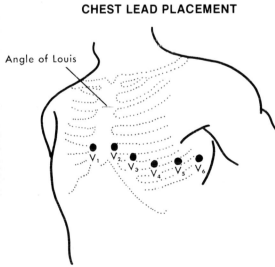

CHEST LEAD PLACEMENT

FIGURE 3-2
Precordial unipolar leads. (From Thelan.)

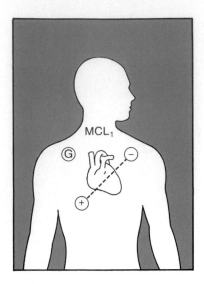

FIGURE 3-3
Modified chest lead. (From Thelan.)

INDICATIONS

To diagnose and monitor: Congenital heart disease
Congestive heart failure
Dysrhythmias
Myocardial infarction
Valvular heart disease
Routine physical examination
Pre- and postoperative evaluation and monitoring

CONTRAINDICATIONS

None

on the upper left chest (Figure 3-3). The lead selected depends on which aspect of the ECG is being monitored. For example, lead II is often used because it produces clear graphs of P wave and QRS complexes. However, in differentiating between right and left premature ventricular contractions, a modified chest lead is preferred.

RECORDING

The ECG tracing is printed on graph paper at a standard speed of 25 mm/sec, with a 0.1 mV electrical impulse producing a 1-mm positive (upward) deflection. On standard ECG graph paper, voltage is measured on the vertical scale, with the smaller 1-mm box equaling 0.1 mV and the larger 5-mm box equaling 0.5 mV. Time is measured on the horizontal axis: 1 mm equals 0.04 seconds and 5 mm equals 0.2 seconds. Thus five large 5-mm grids show 1 second of electrical activity.

NURSING CARE

Ensure electrical safety measures such as grounding.

PATIENT TEACHING

Explain the purpose of the ECG. Describe the procedure, explaining that the ECG is noninvasive and will not cause side effects.

ECG WAVEFORM COMPONENTS

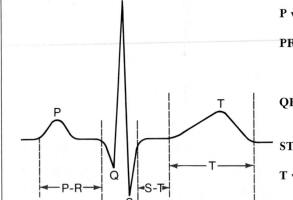

P wave—electrical activity associated with SA node impulse and depolarization of the atria

PR interval—the time the impulse takes to travel through the atria to the AV node, the His-Purkinje system, and through the ventricles
Normal duration: 0.12 to 0.20 second

QRS complex—the electrical depolarization and contraction of the ventricles
Normal duration: .04 to 0.12 second

ST segment—the period between completion of depolarization and the beginning of repolarization of the ventricles

T wave—the recovery, or repolarization, phase of the ventricles

AMBULATORY ELECTROCARDIOGRAPHY (Holter monitor)

The Holter monitor is a portable device that records electrical activity of the heart and produces a continuous electrocardiogram (ECG) on graph paper. Patients keep a diary of their activities and physical symptoms. Symptoms can be correlated with changes in heart rate or rhythm.

The equipment consists of chest electrodes attached to a 2-pound tape recorder that is carried with a belt or shoulder strap. Patients are generally monitored over 12-, 24-, or 48-hour periods (Figures 3-4 and 3-5).

Ambulatory ECG is particulary useful for patients whose clinical symptoms indicate heart disorders but may have normal ECG tracings on standard testing.

INDICATIONS

To diagnose: Suspected dysrhythmias
Unexplained symptoms such as dizziness, syncope, or palpitations
Chest pain episodes
To evaluate: Effectiveness of antiarrhythmic drugs
Pacemaker function

CONTRAINDICATIONS

None

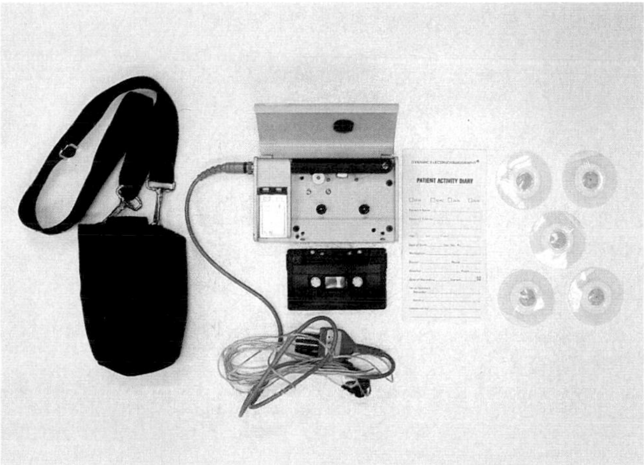

NURSING CARE

The equipment should be inspected to ensure that the lead cable is connected to the monitor and the electrodes are positioned securely. Inspect the patient's skin for signs of irritation from the electrode paste or gel. Be certain that the electrodes are not attached to large muscles to avoid producing artifacts from movement on the ECG.

PATIENT TEACHING

Explain the reason for and purpose of Holter monitoring and stress the importance of continuing with normal activities. Discuss what needs to be included in the written diary (activities, emotional stress, symptoms, and any medications taken, including nonprescription drugs).

Demonstrate how to check the recorder for proper functioning, and have the patient give a return demonstration. Supply instructions on what to do if the equipment malfunctions. Explain that the patient must not get the equipment wet and should forego showers or tub baths during the monitoring period.

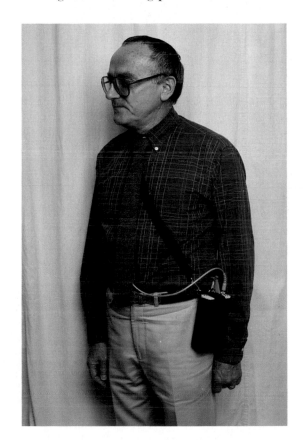

FIGURE 3-5
Patient wearing Holter monitor.

FIGURE 3-4
Equipment for ambulatory electrocardiography (Holter monitor).

EXERCISE STRESS TEST

The exercise stress test (EST) evaluates cardiovascular response to physical stress. The test provides information on myocardial response to increased oxygen demands and determines the adequacy of coronary blood flow. Heart rate, electrical activity, and cardiac recovery time are reflected in the ECG tracing. In addition, the patient's blood pressure and overall clinical response are monitored as the patient exercises (Figures 3-6 and 3-7).

Exercise Testing Protocols

Several exercise testing protocols have been developed. **Single-stage tests** provide some basic information about cardiac function, but they cannot evaluate functional capacity because the workload is constant and the activity is not demanding. For example, in the Master's, or 2-step, test, the patient walks up and down a 2-step staircase while being monitored.

Multistage tests increase cardiovascular workload at regular intervals. The rate, treadmill incline, and length of the test are variables used to increase the workload. For example, the Bruce protocol, a frequently used study, increases the exertion level every 3 minutes by increasing the work level (speed + incline).

Ministress tests are designed to determine the safety of beginning a home walking program for patients recovering from myocardial infarction. The test is usually administered before hospital discharge. The patient walks a treadmill or pedals a stationary bicycle, and the speed or resistance is increased slightly until a predetermined heart rate is reached or the patient develops symptoms.

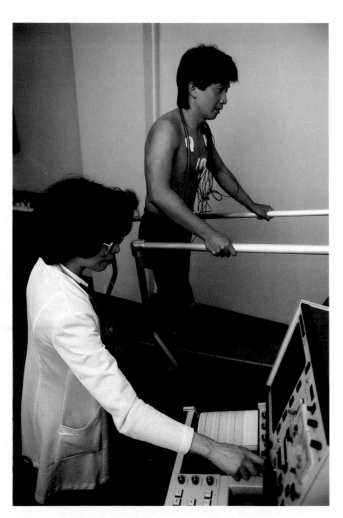

FIGURE 3-6
Patient taking exercise stress test while nurse monitors the ECG response.

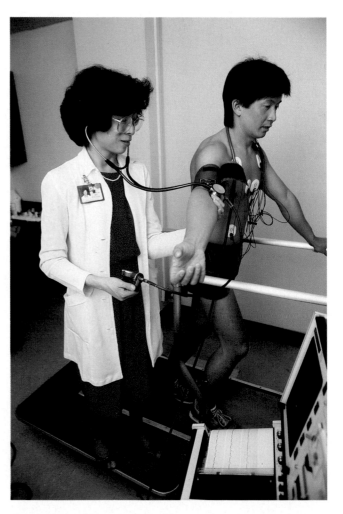

FIGURE 3-7
Nurse monitoring blood pressure response during exercise stress test.

Submaximal stress testing evaluates the effect of exercise that produces less than maximum cardiac exertion. If pulse rate is used as the termination point, this test measures the level of exertion attained at less (usually 70% to 85%) than the age-predicted maximum heart rate. Other methods use a predetermined MET level as the termination point. (MET is a unit of measurement of oxygen consumption by an individual at rest, with 1 MET level = 3.5 ml O_2/kg/min. Tables have been developed that list MET performance based on age.)

Maximal stress testing (or symptom-limited tests) allows the patient to exercise until exhaustion occurs or symptoms develop. These tests evaluate functional capacity of patients 6 to 8 weeks after myocardial infarction or cardiac surgery. Maximal testing is also useful for evaluating cardiovascular fitness before embarking on a fitness program.

Results

The results of stress testing are considered negative if no ECG abnormalities develop and the patient remains free of symptoms. Abnormal findings should be interpreted cautiously, since false-positive results sometimes occur.[13]

INDICATIONS

To diagnose: Chest pain
    Exercise-induced symptoms
    Exercise-induced dysrhythmias
To evaluate: Effectiveness of antiarrhythmic drug therapy
    Cardiovascular fitness prior to starting an exercise program
    Exercise tolerance and functional capacity prior to cardiac rehabilitation program

CONTRAINDICATIONS

Recent myocardial infarction (within 6 weeks)
Unstable angina
Uncontrolled hypertension
Untreated heart failure

NURSING CARE

During stress testing monitor blood pressure, heart rate, and ECG changes such as ST elevation, ST depression, and dysrhythmias.

After the procedure observe the patient for shortness of breath, fatigue, and complaints of chest pain or pressure. If ECG monitoring is continued, monitor for any changes.

PATIENT TEACHING

Explain the procedure and its purpose. Instruct the patient to dress comfortably in gym clothes and athletic shoes. Also instruct the patient not to eat or smoke for 1 to 2 hours before the test and to take prescribed medications as usual, unless instructed otherwise by the physician. Before beginning the test, explain that the patient must report any symptoms immediately during and after the test.

STRESS TESTING ABNORMALITIES

Test	Abnormal results
ECG	Flattening of downslope ≥ 1 mm of the ST segment for at least 0.08 sec at the J point (following junction of QRS and ST segments); development of dysrhythmias (see Figure 3-7)
Blood pressure	Fall of ≥ 10 mm Hg of systolic pressure or rise of diastolic pressure (NOTE: Diastolic pressure should remain constant or decrease slightly)
Heart rate	Bradycardia or heart rate that exceeds predetermined level based on age-predicted maximal heart rate
Symptoms	Chest pain, with or without ST segment depression suggests myocardial ischemia
	Syncope, loss of coordination, mental confusion, or excessive shortness of breath suggests possible valvular or ventricular dysfunction
	Intermittent claudication suggests peripheral vascular disease

ECHOCARDIOGRAPHY

Echocardiography is a noninvasive technique evaluating the internal structures and motions of the heart and great vessels. Ultrasound beams are directed into the patient's chest by a transducer (Figures 3-8 and 3-9). The transducer then acts as a receiver of the ultrasonic waves, or "echoes," to form images.

The images produced from the echoes are transmitted to a monitor. Echocardiography graphically demonstrates overall cardiac performance. It shows the internal dimensions of the chambers, size and motion of the intraventricular septum and posterior left ventricular wall, valve motion and anatomy, direction of blood flow, and the presence of increased pericardial fluid, blood clots, and myomatous tumors.

Modes

Three echocardiographic techniques are used in clinical practice. All use a transducer that emits ultrasonic pulses through the chest wall and receives echoes from the cardiac structures.

M-mode (motion-mode) echocardiography produces an "ice-pick" image of a narrow area within the ultrasonic beam. It shows a one-dimensional, single axis view restricted to the anteroposterior plane. M-mode provides an oscilloscopic presentation that shows position and motion of cardiac structures.

Two-dimensional (2-D) echocardiography produces a cross-sectional view and real time motion of cardiac structures. It allows the ultrasonic beam to move quickly showing the structures and lateral movement. Together this shows the spatial relationship between the heart structures (Figure 3-10).

Numerous views are possible with 2-D echocardiography. The most common views are the apical four-chamber and the parasternal long-axis.

The apical four-chamber view shows the four chambers as well as the mitral and tricuspid valves. In the parasternal long-axis view, a sagittal section of the heart, apex to base, is scanned parallel to the long axis of the left ventricle.

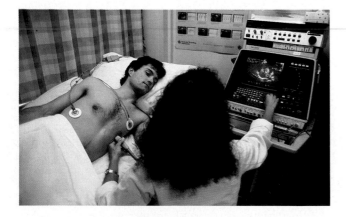

FIGURE 3-8
Clinical laboratory for echocardiography.

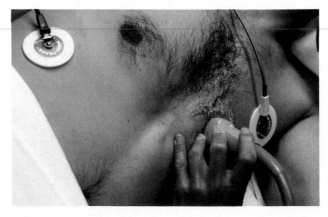

FIGURE 3-9
Close-up of chest leads and placement of transducer on precordium.

INDICATIONS

To diagnose: Valvular heart disease
Congenital heart disease
Cardiomyopathy
Congestive heart failure
Pericardial disease
Cardiac tumors
Intracardiac thrombi

To evaluate: Left ventricular function after myocardial infarction
Presence of pericardial fluid

CONTRAINDICATIONS

None

Doppler ultrasonography provides continuous waves but also uses a sound or frequency ultrasound to record the direction of blood flow through the heart. These sound waves are reflected off red blood cells as they pass through the heart and are referred to as objects. By knowing Doppler frequencies, the velocity of blood can be calculated as it travels through the heart chambers.

Color Doppler mapping is a variation that converts recorded flow frequencies into different colors (Figure 3-11). These color images are then superimposed on M-mode or 2-D echocardiograms, allowing more detailed evaluation of disorders.[13]

NURSING CARE

No specific nursing care is needed for patients undergoing echocardiography.

PATIENT TEACHING

Describe the procedure, stressing that echocardiography is noninvasive and will not cause side effects. Explain that the procedure usually lasts about 1 hour. Explain that a conductive gel will be applied to the chest and the only discomfort may come from pressure of the transducer against the chest. Explain that the patient will be positioned on the left side and may be asked to breathe in and out slowly or to hold the breath. The patient will need to remain quiet during the study.

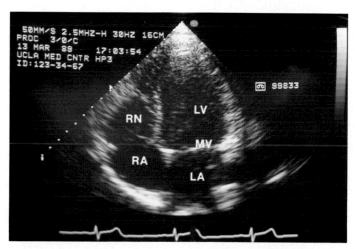

A

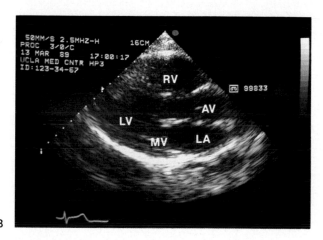

B

FIGURE 3-10
Two dimensional (2-D) echocardiography. **(A)** and **(B)**. (Labels have been added to identify the structures. *RA,* right atrium; *RV,* right ventricle; *LA,* left atrium; *LV,* left ventricle; *MV,* mitral valve.)

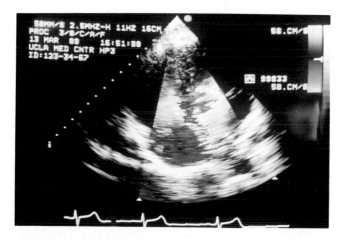

FIGURE 3-11
Color flow Doppler echocardiography. Flow, or signals, moving toward the transducer are recorded in shades of yellow or red. Those moving away from the transducer are recorded as blue.

SCINTIGRAPHY

Scintigraphy or radionuclide angiography is a noninvasive imaging technique that uses radioisotopes to evaluate cardiac structures, myocardial perfusion, and contractility. Radioisotopes emit gamma rays that are detected by a scintillation or scanning camera, which takes a series of images showing the location of the isotopes (Figure 3-12). Two types of radioisotopes are used: those that label the blood vessels and those that label the myocardium. Of the latter type, there are two classes of isotopes: "cold spot" agents that are incorporated into normal myocardial cells and "hot spot" isotopes that bind only to damaged myocardial tissue.

No complications are associated with scintigraphy.

TECHNETIUM-99M PYROPHOSPHATE (99mTc-Pyp) SCINTIGRAPHY

99mTc-Pyp, a standard isotope used in bone scans, binds to calcium. Because calcium crystals are deposited on damaged myocardial tissue, 99mTc-Pyp scintigraphy is ideal for detecting necrosis from acute myocardial infarction. This technique creates "hot spots" that can be detected within 12 hours of myocardial infarction, becoming most apparent between 12 and 48 hours after infarction. Normally, these areas disappear within 1 week. Because areas that persist longer than 1 week suggest ongoing tissue damage, scintigraphy is usually repeated over several weeks to track recurring damage.

99mTc-Pyp also images calcification on valves and great vessels.

INDICATIONS

Recent myocardial infarction
Valve calcifications

CONTRAINDICATIONS

None

NURSING CARE

No specific nursing care is required for 99mTc-Pyp scintigraphy.

PATIENT TEACHING

Explain that 99mTc-Pyp is injected into a vein 2 to 3 hours before scintigraphy is performed. Explain that the scintillation camera passes repeatedly over the patient and that the procedure takes 30 to 60 minutes.

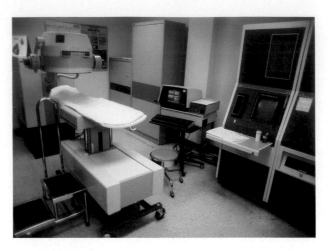

FIGURE 3-12
Clinical setting for scintigraphy.

THALLIUM-201 SCINTIGRAPHY

Thallium-201 or myocardial perfusion scintigraphy is a "cold spot" technique used to diagnose ischemic heart disease. Since the radionuclide concentrates in tissues with normal blood flow, tissue with inadequate perfusion appears as dark areas on scanning (Figure 3-13). Thallium-201 scintigraphy is often used in conjunction with ECG stress testing.

The usual procedure is for the patient to continue the standard ECG treadmill or bicycle ergometer test until chest discomfort, ECG changes, shortness of breath, or fatigue develops. Thallium-201 is then injected and the stress test is resumed for 30 to 60 seconds to allow maximal myocardial uptake. Scintigraphy is performed immediately and repeated 4 hours later.

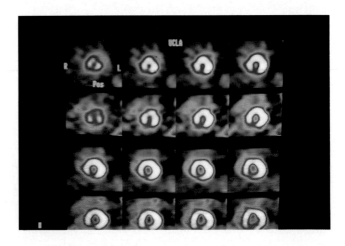

FIGURE 3-13
Thallium-201 scintigraphy produces a series of images of blood flow and tissue perfusion.

INDICATIONS

To diagnose: Coronary artery disease
To evaluate: Myocardial perfusion
                Patency of grafts after bypass surgery

CONTRAINDICATIONS

None

NURSING CARE

No specific nursing care is required for thallium-201 scintigraphy.

PATIENT TEACHING

Explain the procedure. Instruct the patient to take nothing by mouth 3 hours before the test. If done in conjunction with exercise stress testing, explain that the patient must refrain from tobacco, alcohol, and un-prescribed medications for 24 hours before the study.

BLOOD POOL SCINTIGRAPHY

Blood pool scintigraphy or multiple-gated blood pool imaging is used to evaluate ventricular function and left ventricular volume. Human serum albumin or the patient's red blood cells are tagged with technetium-99m pertechnetate and injected intravenously. The scintillation camera records the isotope as it passes through the ventricle. Imaging can be "gated" to the systolic and diastolic events of the cardiac cycle by a device that recognizes the QRS complex of the ECG.

The camera images the heart in at least two views, left and right anterior oblique. A cine film is produced that permits analysis of chamber size, wall motion, filling defects, and ventricular abnormalities (Figure 3-14).

NURSING CARE

No specific nursing care is indicated for blood pool imaging.

FIGURE 3-14
Blood pool imaging.

PATIENT TEACHING

Explain the procedure. If scintigraphy is performed in conjunction with other procedures, provide the appropriate information.

INDICATIONS

To diagnose: Aneurysms of the left ventricle
              Areas of hypokinesis and dyskinesis of the
              left ventricle
To evaluate: Acute myocardial infarction
             Aortic valve insufficiency
             Congestive heart failure
             Intra-aortic balloon counterpulsation
             Ischemic heart disease
             Therapeutic effects of nitroglycerin and ni-
             troprusside

CONTRAINDICATIONS

Pregnancy

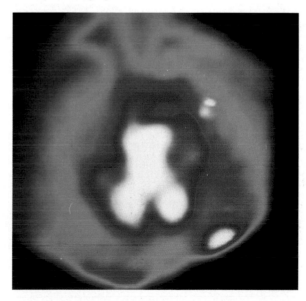

A, Systolic frame.

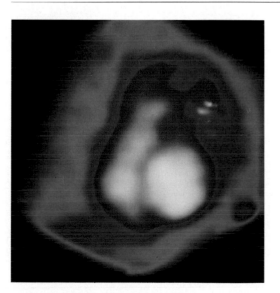

B, Diastolic frame.

CARDIAC CATHETERIZATION AND ANGIOGRAPHY

Cardiac catheterization is an invasive procedure used to visualize the heart's chambers, valves, great vessels, and coronary arteries. In addition, pressure measurements and blood volumes are obtained to evaluate cardiac function and provide information regarding valve patency. The catheterization procedure also is used in a variety of diagnostic and therapeutic procedures, including electrophysiologic studies, hemodynamic monitoring, percutaneous transluminal angioplasty, and palliative procedures for congenital heart defects (Figure 3-15).

Several techniques have been developed that permit assessment of various parameters. The basic procedure involves inserting a flexible, radiopaque catheter through a peripheral vein (right heart catheterization) or artery (left heart catheterization) and guiding it into the heart. Pressures are recorded, blood samples are drawn, and contrast material can be injected through the catheter.

The route of entry may be either by the cut-down or percutaneous method. Because of improvements in catheters, the percutaneous approach has become the more common technique (Figure 3-16). As equipment and techniques have improved, elective cardiac catheterization is associated with a low rate of complications and is often performed on an outpatient basis in low-risk patients.[172]

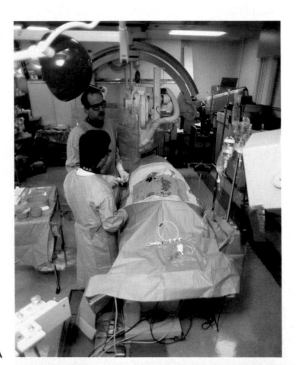

A

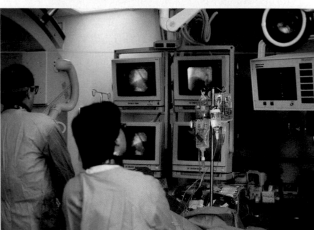

B

FIGURE 3-15
A, Clinical setting for cardiac catheterization. **B,** Monitoring cardiac catheterization procedure.

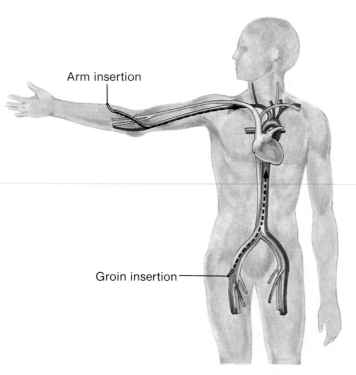

Arm insertion

Groin insertion

FIGURE 3-16
Insertion sites for cardiac catheterization.

RIGHT-SIDED CATHETERIZATION

Right-sided heart catheterization studies include right heart pressure readings, oximetry, shunt studies, calculation of cardiac output, and angiography of the right atrium, right ventricle, tricuspid and pulmonary valves, and pulmonary artery. This technique is also used for continuous hemodynamic monitoring. Catheter insertion is through the basilic or femoral vein.

LEFT-SIDED CATHETERIZATION

Left-sided heart catheterization includes obtaining pressures of the aorta and left-sided chambers. The data obtained provide information regarding left ventricular function and mitral and aortic valve function and shunting. Angiography of the coronary arteries, aortic root, and left ventricle are performed during left-sided catheterization. Catheterization is usually via the brachial or femoral artery.

ANGIOGRAPHY

With the injection of radiopaque contrast material through the cardiac catheter, sequential films can be made to selectively visualize the vessels or chambers. The two standard filming methods are cineangiography and serial angiography. Cineangiography is a technique that produces a motion picture film of the fluoroscopic images. Serial angiography uses a rapid film changer to produce a series of roentgenographic films.

Several different techniques are available to assess cardiac function:

- Aortography identifies structural abnormalities of the aorta and assesses aortic valve competence.
- Coronary arteriography shows any structural abnormalities in the coronary arteries (Figure 3-17).
- Pulmonary angiography detects structural abnormalities in the pulmonary circulation. It is used to evaluate patients with congenital heart disease and pulmonary hypertension and to diagnose pulmonary embolism.
- Ventriculography of the right or left ventricle demonstrates chamber volume, wall thickness, and wall motion. This method detects abnormalities of contraction and AV valve regurgitation.

A
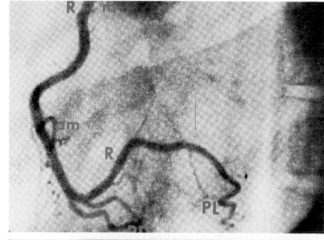

B
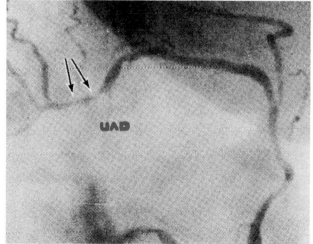

FIGURE 3-17
Coronary arteriography. **A,** Normal filling of right coronary artery. **B,** Obstruction of right coronary artery *(see arrows).*

INDICATIONS FOR RIGHT-SIDED CATHETERIZATION

Intracardiac shunt
Myocardial dysfunction
Pericardial constriction
Pulmonary vascular disease
Valvular heart disease

INDICATIONS FOR LEFT-SIDED CATHETERIZATION

Aortic dissection
Atypical angina
Cardiomyopathy
Congenital heart disease
Coronary heart disease
Pericardial constriction
Post-myocardial infarction complications
Post-heart transplantation
Valvular heart disease

CONTRAINDICATIONS

There are no absolute contraindications to catheterization. Relative contraindications may be considered in the following cases: patients with uncontrollable congestive heart failure, dysrhythmias, infections, drug toxicity, or electrolyte imbalance, or other uncontrolled systemic diseases. In patients with a history of severe reactions to contrast media, angiography should be approached cautiously. Unstable angina, anticoagulant therapy, and pregnancy are relative contraindications. The risk of postponing studies must be weighed against the increased risk of complications in these patients.

COMPLICATIONS

The general complications of catheterization include myocardial infarction, dysrhythmias (i.e., bradycardia, ventricular fibrillation), perforation leading to cardiac tamponade, and adverse reactions to the contrast media. The contrast media used contains iodine, which can produce allergic reactions ranging from a mild rash to anaphylaxis in hypersensitive persons.

The peripheral arterial complications include stroke, pulmonary edema, embolism, thrombosis, aneurysm, infection, and hematoma or hemorrhage at the insertion site.

NURSING CARE

Before the procedure, obtain written informed consent. Determine whether the patient has any allergies to shellfish or iodine or has had an allergic reaction to contrast media in the past. Give nothing by mouth for 6 to 12 hours before the procedure. Withhold routine medications and administer sedative, as ordered. Shave and cleanse the skin at the insertion site.

After the procedure, check vital signs every 15 minutes for the first hour, decreasing in frequency until the patient is stable. Give pain medication as ordered. Encourage fluid intake for the first 6 to 8 hours to help flush out contrast medium.

After arterial puncture, keep the patient in bed with the head elevated at a 20- to 30-degree angle for 6 to 8 hours. Keep the extremity immobile for 2 to 4 hours with a sandbag over the puncture site, applying ice as needed. Compare the peripheral pulse distal to the insertion site with the unaffected site, noting quality, and report any discrepancies. Inspect the area and surrounding skin for redness, swelling, heat, and pain. Observe for development of hematoma at site of insertion, vasospasm of affected extremity (numbness, tingling, loss of pulse), chest pain, or shortness of breath. Notify the physician immediately if systemic or local signs of infection are detected, and obtain blood cultures as ordered.

After venous puncture, maintain the patient on bed rest for 4 to 6 hours. Keep a pressure dressing over the insertion site, and check the site and surrounding area for bleeding, pain, and swelling. Check the peripheral pulses, color, warmth, and feeling of the extremities distal to the puncture site.

PATIENT TEACHING

Before the procedure, explain to the patient and family that the procedure will last 1 to 3 hours. Provide an overview of the procedure. Inform the patient that a local anesthetic will be given in the area where the catheter is to be inserted, that a feeling of pressure may be felt during insertion of the catheter, and that a flushing sensation or nausea when the contrast media is injected. Explain that the patient should cough when instructed by the physician, and that medication will be given if chest pain or other discomfort occurs. Assure the patient that he or she will be closely monitored throughout the procedure. **After the procedure,** instruct the patient to report any signs and symptoms of swelling, increased discoloration, and bleeding at puncture sites.

ELECTROPHYSIOLOGIC STUDIES

Electrophysiologic (EP), or bundle of His, studies are performed to evaluate the electrical conduction system of the heart. Similar to right heart catheterization, an electrode catheter is inserted, usually via the femoral vein, and threaded through the inferior vena cava. It is advanced into the right atrium, through the tricuspid valve, and into the apex of the right ventricle. The patient is monitored continuously with both intracardiac electrocardiograms and external ECG leads to record the cardiac response.

Programmed electrical stimulation (PES) is delivered through the electrode catheter to evaluate the electrical conduction pathways, formation of dysrhythmias, and the automaticity and refractoriness of myocardial cells.[45] PES is administered at different rates and times during the depolarization-repolarization cycle. This procedure is designed to reproduce any dysrhythmias so that the origin of conduction problems can be isolated. In addition, EP studies can be used to evaluate the response to antiarrhythmic agents.

EP studies provide very specific information on each segment of the conduction system, including sinus node, AV node, bundle of His, and the His-Purkinje system of the right and left ventricles.

INDICATIONS

Sinus node disorders
AV block
Intraventricular block
Previous cardiac arrest
Tachycardias >200 bpm
Unexplained syncope

CONTRAINDICATIONS

Underlying cardiac disease that increases the risk of inducing dysrhythmias that can lead to sudden death
Conditions that create findings unrepresentative of the patient's usual state of health, such as electrolyte imbalance or drug toxicity

COMPLICATIONS

Atrial fibrillation
Ventricular tachycardia
Ventricular fibrillation
Cardiac perforation leading to tamponade
Phlebitis
Pulmonary emboli
Thrombosis
Hemorrhage
Infection

NURSING CARE

Before the procedure, obtain written consent and the patient's past and present drug history. Determine whether the patient has any allergies or drug sensitivity. Document symptoms that occur during episodes of dysrhythmia, and ensure that laboratory reports (CBC, PT, PTT, platelet count) and ECG documentation of the dysrhythmia strips are in the patient's chart. Antiarrhythmic agents are discontinued or held prior to the procedure, as ordered. Nothing is given by mouth for 6 to 12 hours before EP studies. Preoperative medications are not usually given, although diazepam may be ordered to reduce anxiety.

After the procedure, check vital signs every 15 minutes for 1 hour and then every 4 hours until the patient is stable. Place the patient on a cardiac monitor as ordered and monitor ECG, documenting rate, rhythm, and any observed changes in frequency of ectopy. Observe the patient for chest discomfort and for therapeutic response to new antiarrhythmic agents used during the procedure. Maintain bed rest for 4 to 6 hours. Keep the extremity immobile during this time. Check the insertion site for bleeding or swelling. Administer analgesics as ordered.

PATIENT TEACHING

Before the procedure, determine the patient's previous experiences with regard to sudden death cardiac arrest, defibrillation, or other EP studies. Explain that the patient will be awake during the procedure and may feel pressure when the catheter is inserted. Tell the patient to report any discomfort during the study. Explain that the patient may be sent to a telemetry or cardiac unit after the procedure for close monitoring.

Before discharge, review the prescribed medications. Discuss possible side effects and how they should be reported. Review symptoms associated with dysrhythmias to report to physician. Make sure the patient has emergency phone numbers. Encourage the patient to carry identification that includes medical history and current medications.

ELECTROPHYSIOLOGIC STUDIES: NORMAL CONDUCTION TIMES

AV interval

A-H interval	Conduction time from the right atrium through the AV node to the bundle of His
	Normal time: 60 to 125 msec
H-V interval	Conduction time from the proximal bundle of His to the ventricular myocardium
	Normal time: 35 to 55 msec

Intra-atrial conduction

P-A interval	Conduction time from the beginning of the P wave to the beginning of the A deflection
	Normal time: 20 to 40 msec

HEMODYNAMIC MONITORING

Hemodynamic monitoring, an invasive technique requiring right heart catheterization, allows close examination of cardiac function in acutely ill patients. Used primarily in critical care units, this procedure allows rapid identification of complications after myocardial infarction, helps differentiate pulmonary disease from left ventricular failure, and guides the management of patients with low cardiac output. Hemodynamic monitoring also provides a direct means of assessing a patient's progress and response to fluid and drug management and permits careful titration of medications.

Several multipurpose catheters with four or five openings, or lumens, have been developed, so that a single catheter can measure four or five parameters. For example, five-lumen catheters can measure right atrial pressure (RAP), pulmonary artery pressure (PAP), pulmonary capillary wedge pressure (PCWP), and cardiac output via thermodilution, with the fifth lumen available for administering drugs or fluids.

Catheters are inserted by either the percutaneous or the cut-down method. The insertion site varies but the internal jugular or subclavian veins are the most common sites.

To keep the pulmonary catheter and arterial pressure lines open, a flushing system consisting of a heparinized solution in 5% dextrose continuously circulates through the catheters. The microdrip heparin flush is infused at higher pressures than the patient's systolic pressure, usually 300 mm Hg.

Standard Measurements

Pulmonary Artery Pressure (PAP) and Pulmonary Capillary Wedge Pressure (PCWP)

The major determinant of left ventricular function is left ventricular end-diastolic pressure (LVEDP), which cannot be measured directly at bedside. However, LVEDP can be assessed indirectly by measuring the pressure in the pulmonary capillaries and by measuring PAP at the end of diastole (PAD).

A catheter is passed through the right side of the heart into the pulmonary artery. There the balloon is inflated, occluding the artery. With the balloon inflated, the catheter is wedged into a distal branch of the pulmonary capillaries. The PCWP reflects left atrial pressure, which corresponds to LVEDP (Figure 3-18).

Intra-Arterial Pressure (Arterial Line)

Placement of an indwelling catheter in a major artery (usually radial) connected to a transducer permits continuous monitoring of systemic arterial pressure. The catheter also provides a ready means of obtaining blood samples for arterial blood gas analysis. The radial artery is the most common site used, although brachial and femoral arteries may be selected for catheter placement. Central artery pressures are more accurate but less often used.

Cardiac Output (CO)

The volume of blood pumped per minute is measured by a calibrated thermistor located near the tip of the pressure catheter. This thermodilution technique is based on the Fick principle and uses blood temperature changes to determine the cardiac output. A measured amount of iced solution is injected through the catheter at a specified rate into the right atrium, and the thermistor records the blood temperature as it passes through the catheter. The difference in temperatures between the solution and the blood is calculated, and the cardiac output is then digitally displayed on a computer. Although standard practice has been to use iced solutions, studies now show that solutions at room temperature produce similar results.

SVR

SVR is the resistance offered by the systemic arterial circulation to LV ejection. Factors or conditions (such as cardiogenic shock) that cause the SVR to increase will also increase the workload of the heart. SVR is calculated as follows:

$$SVR = \frac{MAP - RAP}{CO} \times 80$$

SVo$_2$

To further evaluate cardiac function, it is necessary to assess the adequacy of oxygen supply, i.e., relative to the body's (tissue) demand. Tissue metabolism is determined by measuring the mixed venous oxygen satura-

tion (SVo$_2$), which reflects the overall oxygen utilization by the tissues. Normal SVo$_2$ is between 60% and 80%, 75% being average. SVo$_2$ values are obtained by using mixed venous blood samples from the port of the PA catheter or by a specifically designed fiberoptic PA catheter that permits continuous SVo$_2$ monitoring.

INDICATIONS

To evaluate: The course and management of patients with the following disorders:
Complicated myocardial infarction
Heart failure
Respiratory failure
Shock
To monitor: Intraoperative and postoperative cardiac function
High-risk patients (e.g., trauma victims)

CONTRAINDICATIONS

Radial artery insertion if circulation is inadequate
Right-sided endocarditis (insertion of flotation catheter may cause dislodgement of septic emboli to the lung)
Relative contraindications include:
Bleeding disorders such as severe thrombocytopenia
Severe immunosuppression

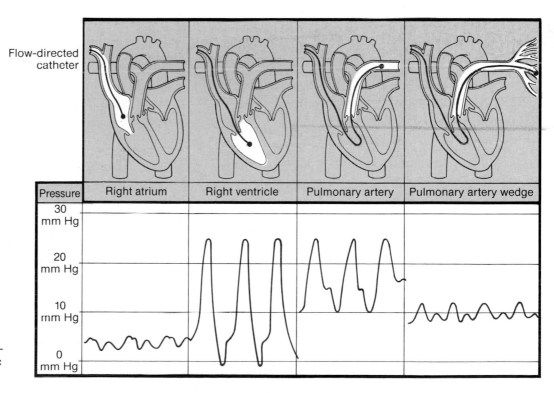

FIGURE 3-18
Sequential placement of balloon-tipped flow-directed catheter with corresponding hemodynamic waveforms.

HEMODYNAMIC PARAMETERS: NORMAL RANGES

Right atrial pressure (RAP)	Mean:	2 to 6 mm Hg
Right ventricular pressure	Systolic:	20 to 30 mm Hg
	Diastolic:	0 to 5 mm Hg
	End-diastolic:	2 to 6 mm Hg
Pulmonary artery pressure (PAP)	Systolic:	20 to 30 mm Hg
	End-diastolic:	8 to 12 mm Hg
	Mean:	10 to 20 mm Hg
Pulmonary arterial wedge pressure (PAWP)	Mean:	4 to 12 mm Hg
Arterial pressure (intra-arterial)	Peak systolic:	100 to 140 mm Hg
	End-diastolic:	60 to 80 mm Hg
	Mean:	70 to 90 mm Hg
Cardiac output (CO)	4 to 8 L/min	
Cardiac index (CO/Body surface area)	2.5 to 4 L/min	
Mixed venous oxygen saturation (SVo_2)	60% to 80%	
Systemic vascular resistance (SVR)	800 to 1200 dynes/sec/cm^5	
Pulmonary vascular resistance (PVR)	37 to 250 dynes/sec/cm^5	

COMPLICATIONS

Pulmonary artery pressure catheters:

Complications that may arise during insertion include pulmonary artery rupture, pneumothorax, dysrhythmias, and kinking of the catheter. Complications that can develop during monitoring include air embolism, dysrhythmias, infection, pulmonary embolism, infarction or perforation, and thrombophlebitis at the insertion site. Patients with left bundle-branch block may develop right bundle-branch block during insertion or monitoring.

Arterial lines:

Complications include hemorrhage, thrombus, infection, diminished or absent pulses distal to insertion site, and hematoma at the insertion site.

NURSING CARE

Before insertion, obtain written informed consent. Measure blood pressure, pulse, and respiration. If the cardiac output is monitored, take the patient's temperature. Connect the patient to an ECG monitor and obtain a baseline rhythm strip. If catheter insertion will be at the bedside, place the patient in a supine or slight Trendelenburg position and assemble the equipment and supplies.

During insertion of the catheter, monitor ECG for ventricular irritability. If entry is via the subclavian vein, observe for signs of pneumothorax. As soon as the procedure is finished, label the catheter and injection ports to prevent confusing the lines.

Throughout hemodynamic monitoring, observe the patient for signs of pneumothorax and pulmonary air embolism (chest pain, dyspnea, or tachycardia). Auscultate for chest sounds every 4 hours, monitor vital signs every 30 to 60 minutes as ordered, and check ECG strip frequently. Check arterial catheter site for signs of decreased circulation (numbness, diminished pulse, decreased color or temperature). Change dressings daily, cleaning insertion sites with antiseptic agent, and check for signs of inflammation. Document all pressure readings as ordered and the patient's position (e.g., head at 30-degree angle). Check pressure catheter waveform for signs of balloon rupture. Administer oxygen therapy and medications as ordered.

Before the pulmonary catheter is removed, make certain that lidocaine bolus and defibrillator are at the bedside. After the pulmonary and arterial catheters are removed, maintain direct manual pressure over the site for 5 to 10 minutes. Check the insertion sites and pulses of the extremity every 2 to 4 hours for the first 24-hour period. Monitor the patient for signs of dysrhythmias, emboli, and infection for 24 hours.

PATIENT TEACHING

Explain to the patient and family the purpose of hemodynamic monitoring. Describe how the catheters will be inserted and briefly explain the monitoring equipment. Offer frequent reassurance and encouragement and answer questions regarding the procedure. Instruct the patient not to move the insertion area after the catheters are in place.

┌───┐
│ **CARE OF HEMODYNAMIC MONITORING EQUIPMENT** │
└───┘

Before the procedure

1. Assemble the necessary equipment and supplies according to hospital policy. Basic equipment includes:

    Monitoring equipment: Pressure catheter, heparin flush solution and closed system tubing, stopcocks, transducer with oscilloscope

    Insertion equipment: Local anesthetic, skin preparation solution, sterile gloves, sterile dressing

2. Calibrate the pressure monitor according to the manufacturer's directions.

    Calibration is essential to ensure accuracy of measurements and avoid erroneous readings caused by temperature changes, which can cause drift of the zero baseline.

3. For PAP readings, the transducer must be calibrated to the level of the right atrium.

During monitoring

1. Calibrate the transducer and monitor q 4 h or as specified by the manufacturer.
2. Relevel the transducer as necessary when the patient changes position to keep the transducer level with the right atrium. Record the position in which readings are taken.
3. Flush all lines q 1-2 h.
4. Check patency of lines and connections q 4-8 h.
5. Check pressure in transfer pack q 4-6 h.
6. Change heparin flush solution and pressure line tubing q 24-48 h.

PROBLEMS OBSERVED IN PRESSURE WAVEFORMS

Observation	Etiologic factors	Interventions
Loss of waveform on oscilloscope	Displacement of catheter	Reposition patient; notify physician
Loss of PAP; PCWP is displayed on monitor	Self-wedging	Instruct patient to cough; obtain x-ray examination
Loss of PWP	Displaced into PAP; balloon rupture	Use diastolic of PAP
Decreased amplitude of waveform (damped wave form)	Damping due to:	
	Clot in catheter	Flush lines: *Do not force if resistance is met*
	Air bubbles	Check all connections for air leaks: flush air bubbles
	Kinking of catheter; occluded catheter; tip against artery wall	Notify physician; reposition patient; have patient cough
Loss of PCWP; no resistance with inflation	Rupture of balloon	Seal off balloon lumen: *Do not allow any injection of air*
Air bubbles in pressure lines; damping of waveform; inaccurate reading;	Air leak in system	Check all connections and secure
Artifacts and inadequate pressure readings	Respiratory interference from handling of pressure equipment during readings	Record pressure at end of exhalation using printed waveform; check for possible interference with tubing during reading
	Inaccurate calibration of equipment	Check for possible interference with tubing during readings
	Faulty equipment	Check electrical system for grounding; check calibration of and level of RA to transducer; check all equipment for proper functioning

From Tucker, S., et al.: Patient care standards, ed 4. St. Louis, 1988, The C.V. Mosby Co.

CHEST ROENTGENOGRAPHY

A chest roentgenogram (x-ray) provides information about the anatomic location and gross structures of the heart, great vessels, and lungs. Chest x-rays also are used to detect and follow progression of disease and to evaluate the response to therapy. A cardiac series consists of four views: posteroanterior (PA), left anterior oblique (LAO), right anterior oblique (RAO), and left or right lateral (Figure 3-19). Anteroposterior (AP) is another view, but it is generally reserved for the use of a bedridden patient. Chest x-rays are taken during deep sustained inspiration with the patient upright.

The PA view is generally used to assess normal radiographic findings. The normal position (situs soltis) is to the left of the sternum, with the heart occupying less than 50% of the thoracic cavity. The cardiac silhouette gives an indication of the relative sizes of the major cardiac structures. From the PA view the right atrium, right ventricle, superior vena caval shadow, aorta, aortic knob, pulmonary artery, and left ventricle can be assessed or evaluated. The oblique views profile specific sections of the heart contours with the body rotated.

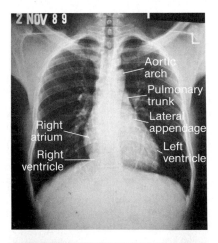

PA view.

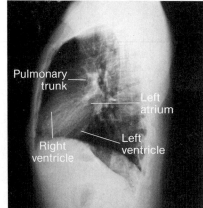

Lateral view.

FIGURE 3-19
Normal chest x-rays.

Pulmonary vascularity can also be assessed on the PA view. Normally, the vessels are more prominent in the lower lobes than the upper lobes when taken with the patient upright. Hilar shadows and the bronchovascular markings formed by the pulmonary arteries and veins are visible.

The cardiac series also shows any calcifications present on the aortic and mitral valves, coronary arteries, and great vessels.

INDICATIONS

To aid in evaluating: Congestive heart failure
Pericardial effusions
Pleural effusions
Pulmonary hypertension

CONTRAINDICATIONS

None, but special precautions must be taken for pregnant women.

NURSING CARE

Ask all women of childbearing age if they suspect they may be pregnant. Have patient remove all neck jewelry and garments with metal objects, buttons, or ornaments above the waist.

PATIENT TEACHING

Explain the procedure and discuss the reasons for having chest roentgenograms.

DIGITAL VASCULAR IMAGING

Digital vascular imaging (DVI) or digital subtraction angiography is an invasive procedure used in conjunction with cardiac catheterization. Contrast material is injected, and a commercial fluoroscopy system with an image intensifer gives a complete view of the arterial supply in the study area. DVI is often used as an adjunct to pulmonary angiography.

DVI has several advantages over other imaging techniques. Because it requires a smaller amount of contrast material, there is less risk of allergic reactions. The procedure is simpler than conventional angiography because the catheter is usually inserted only as far as the right ventricle. This makes DVI ideal for high-risk patients who have pulmonary hypertension, congestive heart failure, renal disease, or sickle cell disease. DVI is often performed on an outpatient basis.

INDICATIONS

Aneurysms
Carotid artery disease
Coarctation of the aorta
Renal artery disease
Pulmonary embolism
Thrombotic/embolic disease of the great vessels

CONTRAINDICATIONS

No absolute contraindications, but relative contraindications are the same as for cardiac catheterization.

COMPLICATIONS

Dysrhythmias, bronchospasm, cardiac perforation, or reaction to the contrast medium may occur during the procedure. Postoperative complications include bleeding at the insertion site, infection, and fever.

NURSING CARE

Obtain written informed consent. The patient is allowed nothing by mouth 4 to 5 hours before the procedure except small sips of water.

After DVI, check vital signs immediately and then as ordered by the physician. Check insertion site for bleeding and keep the patient in bed for 2 to 4 hours.

PATIENT TEACHING

Explain the reason for DVI and that the procedure will last for 1 to 2 hours. Discuss what the patient should expect, including some pressure during positioning of the catheter and a flushing sensation when the contrast medium is injected. Explain that the physician will request that the patient hold the breath for 10 seconds.

If DVI is to be done as outpatient surgery, instruct the patient that bed rest for 2 to 4 hours is recommended and that he should drink at least 1 liter of fluid after the procedure. Instruct the patient to report bleeding or signs of infection.

PLETHYSMOGRAPHY

Plethysmography is a noninvasive technique for measuring peripheral venous flow by recording changes in blood volume and vascular resistance. In venous occlusion plethysmography, two electrodes are applied to the skin to record changes in blood volume. This record is produced on ECG graph paper. A pressure tourniquet is placed on the limb to occlude venous return, and when the tourniquet is released, the filling time is monitored. Venous filling should return to baseline levels within 10 seconds. A delay of more than 10 seconds indicates thrombosis.

INDICATIONS

Deep vein thrombosis
Thrombophlebitis

CONTRAINDICATIONS

None

NURSING CARE

No specific nursing care is required for plethysmography.

PATIENT TEACHING

Explain the purpose of the procedure. Assure the patient that the procedure is painless.

DOPPLER ULTRASONOGRAPHY

Doppler ultrasonography is a noninvasive technique for determining patency of the distal veins and arteries. Ultrasonography emits high-frequency waves (5,000 to 20,000 Hz) and detects the vibrations (echoes) reflected from soft tissues. The echos are converted to electrical potentials and are displayed on an oscilloscope. Doppler ultrasonography amplifies the sounds of peripheral pulses and measures blood flow velocity.

In evaluating venous patency of the lower legs, Doppler ultrasonography is used to determine ankle systolic pressure. The ankle pressure should be equal to or greater than brachial systolic pressure. The measurements are expressed as the ankle/brachial index. Normal ankle systolic pressure is 0.45 to 0.75 mm Hg. It should be $\geq$ brachial systolic pressure. An index of 0.4 indicates claudication, and 0.3 suggests severe arterial insufficiency.

INDICATIONS

Arterial insufficiency
Venous thrombosis

CONTRAINDICATIONS

None

NURSING CARE

No specific nursing care is related to Doppler ultrasonography.

PATIENT TEACHING

Explain the purpose of the procedure. Inform the patient that some discomfort may occur from the pressure of the transducer, but assure the patient that the sound waves are not felt.

PHLEBOGRAPHY (VENOGRAPHY)

Phlebography is an invasive procedure for locating venous thrombi in the extremities. The procedure involves inserting a catheter into the vein, injecting a radiopaque dye, and taking serial x-rays. Dispersion of the contrast material through the vein shows any filling defects caused by a thrombus.

INDICATIONS

Venous thrombosis

CONTRAINDICATIONS

No absolute contraindications, but known allergy to iodine requires proceeding cautiously.

COMPLICATIONS

Allergic reactions to the contrast material, subcutaneous infiltration of the dye, dislodgment of the thrombus leading to embolism, and postoperative infection at the insertion site are complications associated with phlebography.

NURSING CARE

Before the procedure, obtain written consent and determine whether the patient has allergies to shellfish or iodine or a history of allergic reaction to contrast media. Prepare the insertion site and administer sedation as ordered.

After the procedure, monitor the insertion site for bleeding and signs of subcutaneous infiltration of the dye (redness, swelling, and pain). Maintain the patient on bed rest for 2 to 4 hours with the extremity immobile and keep a pressure dressing over the insertion site. Administer analgesics as ordered and encourage the patient to drink fluids.

PATIENT TEACHING

Discuss the purpose of the procedure. Explain that phlebography usually takes 30 to 90 minutes and that a local anesthetic will be injected over the insertion site, which the patient will feel as a "bee sting." Explain that when the contrast material is injected, the patient may feel a warm, flushed sensation and may experience some nausea. Instruct the patient to report any fever, swelling, or bleeding at the puncture site.

125I FIBRINOGEN UPTAKE

^{125}I fibrinogen uptake is a noninvasive procedure for diagnosing and evaluating deep vein thrombosis. Fibrinogen "tagged" with a radioactive material is injected into a peripheral vein, and a series of scintillation scans are performed at intervals over a 24-hour period. A thrombus shows as a "hot spot." A 20% increase of radioisotope in one area over a 24-hour period is considered positive.

INDICATIONS

Deep vein thrombosis

CONTRAINDICATIONS

None

NURSING CARE

Obtain written consent. No specific nursing care is required for this procedure.

PATIENT TEACHING

Explain the purpose of the procedure. Explain that 2 hours after the radioisotope is injected into a vein, a scanning camera will pass over the affected limb and that scanning will be repeated at intervals over the next few days.

Cardiac Diseases and Disorders

In the United States, someone dies of cardiovascular disease every 32 seconds.

Cardiovascular disease is the nation's number one killer, claiming almost as many lives as cancer, accidents, pulmonary infections, and all other causes of death combined. According to 1989 statistics from the American Heart Association (AHA), nearly 1 million deaths from cardiovascular disease were reported, 53.6% of which resulted from heart attacks, 3.1% from hypertensive disease, 0.7% from rheumatic heart disease, and 27.6% from all other cardiovascular diseases.

Mortality tells only part of the story. Of the current U.S. population of 241 million, almost 66 million people have some form of cardiovascular disease—that's one in every four Americans. The AHA estimates that cardiovascular disease cost the nation $88.2 million in physician and nursing services, hospital and nursing home services, prescription medications, and lost productivity resulting from disability. Current morbidity data demonstrate the enormity of the problem:

- There are 1.5 million heart attacks annually, 45% in people under age 65
- Over 60 million people are hypertensive
- Over 2 million people have rheumatic heart disease
- About 25,000 babies are born with congenital heart defects annually
- About 520,000 Americans are living with some form of congenital heart disease

In spite of the high morbidity and mortality rates for cardiovascular disease, death rates are declining, largely through improvements in treatment. In addition, more people are voluntarily adopting healthier life-styles that reduce their risks. And technologic advances now allow not only earlier but also more specific diagnosis of cardiovascular disease.

Optimal treatment of cardiovascular disease usually requires a three-pronged approach. Medical and surgical interventions can improve or even correct many problems. Drug therapy is aimed at maintaining normal physiologic functioning or reducing the symptoms. Finally, eliciting the patient's cooperation in adopting specific health behaviors enhances therapy and reduces the risk of complications.

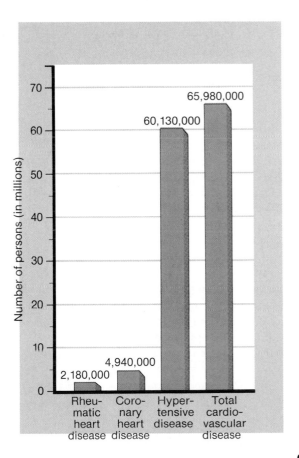

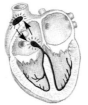

Medulla

Vagus nerve

SA node

AV node

Cardiac Dysrhythmias

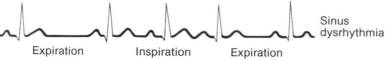

A **dysrhythmia** is a disorder of the heart rate and rhythm caused by a disturbance of the conduction system.

Sinus dysrhythmia

Expiration   Inspiration   Expiration

P   P   P   P

Dysrhythmia with wandering pacemaker

P

SA node

AV node

Left ventricular premature (impulse) contraction

Premature contraction

Dysrhythmias and premature contraction

The most serious consequence of cardiac dysrhythmias is sudden death resulting from electromechanical failure (as in ventricular fibrillation) or from impaired cardiac function. It is estimated that in the U.S., there are 300,000 sudden cardiac deaths annually, which represents approximately 50% of all cardiovascular deaths.[13] And of those deaths attributed specifically to heart attack, 60% occur within the first hour presumably to ventricular dysrhythmias.

Early recognition and treatment are important because various dysrhythmias, such as premature ventricular ectopic beats, may spontaneously become frequent or multifocal. For example, in a patient with myocardial ischemia the ectopic beat may convert to ventricular tachycardia or ventricular fibrillation without warning.

Careful continuous ECG monitoring now enables early detection and prompt treatment of potentially serious dysrhythmias. However, proper treatment involves not only diagnosis but also a thorough understanding of the underlying etiologic factors.

PATHOPHYSIOLOGY

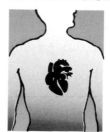

Cardiac dysrhythmias may occur as a result of a primary cardiac disorder, as a secondary response to a systemic problem, or as a complication of drug toxicity or electrolyte imbalance (Table 4-1).

A variety of methods have been developed to classify cardiac dysrhythmias. Most commonly, dysrhythmias have been classified into abnormalities of impulse formation (sinus, atrial, junctional, ventricular), impulse conduction, or a combination of both. Dysrhythmias have also been described on the basis of rate (bradyarrhythmia, tachyarrhythmia) or clinical significance (minor, life threatening). However, to understand the basis of arrhythmogenesis, it is best to examine dysrhythmias according to three basic electrophysiologic mechanisms—re-entry, abnormal enhanced automaticity, and conduction disturbances.

Re-entry and abnormal automaticity account for the

majority of tachyarrhythmias, while conduction disturbances result in the bracydysrhythmias.

Re-entrant mechanism

Re-entrant activity, which accounts for 80% to 90% of tachyarrhythmias, occurs as a result of changes in the transmembrane potential of diseased tissue cells, which alter the conduction pathways and refractoriness of the cell membrane. For re-entry to occur, three conditions must be present: (1) a point at which there are two conduction pathways for an impulse to follow; (2) slow conduction through one portion of the pathways; and (3) unidirectional block at some point along the conduction pathway. During depolarization, the impulse finds one pathway block refractory, permitting it to proceed along the second pathway (limb) of the circuit. If conduction is slow along the second pathway, then a re-entrant circuit (loop) is initiated. Perpetuation of this re-entrant pattern produces a circuitous tachycardia.

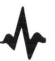

Table 4-1

CAUSES OF CARDIAC DYSRHYTHMIAS

Primary cardiac disorders	Atherosclerosis
	Congestive heart failure
	Myocardial ischemia, infarction
	Cardiomyopathy
	Valvular heart disease
	Hypertensive heart disease
	Congenital heart disease
	Ventricular aneurysm
	Cardiac tumors
	Cardiac trauma
Secondary response to systemic disease condition	Anemia
	Hypothyroidism
	Hypothermia
Drug toxicity	Cardiac agents
	Antiarrhythmics
	Cardiac glycosides
	Antineoplastics
	Adriamycosin
	Phenothiazides
	Sympathomimetics
Electrolyte imbalance	Hypercalcemia/ hypocalcemia
	Hyperkalemia/ hypokalemia
	Hypermagnesemia/ hypomagnesemia
	Hypernatremia/ hyponatremia

Abnormal or Enhanced Automaticity

Normal automaticity occurs in the specialized AV node and the His-Purkinje system by depolarization of the cell membrane to a threshold level. Once the action potential of a cell is reached, self-propagation of depolarization is possible and continues to adjacent cell membranes, spreading throughout contiguous tissue.

In contrast, abnormal automaticity develops when the resting potential of the cell membrane is reduced (e.g., -90 mV to -70 mV). Because of this membrane instability, extraneous stimulation can depolarize the partially depolarized tissue to a threshold potential, causing abnormal automatic rhythms.

Factors contributing to reduced resting membrane potential include ischemia, hyperkalemia, hypoxia, or the effects of drugs.

COMPLICATIONS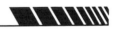

Heart failure	Syncope
Embolic episodes	Sudden death
Ischemia	Cardiac arrest

DIAGNOSTIC STUDIES AND FINDINGS

Diagnostic test	Findings
12-lead electrocardiogram (ECG)	Rate, rhythm, signs of ischemia, atrial or ventricular hypertrophy axis deviation (see pages 64-71, including Figs. 4-1 to 4-17 for ECG characteristics and findings for specific rhythm)
24-hour ambulatory electrocardiogram (Holter monitor)	Rate, rhythm, tachyarrhythmias, conduction abnormalities
Electrophysiologic studies (EPS)	Induced: Ventricular dysrhythmia: ventricular tachycardia, ventricular fibrillation Supraventricular tachycardia (SVT): Wolff-Parkinson White (WPW) Atrial fibrillation, atrial flutter Conduction abnormalities: Atrioventricular heart block Intraventricular conduction delay (IVCD) Sinus node dysfunction
Exercise electrocardiography	Ischemia: ST depression >1 mm (downsloping of ST segment) Dysrhythmias
Laboratory values	Electrolytes: hypokalemia, hyperkalemia, hypoglycemia Chemistries: hypercapnia, acidosis Drug toxicity levels: e.g., digoxin, quinidine, pronestyl

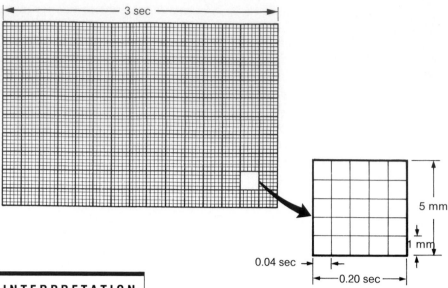

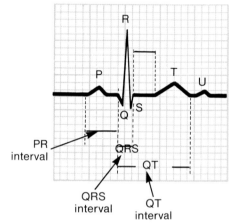

```
ECG INTERPRETATION
```

1. Calculate the heart rate. Calculate the atrial (P wave) rate. Calculate the ventricular (QRS complex) rate.
2. Determine the regularity of rhythm.
3. Determine whether P waves are present. Determine the position of P waves in relation to the QRS complex.
4. Measure the PR interval.
5. Measure the QRS interval.
6. Identify and examine the ST segment and T wave.
7. Determine the origin of the rhythm: Is it sinus, atrial, junctional, or ventricular?

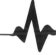

SPECIFIC FINDINGS FOR CARDIAC RHYTHMS

Rhythm characteristics	Etiology	Clinical significance	Management
Sinus tachycardia (Fig. 4-1) Regular rhythm; rate 100-180 bpm (higher in infants); normal P wave; normal QRS complex	Rate increase may be normal response to exercise, emotion, or abnormal stressors such as pain, fever, pump failure, hyperthyroidism, and certain drugs, including caffeine, nitrates, atropine, epinephrine, isoproterenol, and nicotine	May have hemodynamic consequence in patient with damaged heart that is unable to sustain increased workloads (increased MVO_2) brought on by persistent increases in HR	Correcting underlying factors; removing offending drugs

FIGURE 4-1
From Andreoli.[6]

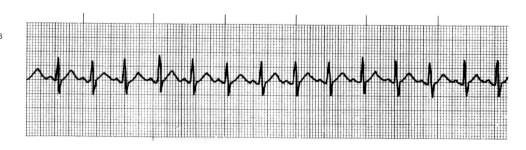

Rhythm characteristics	Etiology	Clinical significance	Management
Sinus bradycardia (Fig. 4-2) Regular rhythm; rate less than 60 bpm; normal P wave; normal PR interval; normal QRS complex	Rate decrease may be normal response to sleep or in well-conditioned athlete; abnormal drops in rate may be caused by diminished blood flow to S-A node, vagal stimulation, hypothyroidism, increased intracranial pressure, or pharmacologic agents such as digoxin, propranolol, quinidine, or procainamide	None unless associated with signs of impaired CO; symptoms: dizziness, syncope, chest pain	Correcting underlying cause; atropine 0.5-1.0 mg IV; transvenous pacemaker

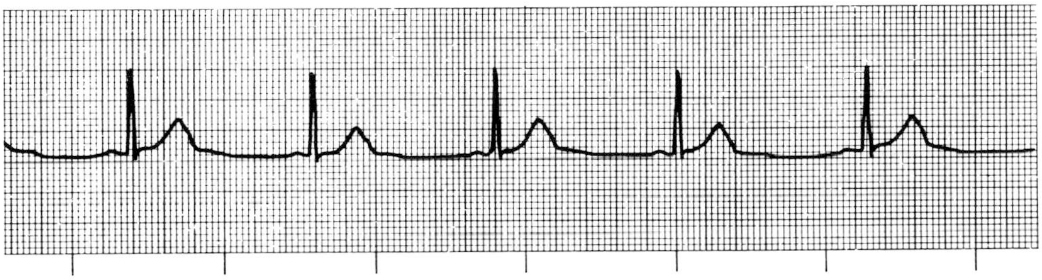

FIGURE 4-2
From Andreoli.[6]

Sinus dysrhythmia (Fig. 4-3) Irregular rhythm; may be phasic with respiration, slowing during inspiration and increasing with expiration; rate 60-100 bpm; normal P-wave; normal PR interval; normal QRS complex	Sinus rhythm with cyclic variation caused by vagal impulses that influence rhythm during respiration; occurs commonly in children, young adults, and the elderly; usually disappears as HR increases	None unless heart rate decreases; symptoms: dizziness with decreased rate	None indicated unless heart rate decreases and symptoms occur

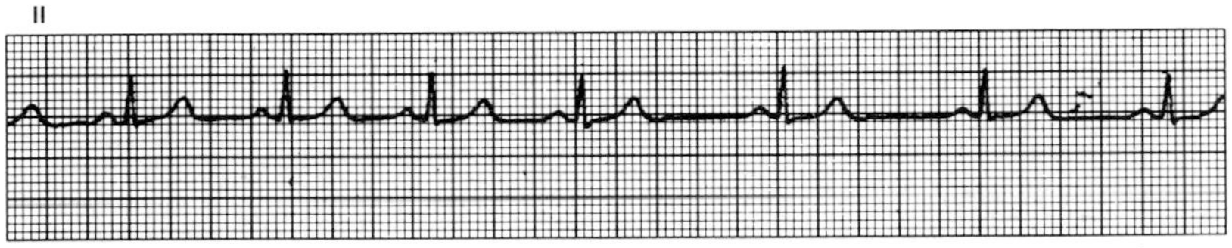

FIGURE 4-3
From Conover.[28]

Atrial premature contractions (APCs, PACs) (Fig. 4-4) Irregular rhythm owing to ectopic beats followed by incomplete compensatory pause; rate normal or increased depending on number of ectopic beats; P wave present but different from normal underlying sinus beat; PR interval may be shorter or longer than normal sinus beat; normal QRS complex	May be precipitated in healthy persons by anxiety, fatigue, caffeine, smoking, and alcohol; observed in patients with ischemia or organic heart disease and those receiving digoxin	May indicate atrial strain or hypoxia; frequent PACs (more than 6/min) reflect atrial irritability and often mark onset of atrial fibrillation	Correcting underlying cause; for frequent PACs, quinidine or pronestyl

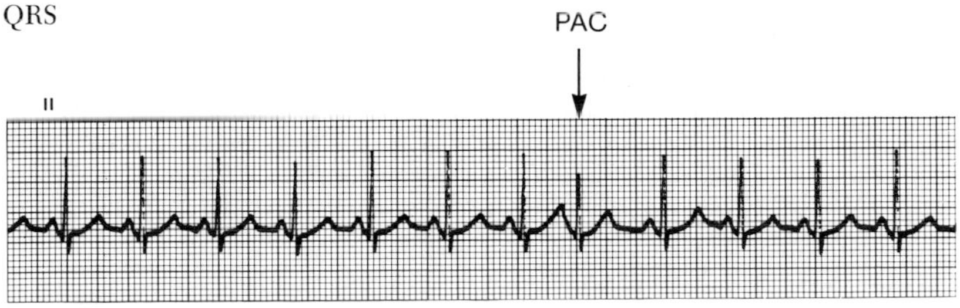

PAC

FIGURE 4-4
From Conover.[28]

Rhythm characteristics	Etiology	Clinical significance	Management
Supraventricular tachycardia (SVT) (Fig. 4-5) Sudden, rapid onset of tachycardia with stimulus originating above AV node; regular rhythm; rate 150-250 bpm; P wave uniform, may or may not be buried in preceding T wave; PR interval may vary, often difficult to measure; normal QRS complex	May begin and end spontaneously or be precipitated by excitement, fatigue, caffeine, smoking, or alcohol	Usually no significant impairment; patient complains of palpitations and shortness of breath; if persistent or occurring in patient with pre-existing organic heart disease, may cause decrease in cardiac output and/or blood pressure resulting in pump failure or shock	Performing vagal stimulation with carotid sinus massage; using Valsalva maneuver to stimulate baroreceptors (may be used in conjunction with carotid sinus massage); decreasing ventricular response with medication to block AV conduction; sedation to reduce sympathetic stimulation; verapamil 5-10 mg IV push; propranolol slowly IV in 1 mg increments up to 4 mg (contraindicated in patients with heart failure); edrophonium, test dose 1 mg followed by 10 mg IV; cardioversion if resistant to preceding

FIGURE 4-5
From Andreoli.[6]

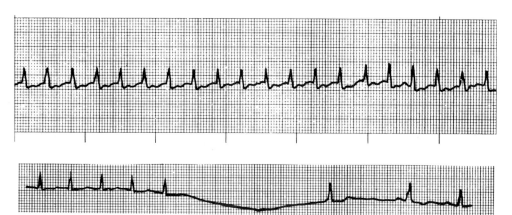

Atrial flutter (Fig. 4-6) Rhythm may be regular or irregular; rate: atrial 250-350 bpm, characterized by saw-tooth flutter waves; ventricular depends on AV conduction, may occur at 2:1, 3:1, or 4:1 ratio; PR interval not measurable; normal QRS complex	Results from rapidly firing ectopic atrial focus; most likely underlying mechanism is localized atrial re-entry phenomenon; seen in patients with organic heart disorders such as CAD and VHD	Patient complains of palpitations, which may be associated with heart failure, and chest pain, particularly in presence of rapid ventricular rates	Cardioversion; digoxin if cardioversion is not used or is unsuccessful; quinidine or procainamide

FIGURE 4-6
From Conover.[28]

II

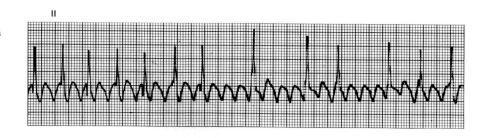

Rhythm characteristics	Etiology	Clinical significance	Management
Atrial fibrillation (Fig. 4-7) Rhythm irregular; rate: atrial > 350 bpm; absence of uniform atrial depolarization produces undulations (f waves); ventricular varies according to AV conduction but may range between 50 and 150 bpm	Results from multiple atrial foci discharging almost simultaneously; atria never uniformly depolarize; reflects organic heart disease; may also occur with digitalis toxicity	With rapid ventricular rates, CO may be impaired, resulting in heart failure, angina, and shock	Determination of underlying cause and whether acute or chronic; cardioversion for rapid ventricular response; digoxin is not used; quinidine; procainamide; verapamil

V₁

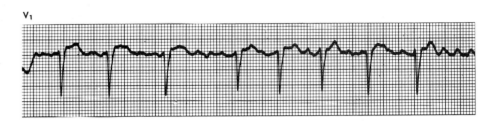

FIGURE 4-7
From Conover.[28]

Junctional escape rhythm (nodal) (Fig. 4-8) Rhythm regular; rate 40-60 bpm; P wave abnormal, may occur before, during, or after QRS complex, may be inverted in leads II, III, and aVF; QRS complex usually normal	Occurs when sinus node is suppressed and atria fail to depolarize AV junction; may be due to digitalis toxicity, vagal stimulation, or ischemic damage to S-A node	Usually none; transient; if condition persists, slow rates may allow foci with rapid rates to take over; may also produce symptoms of diminished CO	Treatment or correction of underlying cause if persistent or if symptoms occur; atropine IV; pacemaker may be indicated

II

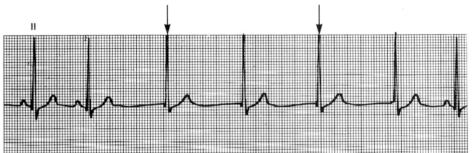

FIGURE 4-8
From Conover.[28]

Premature junctional contractions (Fig. 4-9) Rhythm regular except for junctional beat; rate normal; P wave as described for junctional escape rhythm; PR interval shortened when P wave precedes QRS complex, QRS complex usually normal	Result from increased automaticity of AV junction, causing ectopic focus in AV node to discharge before onset of impulse from sinus node; these ectopic beats usually due to ischemia or digitalis toxicity	Usually none; frequency reflects junctional irritability	None indicated if infrequent; if frequent, quinidine

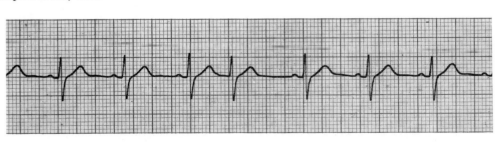

FIGURE 4-9
From Conover.[28]

Rhythm characteristics	Etiology	Clinical significance	Management
Premature ventricular contractions (PVCs) (Fig. 4-10) Rhythm irregular owing to ectopic beats followed by full compensatory pause; rate normal or increased depending on number of ectopic beats; P wave absent in ectopic beat; PR interval absent; QRS complex widened and distorted; T wave is in opposition to R wave	Caused by irritable focus within ventricle, commonly associated with MI; other causes include hypoxia, hypocalcemia, and acidosis	PVCs occurring frequently (more than 6/min) or in pairs indicate increased ventricular irritability	Aimed at suppression of PVCs; if frequent, IV bolus of lidocaine (50-100 mg) followed by continuous IV infusion; additional antiarrhythmic agents in classes I and II may be given

FIGURE 4-10
From Conover.[28]

V₁

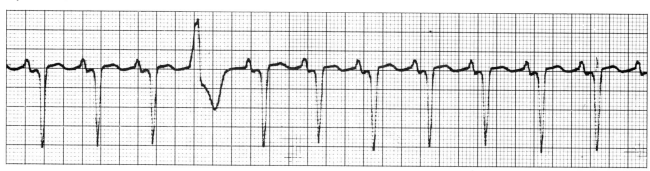

Ventricular tachycardia (Fig. 4-11) Rhythm slightly irregular; rate 100-200 bpm; P wave absent; PR interval absent; QRS complex wide and bizarre, > 0.12 second	Caused by irritable ventricular foci firing repetitively; commonly caused by MI	Often a forerunner of ventricular fibrillation; if persistent and rapid, causes decreased CO owing to decreased ventricular filling time	Most episodes terminate abruptly without treatment; lidocaine bolus 75-100 mg IV followed by continuous intravenous drip; defibrillation

FIGURE 4-11
From Conover.[28]

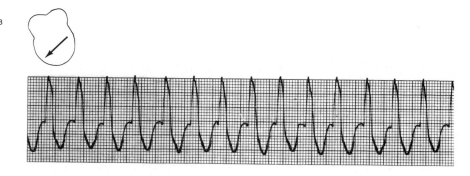

Rhythm characteristics	Etiology	Clinical significance	Management
Torsades de pointes (polymorphous ventricular tachycardia) (Figure 4-12) Atypical ventricular tachycardia occurring in setting of delayed repolarization (prolonged QT interval); rhythm regular or irregular; ventricular rate, 150-300 bpm) PR interval not measurable; QRS complex wide and bizarre in configuration lasting >0.12 second; amplitude and direction of QRS complex vary; QT interval during baseline rhythm >0.46 second or >33% of baseline; T wave during baseline rhythm very broad and flat	Drug toxicity (e.g., quinidine, procainamide, amiodarone); eletrolyte imbalance (e.g., hypokalemia, hypomagnesemia)	Palpitations, which may lead to faintness, syncope; often forerunner of ventricular fibrillation and sudden death	Treatment initiated only if QT prolonged; if present, temporary overdrive ventricular or atrial pacing; IV magnesium sulfate: IV push 2 g over 1-2 min, IV infusion 1-2 g for 4-6 h

FIGURE 4-12
A, Sinus rhythm. T waves are flat, and QT interval is prolonged. Patient's serum potassium level was 3.1 mEq/L. **B,** Taken next day, characteristic torsade. Courtesy Daniel H. Schwartz, South Fallsburg, NY (From Goldberger.)

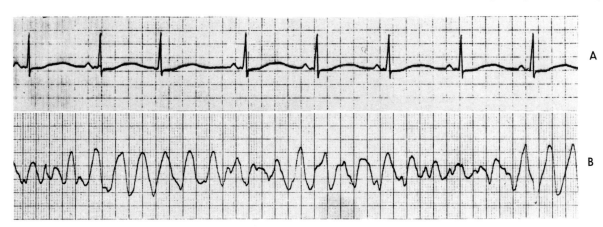

Rhythm characteristics	Etiology	Clinical significance	Management
Ventricular fibrillation (Fig. 4-13) Rhythm irregular; rate: rapid repetitive waves or undulations that have no uniformity and are coarse or fine; P wave, QRS complex, and T wave cannot be identified	Lethal dysrhythmia resulting from electrical stimulation of ventricular muscle, which leads to abrupt cessation of effective blood flow; occurs in severely damaged hearts as with ischemia, drug toxicity, trauma, or contact with high-voltage electricity	Loss of consciousness; decreases in BP and peripheral pulse owing to loss of CO	Cardiopulmonary resuscitation; defibrillation

FIGURE 4-13
From Conover.[28]

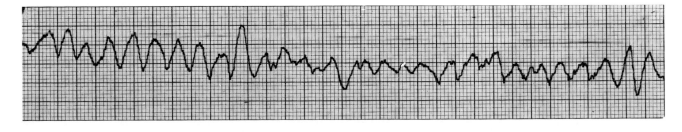

Rhythm characteristics	Etiology	Clinical significance	Management
First-degree AV heart block (Fig. 4-14) Rhythm regular; rate normal; P wave normal; PR interval prolonged to > 0.20 sec; QRS complex normal	Represents delay in impulse conduction through AV node; occurs as a result of increased vagal tone, digoxin administration, or congenital anomalies	No associated symptoms	None indicated; digitalis discontinued if causative factor; observation for development of further AV block

FIGURE 4-14
From Conover.[28]

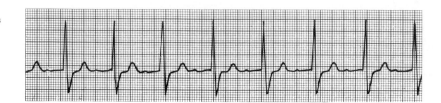

Second-degree AV heart block, Mobitz type I (Wenckebach phenomenon) (Fig. 4-15) Rhythm: atrial regular, ventricular irregular; rate: atrial > ventricular; P wave: multiple P waves before QRS complex; PR interval: progressive prolongation of PR interval until one impulse is completely blocked; QRS complex normal; RR interval becomes progressively shortened until one QRS complex is dropped	Represents progressive decrease in conduction velocity involving AV node and proximal bundle of His; occurs as result of CAD, digitalis toxicity, rheumatic fever, viral infections, or inferior wall MI	No associated symptoms if ventricular rate is adequately maintained	None usually indicated; elimination or correction of underlying cause; observation for progression to higher degree of block

FIGURE 4-15
From Conover.[28]

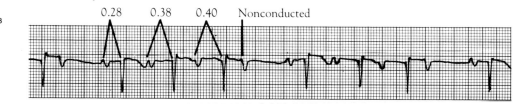

0.28   0.38   0.40   Nonconducted

Rhythm characteristics	Etiology	Clinical significance	Management
Second-degree AV heart block, Mobitz type II (Fig. 4-16) Rhythm: atrial regular, ventricular varies; rate: atrial slow to normal, ventricular may be slow, usually half or one third atrial rate; P wave normal, occurring in multiples before QRS complex; PR interval normal or slightly prolonged, always constant; QRS complex normal or slightly prolonged	Represents block of impulse below level of AV node and within His-Purkinje system; occurs as result of ischemia, digitalis or quinidine toxicity, anterior wall MI	No associated symptoms if ventricular rate is adequately maintained; if rate is slow, CO may be impaired, causing dizziness and weakness	Correction or elimination of underlying cause; tends to be recurrent, may progress to complete heart block, transvenous demand pacing may be required

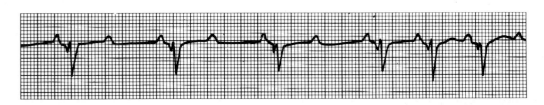

FIGURE 4-16
From Conover.[28]

Third-degree AV block (complete heart block) (Fig. 4-17) Rhythm: atrial and ventricular regular but act independent of each other; rate: atrial 60-90 bpm; ventricular 30-40 bpm; P wave normal but occurs in greater frequency than QRS complex; PR interval: no relationship with QRS complex, therefore never constant; QRS complex normal if ventricular depolarization initiated by junctional escape pacemaker, widened if depolarization initiated by ventricular pacemaker low in conduction system	Represents failure of AV node to conduct impulse to ventricles; block may occur at any point in conduction system at or below level of A-V node; occurs as result of CAD, degenerative fibrosis of conduction system, congenital anomalies, myocarditis, drug toxicity (digitalis, quinidine, procainamide, verapamil), trauma	Symptoms associated with low CO owing to slow ventricular rates; include syncope and signs of ventricular failure	Transvenous demand pacing; while awaiting pacemaker insertion, isoproterenol infusion to accelerate ventricular rate

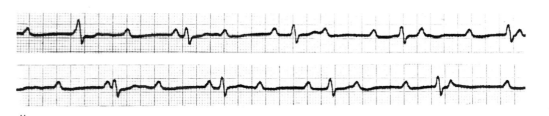

FIGURE 4-17
From Andreoli.[6]

II

MEDICAL MANAGEMENT

GENERAL MANAGEMENT

Diet: Restrictions usually directed to underlying disease process: patients with diagnosed supraventricular tachydysrhythmias instructed to avoid overuse of stimulants such as caffeine.

Smoking: Use of nicotine contraindicated because of its effect on ventricular threshold, which may be basis for dysrhythmias.

Cardiac monitoring: Continuous electrocardiographic monitoring provides most efficient and reliable method of detection of dysrhythmias.

Oxygen therapy: Low-flow oxygen therapy may benefit patient who is dyspneic or patient with chest pain.

DRUG THERAPY

Antiarrhythmic agents:
 Class 1-A Quinidine (Quinidex, Quinaglute, Cardioquin); Procainamide (Pronestyl, Procan SR); Disopyramide phosphate (Norpace)

 Class 1-B Lidocaine (Xylocaine); Phenytoin (Dilantin); Mexiletine; Tocainide (Tonocard); Aprindine

 Class II Propranolol (Inderal); Atenolol; Pindolol

 Class III Bretylium tosylate (Bretylol); Amiodarone

 Class IV Verapamil (Calan, Isoptin)

ADJUNCTIVE THERAPY

Cardiac pacemakers (temporary or permanent): Used to initiate and control heart rate; most common indication for pacemaker is bradyarrhythmias, but advances in technology have broadened its use to suppress supraventricular arrhythmias otherwise resistant to drug therapy.

Electrode catheter ablation: Invasive procedure using intracardiac electrode catheters. Used in the treatment and control of supraventricular and ventricular tachyarrhythmias that are refractory to drug therapy.

Electrical countershock

Cardioversion: Synchronized discharge of electrical impulse used to convert atrial fibrillation, atrial flutter, or supraventricular tachycardia to sinus rhythm.

Defibrillation: Emergency procedure that consists of discharge of unsynchronized electrical impulse; used in treatment of ventricular defibrillation.

Automatic implantable cardioverter defibrillator (AICD): Implantable; used to detect ventricular tachyarrhythmias and to deliver electrical countershock within 15 to 20 sec of sensing the dysrhythmia.

SURGERY

Surgical ablation or resection: Surgical treatment of highly refractory tachyarrhythmias. May be used in treatment of Wolff-Parkinson-White syndrome, since accessory bypass tracts can be excised surgically once located; can also be performed on patients with recurrent ventricular tachycardia through use of programmed stimulation, which allows surgeon to induce ventricular tachycardia, identify dysrhythmogenic site, and excise ectopic focus.

1 ASSESS

ASSESSMENT	OBSERVATIONS
General complaints	Palpitations, dizziness, lightheadedness, chest pain, syncope
Physical examina-tion	Skin: pallor, diaphoresis Arterial pulse: normal with ectopy, tachycardia, bradycardia Rhythm: normal, irregular Hypotension Mental status: confusion
Drug history	Names, dosages of current antiarrhythmic agents Laboratory values: electrolyte imbalance; therapeutic levels of drug

2 DIAGNOSE

NURSING DIAGNOSIS	SUBJECTIVE FINDINGS	OBJECTIVE FINDINGS
Anxiety related to altered heart action	Verbalizes nervousness, fear, uncertainty, helplessness, inability to sleep; complains of palpitations	Restlessness, facial tension, wide-eyed, diaphoretic, constant demands, dyspnea, tachycardia, tachypnea
Decreased cardiac output related to electrical factors (alteration in rate, rhythm, conduction)	Complains of fatigue, SOB, lightheadedness, syncope, "skipped beats," chest pain	Increase or decrease in HR, BP and/or respirations; dyspnea; pale or dusky skin color; breath sounds: crackles (rales); dysrhythmias

Other related nursing diagnoses

Activity intolerance related to diminished cardiac reserve
Ineffective individual coping related to potentially life-threatening events
Noncompliance related to drug regimen

3 PLAN

Patient goals

1. Patient will exhibit a decrease in anxiety.
2. Patient will exhibit normal or controlled heart rate and rhythm.
3. Patient will maintain a stable CO.
4. Patient and family or significant other will demonstrate an increased understanding of the disease process and self-care management.

4 IMPLEMENT

NURSING DIAGNOSIS	NURSING INTERVENTIONS	RATIONALE
Anxiety related to altered heart action	Assess level of anxiety and degree of understanding noting both verbal and nonverbal expressions regarding diagnosis, procedures, and treatments.	To determine sources of anxiety and fear; to identify and clarify any misconception. The level of anxiety varies in intensity and expression and may be influenced by previous experiences such as having survived sudden death episode. Extreme or severe anxiety can lead to activation of sympathetic nerve fibers and release of epinephrine, which further influences automacity causing dysrhythmia.
	Provide continuous explanation for the various diagnostic and/or monitoring devices in use, explaining which are routine or part of unit protocol.	Various procedures and equipment may be perceived as indicators of severity of illness; information-giving alleviates anxiety and increases patient's sense of control.
	During periods of heightened anxiety, remain with patient, offering realistic assurances, refrain from performing nonessential procedures and decrease sensory stimulation by using short, simple explanations.	Remaining with patient provides a sense of consistency and increases sense of trust, reassurance, and comfort that staff is available.
	Evaluate usual coping mechanisms used during stressful situations.	Established coping defense may be inadequate or inappropriate in dealing with this potential life-threatening situation.
Decreased cardiac output related to electrical factors	Assess patient's level of consciousness, changes in baseline ECG, HR, and BP according to unit policy or as indicated by clinical picture.	Changes in clinical status, which may be sudden, may reflect decrease in CO, response to antiarrhythmic agents, response to nonpharmacologic treatment.
	Monitor heart rate and rhythm.	To identify dysrhythmias.
	Document any changes or development of dysrhythmias with rhythm strip.	To use as baseline in evaluating response to treatment.
	Assess for signs of ventricular failure: auscultate lung and heart sounds q 8 h.	Ventricular function may be decreased by persistent tachyarrhythmias, which can further impair ventricular functioning.
	Administer antiarrhythmic agents as ordered, following serum blood levels as guide for dosage. Monitor patient's response: ECG, clinical status.	To maintain therapeutic drug levels that maximize effect and avoid drug toxicity and unnecessary side effects.
	Monitor laboratory data daily or more frequently as indicated, especially potassium.	Potassium influences repolarization of myocardial cell; any increase or decrease can lead to dysrhythmias. Hypokalemia increases risk of digitalis toxicity.

NURSING DIAGNOSIS	NURSING INTERVENTIONS	RATIONALE
	Monitor drug levels as indicated.	Many drugs, including antiarrhythmic agents, can lead to dysrhythmias, particularly if there are other organ system failures (e.g., liver) or if used in combination with other drugs.
	Maintain quiet environment, administer sedation or pain medication as ordered.	Increased stimulation and pain can lead to increased release of catecholamines.
	Administer oxygen therapy as ordered.	To treat hypoxia, which can lead to myocardial ischemia.

	Initiate prompt treatment of life-threatening dysrhythmias per unit protocol:
	  Defibrillation
	  CPR
	  Parenteral drug therapy
	  Preparation for pacemaker insertion
		Quick, immediate assessment of and action for life-threatening events are required to ensure adequate CO.

Knowledge deficit	See Patient Teaching.	

5 EVALUATE

PATIENT OUTCOME	DATA INDICATING THAT OUTCOME IS REACHED
Anxiety level is reduced.	Patient appears calm and relaxed. Patient is able to identify anxiety in self and uses adaptive coping strategies to deal with stress.
Heart returns to baseline rhythm.	ECG tracing reflects baseline rhythm; BP and HR are within normal limits. There is no ectopy.
CO is adequate to maintain cerebral perfusion.	Patient is alert and has no dizziness, syncopal episodes, or chest pains. Vital signs are stable. Peripheral perfusion is good.
Patient's knowledge level is increased.	Patient demonstrates understanding of dysrhythmia, actions to take when experiencing signs and symptoms of dysrhythmias, and knowledge regarding drug therapy; Patient demonstrates pulse-taking technique.

PATIENT TEACHING

Instruction for a patient with a cardiac dysrhythmia begins with the initial phase of care, whether in a coronary care unit or in an outpatient setting. The following points should be included.

1. Briefly describe the disease etiology and/or the rhythm disturbances and associated symptoms.
2. Explain any diagnostic and treatment procedures that are planned.
3. Explain the monitoring equipment that may be used.
4. Explain any dietary restrictions that may be prescribed—need to avoid products that have caffeine (e.g., coffee, certain teas, soft drinks, chocolate).
5. Explain importance of avoiding or stopping smoking or use of nicotine products.

6. Instruct the patient regarding drug therapy and its purpose, desired effects, and dosage and the side effects to report to the physician.
7. Explain the reasons for and method of taking pulse rate and rhythm.
8. Explain the need to exercise to tolerance, to avoid strenuous and/or isometric activity, and to check with physician regarding limitations and allowances.
9. Instruct the patient regarding energy conservation for ADLs:
   - Take regular rest periods: between activities and for 1 hour after meals.
   - When possible, sit rather than stand when performing a task.
   - Stop activity or task if symptoms begin to appear: fatigue, dyspnea, palpitations.

Coronary Artery Disease

Coronary artery disease is a disorder of the coronary arteries that ultimately leads to an interference in blood supply to the myocardium. Permanent disruption of blood flow causes myocardial dysfunction, including sudden death.

Coronary artery disease (CAD) and its clinical sequelae, myocardial infarction, remains the leading cause of morbidity and mortality in the United States. It is estimated that CAD is responsible for half a million deaths each year, with 45% of all heart attacks occurring in patients under age 65 and 5% under age 40. As a chronic condition, it has been further estimated that there are nearly 5 million persons with evidence of CAD.

EPIDEMIOLOGY

The etiology of CAD is complex. While there are other causes of coronary obstruction, atherosclerosis remains the leading contributor to CAD. At this time, researchers do not know how atherosclerosis begins. But as a result of several large-scale studies, such as the Framingham study started in 1950, several factors have been identified as increasing the risk of developing coronary atherosclerosis.[79] These risk factors include heredity, age, sex, hypertension, lipid levels, obesity, smoking, a sedentary life-style, and psychosocial factors.

Heredity. Although the association is not clear, genetic factors appear to play a role in the development of CAD. Apparently a tendency toward hypertension, hyperlipidemia, and diabetes exists in some families. However, it is unknown whether the tendency is inherited or simply the result of life-style patterns that are passed down from generation to generation. If the latter is true, these major risk factors may be altered favorably.

Age and sex. CAD is more prevalent in older men. Deaths from CAD are reported to be five times as frequent for men as for women in the 35- to 40-year-old

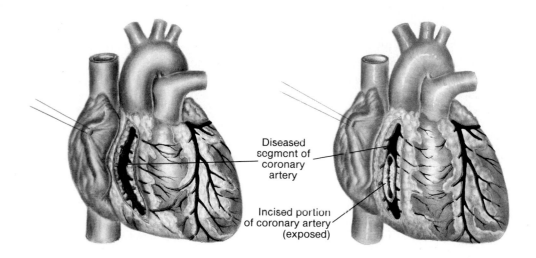

Diseased
segment of
coronary
artery

Incised portion
of coronary artery
(exposed)

group and two to three times as frequent in those 60 years and older. These differences have been attributed to female sex hormones, since this female advantage declines rapidly after menopause. In recent years, however, these age differences appear to have changed, probably because of increased social and economic pressures on women and changes in their life-styles, including an increased incidence of smoking and use of oral contraceptives. Estrogen-based oral contraceptives have been shown to be associated with increased risk of CAD and acute MI in women 45 years and younger, particularly if they also smoke and have high blood pressure. These findings result from studies that have demonstrated high serum cholesterol and triglyceride levels in women taking oral contraceptives.[115,143] The occurrence of CAD in persons less than 30 years of age is usually associated with hyperlipidemia, hypertension, and smoking.[2]

Hypertension. Although diastolic hypertension is the major criterion for defining high blood pressure and is better correlated with cardiovascular disease, elevations in both systolic and diastolic pressure correlate with the development of ischemic heart disease. Systolic pressures greater or equal to 140 mm Hg or diastolic pressures greater than or equal to 90 mm Hg are considered a significant risk factor for heart attacks, particularly when present in younger persons.[76,167]

Lipids and lipoproteins. Of the various types of circulating lipids, lipoproteins, cholesterol, and triglycerides are most commonly associated with CAD. Hyperlipidemia may be a primary disorder or may occur as a result of diabetes, myxedema, or alcoholism. Lipoproteins can be measured separately to determine which levels are atherogenic. Low-density lipids (LDLs) carry a high percentage of cholesterol and plasma and in high levels promote the production of atheromas. Conversely, high-density lipids (HDLs) are mostly protein and carry a smaller percentage of cholesterol, thereby assisting in the removal of lipids from the cell, primarily through liver metabolism. Recent studies show that the ratio of HDLs to LDLs is lower in patients with CAD and that a high ratio of HDLs helps reduce vascular disease.[101] The formation of HDLs is stimulated through exercise, fat-controlled diets, and estrogens.[13]

Obesity. Studies have demonstrated that an increased food intake is associated with elevations in LDLs. Obese people also have a tendency toward hypertension and glucose intolerance. Obesity is defined to be a body-mass index (weight/height squared) greater than 20% above ideal weight.

Smoking. Cigarette smoking is a major risk factor leading to death from CAD. Male smokers have a 70% higher mortality rate than male nonsmokers. In women under 50 years who smoke 35 cigarettes or more per day, the risk of having an MI is 20 times greater than those who never smoked.[115] Primarily through adrenergic stimulation, nicotine contributes to hemodynamic changes including increases in heart rate, stroke volume, cardiac output, and blood pressure. Nicotine also causes peripheral vasoconstriction and, in persons with decreased blood flow, enhances ischemic changes. Furthermore, smoking decreases the threshold for ventricular fibrillation through its interference with oxygen binding with hemoglobin, thus impairing oxygen diffusion into mitochondria.

Sedentary life-style. Although precise documentation of the positive effects of exercise on the risk of CAD is difficult, studies do support a decreased risk of

CAD among well-conditioned persons such as joggers and marathon runners. Inactivity is associated with decreases in HDLs.

Psychosocial factors. The coronary-prone, or type A, personality has been demonstrated to be more characteristic of persons in whom CAD will develop. The characteristics of this personality trait include aggressiveness, competitiveness, and an urgent sense of time. When the type A personality is combined with other risk factors such as age, high lipid levels, and smoking, the risk of heart disease increases.

Diabetes. Apart from the preceding factors that have been studied and strongly implicated in CAD, glucose intolerance as evidenced in diabetes mellitus has been identified as a strong cardiovascular risk factor, especially among women.[4,115]

PATHOPHYSIOLOGY

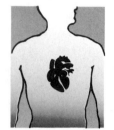 Atherosclerosis, the basic underlying disease affecting coronary lumen size, is characterized by changes in the intimal lining of the arteries. It begins as an irregular thickening process producing fatty streaks. This advances to a more severe form involving the combination of large amounts of lipids with collagen to produce fibroblasts that ultimately lead to fibrous atherosclerotic plaques (Figure 4-18).

The severity of the disease is measured by the degree of obstruction within each artery and by the number of vessels involved. Obstructions exceeding 75% of the lumen of one or more of the three coronary arteries increase the risk of death. The annual mortality of persons with one-vessel disease is 1% to 3%. Three-vessel disease increases the risk to 10% to 15%. Among persons with 75% obstruction of the left main artery, however, the annual mortality is 30% to 40%.

Myocardial Perfusion

The basic physiologic changes occurring as a result of the atherosclerotic process are problems of myocardial oxygen supply and demand. When myocardial oxygen demand exceeds the supply delivered by the coronary arteries, ischemia results. Myocardial metabolism is oxygen dependent (aerobic), extracting up to 80% of the oxygen from the coronary blood supply. Coronary blood flow to the myocardium occurs primarily during diastole. The factors influencing supply include cardiac output, intramyocardial tension, aortic pressure, and coronary artery resistance. Coronary blood flow can be increased by increasing the cardiac output and aortic pressure and decreasing coronary artery resistance and intramyocardial tension.

The factors determining myocardial oxygen demand are heart rate, myocardial wall tension, and contractile state of the myocardium. As the heart rate increases, so does the demand for oxygen to the myocardial cells. Myocardial wall tension occurs during contraction and is influenced by ventricular and systolic (arterial) pressure. Myocardial contractility is stimulated through the release of catecholamines or sympathetic stimulation. Combined, these increase wall tension and thereby increase energy or oxygen demands.

Myocardial ischemia is the result of impaired myocardial perfusion. In the setting of CAD, it is the consequence of coronary atherosclerotic heart disease. The narrowing or obstruction varies in degree and may be well tolerated as long as the myocardial oxygen demand is minimal. As the demand increases and the obstruction persists or advances, ischemic changes result. Coronary blood vessel distribution is also important in providing oxygen to the myocardium. The coronary arteries sit on the epicardial surface of the heart. Blood travels inward toward the endocardium. The inner subendocardial layers of the myocardium therefore are particularly susceptible to ischemia. Increases in heart rate and wall tension can reduce flow to the endocardium.

In addition to ventricular perfusion, the coronary arteries supply major conduction structures within the myocardium. The right coronary artery (RCA) supplies the sinus node in 55% to 60% of persons, whereas in the remainder it is supplied by a branch of the circumflex artery. The RCA also supplies the A-V node in 85% of persons, whereas in the remaining 15% the left coronary artery does. The septum is supplied primarily by the left anterior descending (LAD) artery, although a portion of the posterior wall is supplied by the RCA. An obstruction or impedance to flow in any of the major arteries or their branches results in ischemia to the portion of myocardium nourished by that vessel. Obstruction of the LAD results in ischemic changes of the anterior wall of the ventricle.

Inferior and posterior MIs result from RCA obstruction. Occlusion of the RCA also is responsible for right ventricular injury. The degree of obstruction and number of coronary arteries involved dictate the severity of the disease. CAD is commonly described as single-, double-, or triple-vessel disease, the last referring to three major arteries. When a major obstruction occurs in the initial branch of the left coronary artery or the left main artery before bifurcation, the risk for a major infarction and death rises. This is referred to as left main disease.

The major clinical manifestations of ischemia are chest pain and ECG changes. The associated symptoms occur as a result of secondary effects brought on by compromised cardiac function.

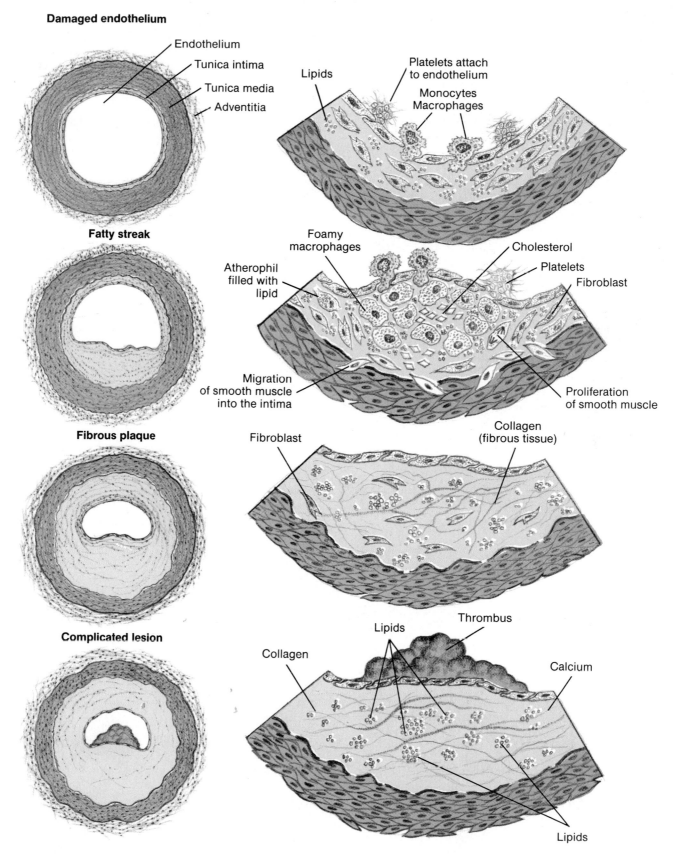

FIGURE 4-18
Progression of atherosclerosis. (From McCance.)[107a]

Angina Pectoris

The term **angina pectoris**, which means chest pain, is used to describe pain as a symptom of myocardial ischemia. Myocardial ischemia is the result of an imbalance between myocardial oxygen supply and demand. It occurs most commonly in the setting of coronary atherosclerosis but can also occur in patients with normal coronary arteries. For example, patients with aortic stenosis, hypertension, and hypertrophic cardiomyopathy may have clinical symptoms of angina pectoris. In these patients, myocardial work is increased but perfusion of the hypertrophied muscle is inadequate, resulting in myocardial ischemia despite normal coronary arteries.

Various terms have been used to describe the clinical syndromes associated with myocardial ischemia. The following are commonly used to describe chest pain that is transient and associated with myocardial ischemia.

Stable angina pectoris is characterized by effort-induced chest discomfort, with or without radiation, that lasts from a few seconds to 15 minutes. It is generally relieved by rest, removal of provoking factors, or sublingual vasodilators.

Unstable angina pectoris is characterized by pain that lasts longer, occurs more frequently, and may be precipitated by factors other than effort or activities. Various names are used to describe this syndrome, such as crescendo angina, preinfarction angina, angina decubitus, and nocturnal angina.

Variant (Prinzmetal's) angina is characterized by chest pain that occurs at rest in the early hours of the morning and is often associated with ST elevations on the ECG. The underlying cause is thought to be coronary artery spasm. Unlike angina pectoris, variant angina is due to a sudden reduction in coronary blood flow brought on by spasm and not by an increase in myocardial oxygen demand. It has been suggested that the decrease in myocardial consumption occurring during sleep or rest may lead to coronary artery vasoconstriction and is responsible for the spasm.[198]

The etiology of spasm is not clearly understood, but researchers have postulated a correlation with stimulation of alpha (vasoconstriction) and beta (vasodilation) adrenergic receptors.[197] Other studies have suggested various mechanisms involved in the genesis of spasm, including an increase in the level of free calcium ions and possibly local abnormalities of vascular smooth muscle.[14]

Myocardial Infarction

Myocardial infarction (MI) is the development of ischemia and necrosis of myocardial tissue. It results from a sudden decrease in coronary perfusion or an increase in myocardial oxygen demand without adequate coronary perfusion.

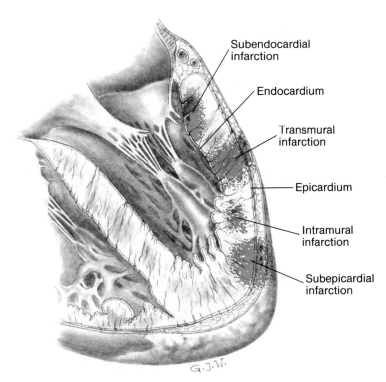

Subendocardial infarction

Endocardium

Transmural infarction

Epicardium

Intramural infarction

Subepicardial infarction

FIGURE 4-19
Location of infactions in ventrical wall. (From Thelan.)[169]

Infarctions are frequently described according to the myocardial layers involved (Figure 4-19). Subendocardial infarction is generally confined to small areas of myocardium, particularly within the subendocardial wall of the ventricle, the ventricular septum, and papillary muscles. Transmural, or full-thickness, infarction is widespread myocardial necrosis extending from the endocardium through to the epicardium. The majority of MIs involve the left ventricle (LV). However, because of serious hemodynamic consequences, right ventricular (RV) infarctions usually occur as a complication of a transmural inferior-posterior LV wall MI. Studies show the frequency of occurrence to be between 24% for posterior MI and 40% for patients with inferior wall MIs. RV infarction can occur as an isolated event, but this is rare with a reported incidence rate of 2.5%.[73]

Myocardial tissue death is usually preceded by a sudden occlusion of one of the major coronary arteries. Coronary thrombosis is the most common cause of infarction, but many interrelated factors may be responsible. These include coronary artery spasm, platelet aggregation and embolism from a mural thrombus, a thrombus on a prosthetic mitral or aortic valve, or a dislodged calcium plaque from a calcified aortic or mitral valve.

Persistent cellular ischemia interferes with myocardial tissue metabolism, causing a rapid development of irreversible cellular damage. In the initial phases of the infarction there are three zones of tissue damage. The first is a central area consisting of necrotic myocardial cells, capillaries, and connective tissue. Surrounding this necrotic tissue is a second zone of "injured" myocardial cells that are potentially viable if adequate circulation is quickly restored. The third zone, called ischemia, is also viable and can be expected to recover unless the ischemia persists or worsens. The severity or extension of a myocardial infarction often depends on the fate of the injured and ischemic zones. Without appropriate interventions, ischemia may progress to necrosis. Since the infarction process may take up to 6 hours to complete, restoration of adequate myocardial perfusion is important if significant necrosis is to be limited.

COMPLICATIONS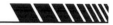

Dysrhythmias	Papillary muscle rupture
Heart failure	Ventricular septal defect
Extension of MI	Ventricular aneurysm
Cardiogenic shock	Cardiac arrest

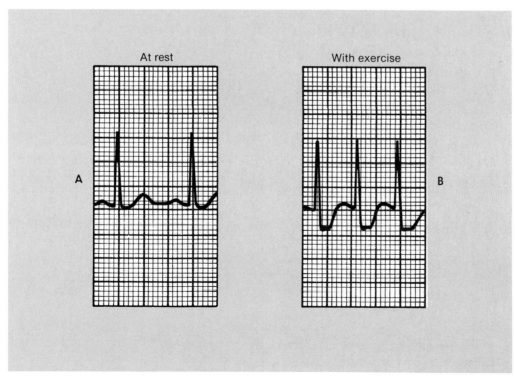

ECG changes with exercise. **A,** At rest. **B,** Demonstrates 3 mm ST depression during exercise stress test.

DIAGNOSTIC STUDIES AND FINDINGS

Diagnostic test	Findings			
	Stable angina pectoris	Variant (Prinzmetal's) angina	Unstable angina pectoris	Myocardial infarction
Electrocardiogram (ECG)	Changes usually seen during anginal episodes; 50%-70% of patients have normal ECG during pain-free episodes; ischemia determined by horizontal ST segment or downsloping with depression of >1 mm; T wave inversion represents impaired repolarization caused by ischemia	Ischemia appears as ST elevation during anginal attack but regresses as pain subsides; ECG changes may be seen before patient complains of chest pain or may be recorded in absence of pain; A-V conduction defects may occur, particularly when right coronary artery is involved, and include Mobitz type II and complete A-V block; ventricular irritability such as premature ventricular contractions, ventricular tachycardia, or fibrillation can occur, particularly during ischemic attack	Ischemia determined by horizontal ST segment or downsloping with depression of >1 mm; T wave inversion represents impaired repolarization caused by ischemia; ventricular irritability such as premature ventricular contractions, ventricular tachycardia, or fibrillation	Changes are evolutionary and indicate progression of infarction; in acute stage, ST elevations with subsequent T wave inversion and Q wave formation; Q waves indicate necrosis and are considered pathologic if they are 0.04 second or greater in duration, 0.4 mm or greater in depth, or present in leads that do not normally have Q waves; ST elevations reflect myocardial injury that interferes with polarization of cells, are seen in leads facing injured area, and return to normal (isoelectric) within days; ST elevations beyond 4-6 wk should raise suspicion of ventricular aneurysm; infarction location determined by identifying leads that demonstrate characteristic ECG changes; such leads are those with positive terminals that face injured site of heart; reciprocal changes, seen in leads that face *opposite* surface of damaged heart, are absence of Q wave, increase in R wave amplitude, depressed ST segment, upright tall T wave *RV infarction:* ST elevation in right precordial leads (V_1, V_3R-V_6R). V_4R-V_6R may be more sensitive indicators
Laboratory tests Enzymes	No elevation; checked to rule out MI	No elevation; checked to rule out MI	No elevation; checked to rule out MI	*Onset* / *Peak* / *Return to normal*
				SGOT 6-12 h / 36 h / 3-4 days
				CPK-MB 4-12 h / 24 h / 3-4 days
				LDH (iso-enzyme) 24-48 h / 3-6 days / 8-14 days
				LDH_1 to LDH_2 ratio > 1.0
Complete blood count (CBC)	No elevation; checked to rule out anemia-induced angina	No elevation; checked to rule out anemia-induced angina	No elevation; checked to rule out anemia-induced angina	Elevated WBC and ESR reflect tissue necrosis
Glucose	No elevation	No elevation	No elevation	Transiently elevated owing to adrenergic response
Lipid levels (triglycerides, cholesterol, high- and low-density lipids)	Checked to determine any lipoprotein abnormalities	Checked to rule out presence of atherosclerotic process	Checked to determine any lipoprotein abnormalities	Checked to determine any lipoprotein abnormalities. Total cholesterol and HDL may drop 48 hours after admission

Test				
Chest x-ray	Normal	Normal	Normal; may show signs of cardiomegaly or signs of left ventricular failure	Same as unstable angina
Exercise stress test (EST)	Chest pain; horizontal ST segment or downsloping of 1 mm or more; failure of systolic blood pressure to rise or drop; ST elevations	Normal stress test done to differentiate between variant and classic angina; ST elevation with or without associated chest pain occasionally develops	As in stable angina pectoris; should not be done until patient has been stable and pain free for 24 hours	Not done in presence of documented MI, low-level test may be performed before discharge from hospital
Echocardiography	Limited use, but performed after EST may detect wall motion abnormalities		2-dimensional: may show transient abnormalities of ventricular wall motion	Identifies area of abnormal regional wall motion; aids in detecting complications associated with acute MI: papillary dysfunction, septal rupture; visualizes LV thrombus RV *infarction*: dilated RV, abnormal RV wall motion
Thallium 201 scintigraphy	Ischemic areas appear as "cold" areas, reflecting reduced thallium uptake; when ischemia relieved, "cold" areas show normal thallium uptake	Ischemic "cold" areas may be demonstrated once involved coronary artery has been identified	Similar to stable angina pectoris	Similar to stable angina pectoris
Radionuclide blood pool imaging with technetium 99m			Positive findings suggest recent (previous) minor degrees of subendocardial necrosis or infarction	Confirms myocardial damage by localizing and permitting estimation of size of transmural infarction; must be done within 2-6 days after acute infarction; determines wall motion abnormalities; permits estimation of ventricular function by determining ejection fractions
Magnetic resonance imaging (MRI)				Differentiates ischemic, infarcted and normal myocardial tissue; used in early detection of MI to assess areas of perfusion and to detect jeopardized or vulnerable tissue
Cardiac catheterization and coronary angiography	Determines number and location of obstructive lesions, "graftability" of artery distal to obstructive lesion, and ventricular function	Distinguishes spasm in normal coronary arteries from those with severe obstructive lesions; intravenous injection of ergonovine maleate provokes coronary artery spasm in patients with variant angina	As in stable angina pectoris; used in conjunction with PTCA	Generally not performed as diagnostic procedure during acute period unless done in conjunction with intracoronary thrombolysis

MEDICAL MANAGEMENT

GENERAL MANAGEMENT

Admission to coronary care unit (CCU): Indicated for patients with acute chest pain for evaluation, surveillance, and management.

Electrocardiogram (ECG): Used to detect conduction change reflecting myocardial ischemia vs infarction. Continuous cardiac monitoring aids in detecting serial changes, extension of MI, and onset of dysrhythmias.

Hemodynamic monitoring: Used to assess and monitor signs of life-threatening complications associated with severe myocardial ischemia and/or necrosis.

Oxygen therapy: Oxygen tension (Pa_{O_2}) is measured on admission to CCU; if normal, oxygen therapy may be omitted; hypoxemic patients receive 2 to 4 L/min of oxygen by mask or prongs for 2 to 3 days; serial arterial blood gas determinations to monitor effectiveness of therapy.

Diet: Admission diet will depend on clinical status; during acute phase, patient may remain NPO or on clear liquids progressing to 1500 calorie soft, low-fat, 2 g sodium diet. Iced beverages limited to 600-800 ml; caffeine products avoided.

Physical activity: Bed rest progressing toward ambulation. Uncomplicated MI—bedrest for first 24 h, assist with use of bedside commode; after second day may be up in chair for short period of time; ambulation using structured progressive levels of activities. Complications occur within first 5 days in 50% of patients with acute MI.

DRUG THERAPY

Vasodilators: Nitrates: Short-acting nitrates (sublingual nitroglycerin, isosorbide dinitrate); Long-acting oral nitrates (isosorbide dinitrate); Topical 2% nitroglycerin ointment

Beta-adrenergic blocking agents: Propranolol (Inderal); Nadolol (Corgard); Timolol; Atenolol

Calcium antagonists: Nifedipine (Procardia); Verapamil (Calan, Isoptin); Diltiazem (Cardizem)

Antihyperlipidemic agents: Cholestyramine (Questran); Neomycin sulfate; Clofibrate (Atromid-S); Gemfibrozil (Lopid); Niacin (nicotinic acid)

Antiplatelets: Aspirin (acetylsalicylic acid, ASA); Dipyridamole (Persantine, Persantin)

Stool softeners: Dioctyl sodium sulfosuccinate

ADJUNCTIVE THERAPY

Percutaneous transluminal coronary angioplasty (PTCA): Restores luminal patency by compressing atheromatous plaques within the coronary vessel. (See page 235.)

Thrombolytic therapy: Nonsurgical reperfusion procedure used to stop progression of MI and limit infarct signs. Improvement of the ischemic area can be achieved if therapy is initiated within 4-6 h from onset of infarction. (See page 243.)

Intra-aortic balloon counterpulsation (IABP): Used to achieve hemodynamic stability after acute MI. Supports diastolic pressure, which aids in improving coronary perfusion.

SURGERY

Coronary artery bypass graft (CABG): Myocardial revascularization aimed at increasing myocardial coronary blood flow.

1 ASSESS

ASSESSMENT	OBSERVATIONS			
	STABLE ANGINA PECTORIS	**VARIANT (PRINZMETAL'S) ANGINA**	**UNSTABLE ANGINA PECTORIS**	**MYOCARDIAL INFARCTION**
Chest pain **Quality**	Aching, sharp, tingling, or burning sensation or pressure	Similar to stable angina pectoris	Similar to stable angina pectoris but may be more severe	Crushing, squeezing, stabbing, oppressive sensation or as if a heavy object is sitting on chest
Location and radiation	Substernal with radiation to left shoulder, down inner aspect of left arm or both arms; neck, jaw, and scapula may be additional sites of radiation	Similar to stable angina pectoris	Similar to stable angina pectoris	Retrosternal and left precordial, radiating down left arm and to neck, jaws, teeth, epigastric area, and back
Precipitating factors	Onset classically associated with exercise or activities that increase myocardial oxygen demand, e.g., physical exercise, heavy lifting, emotional stress, cold temperatures	Onset at rest; pain is cyclic, often occurring during sleep (most common in early morning hours)	Pain may be brought on with less than usual exertion; may occur at rest	May occur at rest or during exertion
Duration and alleviating factors	3-15 min; relieved by rest, stopping pain-inducing activities; taking sublingual nitroglycerin (NTG) tablet	Characteristically, pain intensifies quickly, tends to last longer than angina, and subsides with exercise	Prolonged and not usually as quickly relieved by rest or taking NTG	Described as continuous, lasting more than 30 min, unrelieved by rest, position change, or taking NTG tablets

→ > >

ASSESSMENT	OBSERVATIONS			
	STABLE ANGINA PECTORIS	VARIANT (PRINZMETAL'S) ANGINA	UNSTABLE ANGINA PECTORIS	MYOCARDIAL INFARCTION
Associated signs and symptoms	During anginal attack, dyspnea, anxiety, diaphoresis, cool clammy skin	Similar to stable angina pectoris	Similar to stable angina pectoris but symptoms may be more prominent and may persist; may be associated with nausea	Anxiety, restlessness, weakness, associated profuse diaphoresis, dyspnea, dizziness; signs of vasomotor response including nausea, vomiting, faintness, and cold clammy skin; hiccough and other gastrointestinal distress may be present; low-grade temperature elevations common for first 24-48 h but may last several days
Physical examination	Normal during asymptomatic periods; during anginal attacks, increased HR, pulsus alternans, and transient abnormal findings including precordial bulge and atrial and ventricular gallops (S_3, S_4)	Similar to stable angina pectoris	Similar to stable angina pectoris; may also demonstrate irregular pulse, hypotension, or signs of LV dysfunction	May be unremarkable unless signs of ventricular failure or cardiogenic shock are present; BP normal, elevated, or decreased (initially elevated when pain is present but usually decreases in first few days); Cheyne-Stokes respiration owing to CNS hypoperfusion or opiate therapy; initial tachypnea returns to normal once pain subsides;

ASSESSMENT	OBSERVATIONS			
	STABLE ANGINA PECTORIS	VARIANT (PRINZMETAL'S) ANGINA	UNSTABLE ANGINA PECTORIS	MYOCARDIAL INFARCTION
				heart sounds: S_3, S_4 gallops indicative of ventricular dysfunction; systolic murmurs reflecting papillary muscle dysfunction; diminished heart sounds and pericardial friction rub may occur; with LV dysfunction: pulmonary crackles, decreased urine output, increased amplitude of "a" wave in jugular vein; with RV dysfunction: increased jugular venous distention, peripheral edema, liver tenderness; pulse often within normal limits; bradycardia present with inferior wall MI; tachycardia with rates > 100 bpm may reflect compromised ventricle
Hemodynamic parameters				Increased PAP, PCWP, SVR; Decreased CO/CI *RVInfarction:* Increased RAP, SVR; Decreased PAP, PCWP, CO/CI

2 DIAGNOSE

NURSING DIAGNOSIS	SUBJECTIVE FINDINGS	OBJECTIVE FINDINGS
Pain (chest) related to imbalance of myocardial oxygen supply and demand	Complains of pain, discomfort, nausea	Guarded behavior—holding chest Impaired thought processes Distracted behavior, e.g., moaning, restless Facies: grimace Autonomic responses: pallor, diaphoresis, tachycardia, tachypnea
Decreased cardiac output related to electrical factors (dysrhythmias), decreased myocardial contractility, and structural defects (e.g., papillary muscle dysfunction and ventricular septal rupture)	Complains of fatigue, weakness, dyspnea, activity intolerance, syncope, restlessness, altered mentation	Hypotension, tachycardia, irregular heart rhythm, decreased peripheral pulses Elevated temperature Skin: cold, clammy, diaphoresis, pallor, cyanosis Urine output: < 30 ml/h Breath sounds: crackles (rales) and wheezes (rhonchi) Heart sounds: S_3, S_4; murmurs Increased PAP, PCWP, SVR; decreased CO/CI
Anxiety related to perceived or actual threat to biologic integrity	Verbalizes vague diffuse feelings; Verbalizes feelings of fear, uncertainty, panic, jitteriness	Poor eye contact, dilated pupils Facies: wide-eyed, increased alertness Autonomic response: flushed face, tachycardia, diaphoresis, tachypnea, dry mouth

Other related nursing diagnoses

Potential impaired gas exchange related to increased pulmonary capillary pressure
Potential fluid volume excess related to reduced renal blood flow
Activity intolerance related to decreased cardiac reserve

3 PLAN

Patient goals

1. Patient will verbalize relief of pain.
2. Patient will demonstrate stable or improved cardiac performance.
3. Patient will demonstrate reduced anxiety level.
4. Patient will demonstrate increased understanding of disease process and need to alter life-style.

4 IMPLEMENT

NURSING DIAGNOSIS	NURSING INTERVENTIONS	RATIONALE
Pain (chest) related to imbalance of myocardial oxygen supply and demand	*Acute care*	
	Assess original pain: location, duration, radiation, and onset of new symptoms.	Prolonged episodes of myocardial ischemia are associated with acute MI. In patients with MI, continuous pain suggests extension of infarction.
	Assess and describe angina and activity prior to onset of pain.	To determine precipitating factors.
	Obtain 12-lead ECG during anginal pain episode.	To document signs of ischemia vs infarction. To determine extension of infarction.
	Assess for signs of hypoxemia; administer oxygen therapy as indicated.	Hypoxemia may result from ventilation-perfusion abnormalities. In absence of hypoxemia, providing additional inspired oxygen does not ensure increased oxygen delivery to myocardium.
	Administer medications as indicated: Nitrates (short acting), IV nitroglycerin, morphine sulfate, 4-8 mg IV. Assess and record the response.	Nitrates relieve pain through venoarterial dilatation. Morphine relieves pain by reducing the autonomic response.
	Maintain bed rest for first 24-30 h during episode of pain.	To conserve myocardial oxygen consumption.
	Obtain BP, pulse, and respiration during pain episode and after receiving drug therapy.	To monitor for signs of hypotension, which may reflect hypoperfusion or side effects of nitrates.
	Convalescent care	
	Administer long-acting nitrates as ordered. Increase activity as tolerated; assist patient to identify and limit activities that elicit pain.	To control anginal pain.
Decreased cardiac output related to electrical factors (dysrhythmias), decreased myocardial contractility, and structural defects	Assess and report signs of decreased CO.	Incidence of mortality and morbidity due to MI is greatest in the first 24 h.
	Monitor and record ECG continuously to assess rate, rhythm, and any changes q 2-4 h as indicated. Use MCL_1 and obtain 12-lead ECG.	Ventricular fibrillation, the primary cause of death from acute MI occurs within the first 4-12 h from onset of attack. MCL_1 differentiates ventricular ectopy from aberrancy. The 12-lead ECG confirms and identifies location of MI.
	Assess and monitor vital signs and hemodynamic parameters q 1-2 h or as indicated by clinical status.	To detect onset of myocardial dysfunction due to complications.
	Maintain bed rest with head of bed elevated 30 degrees for first 24-48 h.	To reduce myocardial oxygen demand.

→ › ›

NURSING DIAGNOSIS	NURSING INTERVENTIONS	RATIONALE
	Initiate a patent IV line.	To provide ready access for administration of intravenous drug therapy.
	Administer medications as ordered—antiarrhythmics, nitrates, and beta-blockers.	Antiarrhythmics correct dysrhythmias. Nitrates reduce afterload. Beta-blockers reduce ischemia by decreasing myocardial contractility and reducing workload of heart.
	Prepare and/or initiate thrombolytic therapy as ordered.	To limit infarction size by reperfusing ischemic heart muscle.
	Convalescent Care Continue to assess and monitor for signs of decreased CO. Auscultate breath sounds and heart tones q 4-8 h.	To monitor for signs of early complications; e.g., extension of MI, cardiogenic chock, heart failure, myocardial rupture, which may occur up to 10 days from onset of attack.
	Increase activity level as indicated by clinical status. Monitor BP and HR response as patient increases activities. (In uncomplicated MI, patient may be up in chair after 24-48 h.)	Careful monitoring is necessary to detect hypotension and dysrhythmias and to pace the activity level appropriately.
Anxiety related to perceived or actual threat to biologic integrity	Assess for signs and verbal expressions of anxiety.	Anxiety levels progressing to panic stimulate sympathetic response by releasing catecholamines, which contribute to increased myocardial oxygen demand.
	Initiate measures to reduce anxiety levels. Provide a quiet, restful environment. Administer sedation as ordered.	To decrease unnecessary external stimuli.
	Stay with patient during periods of highest anxiety offering reassurance; use calm, but concerned voice.	Empathetic understanding is therapeutic and may enhance patient's coping abilities.
	Permit family members to assist patient whenever possible; refer to spiritual advisor.	Use of patient's support system can increase comfort level and reduce tension due to uncertainty of surroundings.
	Provide brief explanations for all procedures and treatments.	Providing information prior to procedures and treatments increases sense of control and decreases uncertainty.
	Encourage expression of feelings; permit crying.	Acceptance of emotional expressions contributes to patient ability to deal with uncertainty and dependence.
	Initiate relaxation techniques, e.g., deep breathing, visual imagery, soft rhythmic music.	To distract patient from immediate events.
Knowledge deficit	See Patient Teaching.	

5 EVALUATE

PATIENT OUTCOME	DATA INDICATING THAT OUTCOME IS REACHED
Patient is free from pain.	Patient verbalizes absence of pain. BP and HR are within normal limits. Patient engages in hospital routines and activities without pain. Patient appears relaxed. Patient verbalizes appropriate measures to relieve pain.
CO in improved/ maintained.	ECG rate and rhythm are normal; dysrhythmias are controlled or absent. BP, HR, respiration, and urine output are within normal limits, demonstrating hemodynamic stability. Skin is warm and dry.
Anxiety level is reduced.	Patient appears relaxed; verbalizes sense of calm.
Patient's knowledge level is increased.	Patient demonstrates understanding of disease process, is able to verbalize risk factors for CAD, and reports appropriate changes in life-style.

PATIENT TEACHING

1. Explain atherosclerotic disease process and its different clinical manifestations: angina pectoris and heart attack. Discuss signs and symptoms of angina vs MI pain. Explain importance of notifying physician if chest pain lasts longer than 20 minutes.
2. Discuss contributing risk factors, identifying which are specific to patient and methods to modify them.
3. Review importance of smoking cessation and avoiding use of all tobacco products.
4. Explain activity allowances and limitations:
    Explain importance of planned rest periods and avoiding or modifying activities after heavy meals, after alcohol consumption, or after periods of emotional distress.
    For MI patients, explain that because the healing process takes approximately 6 to 8 weeks, activities such as driving, return to work, traveling, and sexual activity will be limited. Explain the need to avoid isometric-type activities such as heavy lifting and pushing.
    Refer to cardiac rehabilitation program to assist with progressive increase in activity levels.

5. Teach the patient to avoid foods high in sodium, saturated fats, and triglycerides. Review alternative ways of seasoning foods to avoid cooking with salt and salt products. Explain need to limit intake of eggs, cream, butter, and foods high in animal fat. Discuss need to follow calorie reduction diet to maintain ideal body weight.
6. Explain the name, purpose, side effects, and method of administration of drugs.
7. For women: if the patient is using oral contraception, refer her to a gynecologist to seek alternative methods.
8. Refer the patient to social support groups as indicated.

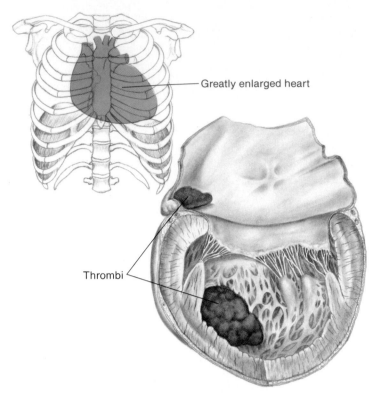

Greatly enlarged heart

Thrombi

Greatly enlarged and hypertrophied heart,
Thrombi in left ventricle and left atrium

Cardiomyopathy

The term **cardiomyopathy** is applied to diseases that diffusely affect the myocardium, resulting in enlargement or ventricular dysfunction.

In the past three decades, great advances in the understanding of this complex disorder have been made, particularly with regard to pathophysiology, diagnosis, and treatment. To distinguish the various forms and causes of the myopathies, several classifications have been proposed. Two are discussed here. First, in classifications according to cause, terms such as idiopathic cardiomyopathy and myocardiomyopathy have been used to describe primary myocardial disease not caused by coronary artery, valvular, or congenital heart dis-

ease. Types of idiopathic cardiomyopathy are listed in the box below.

Secondary cardiomyopathies occur as a result of a generalized disease process that affects other parts of the body before or after the myocardium is involved. Examples of such conditions are listed in the box on page 93.

PATHOPHYSIOLOGY

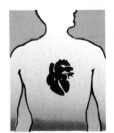

There are three basic types of cardiomyopathy—dilated (also known as congestive), hypertrophic, and restrictive (Figure 4-20).

Dilated Cardiomyopathy (Idiopathic Dilated Cardiomyopathy)

The most common form of cardiomyopathy is characterized by gross dilation of the heart, interference with systolic function, and damage to myofibrils. Unlike hypertrophic cardiomyopathy, in which ventricular filling is impaired, dilated cardiomyopathy is characterized by impaired systolic ejection function, with both the end-diastolic and end-systolic volumes increased.

On gross examination the heart is globular with enlargement and dilation of all four chambers (Figure 4-

---

TYPES OF IDIOPATHIC CARDIOMYOPATHY

Endocardial fibroelastosis
Hypertrophic obstructive cardiomyopathy
Primary myocardial disease
Familial cardiomyopathies
   Metabolic storage diseases
      Pompe's disease (glycogen)
      Fabry's disease (glycolipid)
   Muscular dystrophies
   Friederich's ataxia
   Sickle cell anemia

SYSTOLE   DIASTOLE

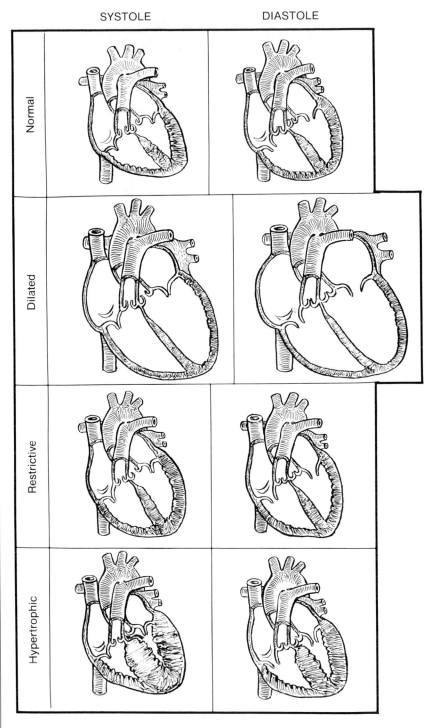

TYPES OF SECONDARY CARDIOMYOPATHY

Inflammatory
  Infectious
    Viral (e.g., coxsackievirus, rubella)
    Rickettsial (typhus, Q fever)
    Bacterial (streptococcal)
    Spirochetal (leptospirosis, syphilis)
    Fungal (histoplasmosis, coccidioidomycosis)
    Parasitic (Chagas' disease, schistosomiasis)
  Noninfectious (collagen)
    Rheumatic heart disease
    Scleroderma
    Systemic lupus erythematosus
    Polyarteritis
    Löffler's disease
    Dermatomyositis
Infiltrative
  Sarcoidosis
  Amyloidosis
  Neoplastic
Metabolic
  Endocrine disorders
    Thyrotoxicosis
    Myxedema
  Nutritional
    Starvation, malnutrition
    Beri-beri
Toxic
  Alcohol
  Carbon monoxide
  Arsenic
  Immunosuppressive drugs (e. g., doxorubicin)
  Emetine
Miscellaneous
  Postpartum
  Radiation

FIGURE 4-20
Types of cardiomyopathies. (From Thelan.)[169]

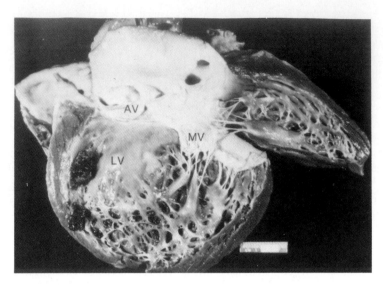

FIGURE 4-21
Heart with idiopathic dilated congestive cardiomyopathy. Opened left ventricle, *LV,* has dilated and globular configuration. Aortic valves, *AV,* and mitral valves, *MV,* are normal. (From Thompson.)[171]

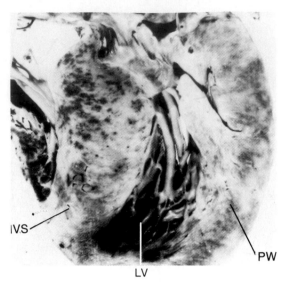

FIGURE 4-22
Heart with hypertrophic cardiomyopathy. Interventricular septum, *IVS,* is thicker than posterior wall, *PW.* (From Bulkley.)[16]

21). Although the heart may weigh up to 700 g (normal 350 g), the wall thickness may be normal or decreased. Left ventricular filling pressures are generally elevated as a consequence of poor contractile function. The cardiac valves are intrinsically normal, as are the coronary arteries. Endocardial thrombi are common, particularly in the ventricular apex. Failure occurs as a result of decreased systolic ejection fraction.

Histologic examination reveals nonspecific changes, including cellular hypertrophy and extensive interstitial and perivascular fibrosis.

The cause of this disorder is not clear, but it has been linked etiologically to various factors that predispose to the development of cardiomyopathy, including alcohol, pregnancy, infections, toxins, and immunologic abnormalities. It is also thought to be familial. It may occur as result of ischemia.

Hypertrophic Cardiomyopathy

Hypertrophic cardiomyopathy is a form of myocardial disease whose pathophysiologic, etiologic, and clinical features have received wide attention. As a result, it has acquired an extensive list of identifying terms that generally describe features of the disease not present in all cases. These include idiopathic hypertrophic subaortic stenosis (IHSS), asymmetric septal hypertrophy (ASH), and hypertrophic obstructive cardiomyopathy (HOCM). Hypertrophic cardiomyopathy (HCM) is the preferred term. HCM may be genetically transmitted and has been observed in relatives who remain asymptomatic.[180] It tends to occur equally in men and women. It is also seen in young adults.[197]

HCM is characterized by a distinctive pattern of hypertrophy, with disproportionate thickening of the interventricular septum when compared with the free wall of the left ventricle (Figure 4-22). The overgrowth of muscle mass renders the ventricular walls rigid, increasing resistance as blood enters from the left atrium. Obstruction to left ventricular outflow is another characteristic of HCM. Consequently, left ventricular ejection is impeded throughout systole. Contributing to outflow obstruction is the obstruction produced by opposition of the anterior mitral leaflet against the hypertrophied septum during midsystole. Systolic motion of the anterior mitral leaflet has been used to determine the severity of outflow obstruction. Elevated systolic pressure gradients occur in the range of 70% to 90% of left ventricular volumes.[16, 197] Failure occurs as resistance to diastolic filling increases as the result of a stiff, noncompliant left ventricle.

On gross examination of these hearts, there is massive overgrowth of myocardial tissue with small ventricular cavities. The atria are also hypertrophied and dilated, reflecting the high resistance to ventricular filling.

Histologically the heart muscle may show myocardial fiber disarray. First described in 1958 by Donald Teare, this form of HCM is thought to reflect an underlying genetic defect that manifests itself in abnormal cardiac structure. This feature of disorganized cellular architecture is not considered to be pathognomonic of HCM. Similar disorganization has been seen in some cases of acquired or congenital heart disease.[16]

Restrictive Cardiomyopathy

A less common form of cardiomyopathy, restrictive cardiomyopathy is characterized by abnormal diastolic (filling) function and excessively rigid ventricular walls. Contractility, however, is relatively unimpaired with normal systolic emptying of the ventricles. Hemodynamically, this group of cardiomyopathies resembles constrictive pericarditis.

The abnormal diastolic filling occurs as a result of infiltration of the endocardium or myocardium with fibroelastic tissue similar to that seen in Löffler's endocarditis, endomyocardial fibrosis, and amyloidosis.

COMPLICATIONS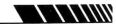

Dilated cardiomyopathy
  Congestive heart failure
  Dysrhythmias
Hypertrophic cardiomyopathy
  Syncope
  Congestive heart failure
  Cardiac arrest
  Sudden death
Restrictive cardiomyopathy
  Congestive heart failure

DIAGNOSTIC STUDIES AND FINDINGS

Diagnostic test	Findings		
	Hypertrophic cardiomyopathy	Dilated cardiomyopathy	Restrictive cardiomyopathy
Chest roentgenogram	Enlarged cardiac silhouette (mild to moderate)	Enlarged cardiac silhouette; prominence of LV (moderate to marked); interstitial or alveolar edema	Cardiac (biatrial) enlargement (mild); pulmonary venous congestion and pleural effusions
Electrocardiogram (ECG) (24-hour ambulatory monitor)	LV hypertrophy; ST segment and T wave changes; Q waves may be seen in precordial leads; atrial dysrhythmias	LV hypertrophy; sinus tachycardia; atrial and ventricular dysrhythmias; ST segment and T wave changes; conduction disturbances; LBBB	Low-voltage; conduction disturbances; high degree AV block
Echocardiogram (2-D)	Narrow LV outflow tract; abnormal thickened septum; systolic anterior motion of mitral valve; decreased internal dimension of LV; LV hypertrophy	LV dilation; abnormal diastolic mitral valve motion; enlarged atria; decreased ejection fraction	Increased LV wall thickness and mass; small or normal LV cavity; normal systolic function; pericardial effusion
Radionuclide studies	Hyperdynamic systolic function; Technetium shows decreased LV volume; Thallium 201 shows increased muscle mass, ischemia; gated-blood pool imaging evaluates size and motion of septum and LV	LV dilation and hypokinesis; decreased ejection fraction	Myocardial infiltration; small or normal LV cavity; normal systolic function; Computerized axial tomography and MRI define pericardial thickness
Cardiac catheterization	Decreased LV compliance; mitral regurgitation; hyperdynamic systolic function; LV outflow obstruction; increased LVEDP	LV enlargement and dysfunction; mitral and tricuspid regurgitation; increased LVEDP; decreased CO/CI	Decreased LV compliance; normal systolic function; increased LVEDP
Endocardial biopsy	May be used to confirm diagnosis	May be used to determine etiology and confirm diagnosis	Confirms restrictive or infiltrative cardiomyopathy; rules out constrictive pericarditis

MEDICAL MANAGEMENT

GENERAL MANAGEMENT

Physical activity: Restricted during acute phase; allowances and limitations guided by clinical condition.

Diet: Restrict sodium and fluid intake.

Oxygen therapy: As indicated by clinical status.

Hemodynamic monitoring: Initiated as means of assessing LV function and CO.

Intraaortic balloon counterpulsation: Used to sustain severely depressed ventricular function by decreasing afterload and increasing coronary artery perfusion.

Cardiac monitoring: Used to determine presence of atrial or ventricular dysrhythmias or conduction defects and to assess effectiveness of antiarrhythmic agents.

Cardioversion: Used in treatment of atrial fibrillation with rapid ventricular response.

DRUG THERAPY

Dilated cardiomyopathy: Pharmacologic interventions directed largely by symptoms, to maximize cardiac function; as with any patient in congestive heart failure, digitalis, diuretic, and vasodilator therapy used; antiarrhythmics used to treat dysrhythmias.

Hypertrophic cardiomyopathy: Goals of drug therapy are to decrease ventricular contractility and increase ventricular volume and LV outflow.

Cardiac glycosides—Digitalis: Not favored in management of hypertrophic cardiomyopathy because it increases contractility and therefore degree of obstruction; used in presence of atrial fibrillation with rapid ventricular rates or LV dysfunction without obstruction.

Beta-adrenergic blocking agents—Propranolol (Inderal): Indications: principal mode of therapy; has negative inotropic effects on myocardial contractility and thus is believed to prevent increase in outflow obstruction, decrease myocardial oxygen consumption, and exert antiarrhythmic actions.

Calcium antagonists—Verapamil (Calan): Indications: decreases LV contractility which then reduces outflow tract obstruction; reduces symptoms; increases exercise tolerance; Nifedipine (corcard)—improves LV relaxation and filling; may provide symptomatic relief for chest pain.

Antiarrhythmic drugs—Amiodarone: Indications: supraventricular and ventricular dysrhythmias; for symptomatic relief and increased exercise tolerance.

Restrictive cardiomyopathy: Pharmacologic agents directed by underlying disorders; digitalis and diuretics often employed to treat dysrhythmias and signs of failure, but their effectiveness is limited.

SURGERY

Myotomy-myectomy: for patient with HCM who has intractable symptoms and severe obstruction; hypertrophied septum is excised, which diminishes left ventricular gradient and mitral regurgitation; procedure improves symptoms but has not been reported to prolong life.

Excision of fibrotic endocardium: Successful in limited number of cases of restrictive cardiomyopathy; procedure apparently decreases ventricular filling pressures and increases CO.

Cardiac transplantation: Increasingly becoming surgical intervention for patients with dilated cardiomyopathy that is refractory to medical therapy.

Other surgical interventions: Valve replacement is considered in individual cases, but is generally not favored.

1 ASSESS

ASSESSMENT	OBSERVATIONS		
	HYPERTROPHIC CARDIOMYOPATHY	DILATED CARDIOMYOPATHY	RESTRICTIVE CARDIOMYPATHY
General complaints	Dyspnea; SOB; angina pectoris; fatigue; palpitations; syncope (may be exertional)	Dyspnea; fatigue; complaints associated with biventricular failure; chest pain	Dyspnea; fatigue; exercise intolerance; complaints associated with RV failure
Arterial pressure		Normal or low systolic; narrowed pulse pressure	Narrowed pulse pressure
Arterial pulse	Brisk carotid upstroke followed by decline in midsystole; pulsus bisferiens	Low amplitude and volume; pulsus alternans	
Jugular venous pressure	Dominant a wave	Distended; prominent a and v waves	Distended
Palpation	Apical and LSB systolic thrill and heave, does not radiate	Apical impulse displaced laterally; parasternal impulses and heaves; pulsatile liver	Apical impulse difficult to palpate; pulsatile liver
Auscultation	Systolic murmur at lower LSB increasing in intensity with Valsalva maneuver; S_4 gallop	Murmurs of mitral and tricuspid regurgitation; S_3 and S_4 gallops; pulmonary crackles (rales)	Murmurs of mitral regurgitation; S_3 and S_4 gallops; heart sounds distant
Hemodynamic parameters			
RAP	Slightly increased	Increased	Increased
PAP	Increased	Increased	Increased
PCWP	Increased	Increased	Increased
SVR	Increased	Increased	Increased
CO/CI	Normal; may be decreased in patients with severe gradients	Decreased	Decreased

➜ ❯ ❯ ❯

2 DIAGNOSE

NURSING DIAGNOSIS	SUBJECTIVE FINDINGS	OBJECTIVE FINDINGS
Decreased cardiac output related to mechanical factors (preload, afterload, or contractility)	Complains of fatigue, DOE, chest pain, syncope, SOB	Restlessness Skin: cool, clammy, cyanosis; jugular venous distention; dependent edema; decreased peripheral pulses; tachypnea, tachycardia Breath sounds: crackles, wheezes Heart sounds: murmurs, S_3, S_4, summation gallop
Fluid volume excess related to increased levels of aldosterone, sodium retention, and antidiuretic hormone	Complains of SOB, weight gain	Bounding pulse, tachypnea, jugular venous distention, dependent edema Breath sounds: crackles, wheezes Heart sounds: S_3
Activity intolerance related to diminished cardiac reserve	Complains of fatigue, weakness, SOB, activity intolerance, DOE, chest pain	Response to activity: exertional tachycardia, tachypnea, hypotension, irregular heart rhythm; ECG: dysrhythmias during or following activity
Ineffective individual coping related to inability to deal with multiple stressors (anxiety, fear of death, sense of helplessness) and progressive deterioration with health status	Verbalizes feelings of helplessness, apathy, preoccupation with self	Physical signs and symptoms— tachycardia, anorexia Emotional and cognitive—depression, tearful, inaccurate appraisal of situation, inability to meet role expectations, inability to problem solve, inappropriate use of defense mechanisms, social withdrawal

Other related nursing diagnoses

Impaired gas exchange related to alveolar-capillary membrane changes due to increased pulmonary capillary pressure

Altered nutrition: less than body requirements related to impaired absorption of nutrients

Pain (chest) related to low cardiac output (HCM)

3 PLAN

Patient goals

1. Patient will demonstrate improved cardiac output.
2. Patient will demonstrate normovolemic balance (dilated cardiomyopathy).
3. Patient will demonstrate understanding of factors that cause activity intolerance and progress toward optimum levels of activity for age and physiologic limitations.
4. Patient will demonstrate awareness and realistic perception of stressors and develop adaptive long-term coping responses that reduce stress.
5. Patient will demonstrate increased knowledge regarding cardiomyopathy and the effect on his or her life-style.

4 IMPLEMENT

NURSING DIAGNOSIS	NURSING INTERVENTIONS	RATIONALE
Decreased cardiac output related to mechanical factors (preload, afterload, or contractility)	Assess and monitor for signs and symptoms indicating reduced CO.	To detect early and/or progressive signs of diminished CO.
	Encourage bed rest during acute phase. Limit self-care activities as indicated.	To conserve energy and decrease oxygen demand.
	HCM: avoid activities that elicit Valsalva maneuvers.	Valsalva manuevers increase MV_{O_2} and in presence of outflow obstruction, the heart may be unable to respond and CO drops.
	Monitor arterial pressure, RAP, PAP, PCWP, CO/CI q 2-4 h as indicated.	To determine degree of failure and to assess response to unloading therapy.
	Observe for and record dysrhythmias q 4 -8 h as indicated.	Presence of uncontrollable dysrhythmias can lead to further reduction in CO.
	Administer medications as ordered: unloading agents and inotropic agents	To improve ejection, reduce preload, and improve contractility.
	Administer calcium antagonists as ordered.	To decrease LV outflow obstruction and increase LV compliance, thus improving ventricular filling.
	HCM: Avoid use of nitrates, beta adrenergics, and cardiac glycosides.	Vasodilators and positive inotropic agents increase contractility and thus increase the obstruction.
	Monitor intake and output q 4 to 8 h limiting IV and PO fluids as indicated.	To assess response to therapy and to assess degree of circulating volume.
	Convalescent care Progressively increase activity level as indicated by improvement in clinical status.	Gradual increase in activities will minimize sudden, excessive increase in myocardial oxygen workload and demand.
	Monitor vital signs and report any changes in HR or BP.	Changes in HR or BP are early indicators of myocardial oxygen deprivation; any changes may require changes in medication or modification of activities.
	HCM: Instruct patient to avoid strenuous exercise and to avoid competitive sports. Refer family for instruction in CPR.	The high mortality rate associated with HCM is attributed to sudden unexpected death.

→ 〉 〉

NURSING DIAGNOSIS	NURSING INTERVENTIONS	RATIONALE

Fluid volume excess related to increased levels of aldosterone, sodium retention, and antidiuretic hormone	Assess and monitor the following:
	  Increase in jugular venous distention.
	  Intake and output; report output of <30 ml/m or intake > output on daily basis.
	  Auscultate heart sounds (S_3, S_4) and lung sounds q 4-8 h.
	  Monitor and obtain RAP, PAP, and PCWP as indicated.
		To detect signs of fluid retention, increased congestion, and/or response to therapy.

	Weigh daily using same amount of clothing and same time of day.	To determine response to therapy and/or continued fluid retention. Daily weight fluctuations are often due to water loss or gain.
	Administer medications as ordered— diuretics and positive inotropic agents (except for HCM).	To decrease circulating volume.
	Monitor serum electrolytes, especially sodium and potassium.	Potassium is lost with loop diuretics, and hypokalemia results in ventricular ectopy.
	Restrict sodium and fluid intake as indicated.	To control sodium resorption and fluid retention due to excessive aldosterone secretion.
Activity intolerance related to diminished cardiac reserve	Assess and monitor patient's tolerance to activities, noting which activities are aggravating factors.	Dysfunctional myocardium may be unable to meet MV_{O2} demand and therefore activities should be evaluated and/or modified.
	Check BP, HR, and respiration before and after activity.	To observe for orthostatic changes associated with prolonged rest and to identify signs of unmet oxygen demand.

	Coordinate care to promote rest:
	  Provide scheduled periods of rest and sleep.
	  Coordinate treatment activities so as to not interfere with scheduled rest periods.
		To ensure periods of complete and uninterrupted rest, which helps to restore physical and psychologic well-being.

	Increase activities gradually; assist as needed. Instruct patient to perform activity at own rate. Monitor vital signs before, during, and after activity.	To permit neurovascular compensatory adjustment to increased demands. Activity should be discontinued if symptoms appear (e.g., chest pain, dyspnea, cyanosis, dizziness, hypotension, sustained tachycardia).
	Instruct patient in energy conservation methods: schedule regular rest periods during day, and prior to engaging in new or strenuous activities; rest after meals; where possible, sit to perform task; stop task or activity if signs of cardiac hypoxia are present (rapid pulse, fatigue, DOE, SOB, chest pain).	To limit or reduce energy expenditure, thereby avoiding increases in myocardial oxygen demand.

NURSING DIAGNOSIS	NURSING INTERVENTIONS	RATIONALE
Ineffective individual coping related to inability to deal with multiple stressors (anxiety, fear of death, sense of helplessness) and progressive deterioration of health status	Assess patient's cognitive appraisal of illness and factors that may be contributing to patient's inability to cope. Determine baseline knowledge of disease, current events, and future outcome.	Primary appraisal of threat, which involves how threat is perceived and interpreted, may be further influenced by past experiences, level of understanding, previous coping mechanisms in dealing with stressful events, inner belief or strength to deal with situation; type/amount of supportive resources, (e.g., family or financial).
	Provide factual information about disease treatments and future health status.	To clarify any misinformation or confusion.
	Provide time to listen to patient's feelings; encourage expression of feelings of hopelessness and fears.	Listening will assist in providing insight to patient's perception of threat, will identify any misconceptions, and will provide patient with feelings that staff cares about what is happening and a sense of comfort.
	Encourage and assist patient to participate in decision-making process with regard to adjustments in life-style.	Helps patient to regain a sense of power and control in self care and in routines of daily living.
	Assist patient to develop appropriate coping strategies that are based on personal strengths, previous positive experiences in dealing with stress, and situational supports.	To enhance patient's perception of his/her strengths that can help in maintaining hope.
	Offer assistance in exploring alternative strategies that enhance coping skills: role playing, rehearsal to practice new approaches to problems, giving positive reinforcement.	To develop new coping skills.
	Refer to support groups and/or counseling as indicated.	Support groups provide patient with feeling of being less alone and isolated.
Knowledge deficit	See Patient Teaching.	

5 EVALUATE

PATIENT OUTCOME	DATA INDICATING THAT OUTCOME IS REACHED
Ventricular function is improved or maintained: **Hypertrophic—** outflow obstruction is decreased. **Dilated—LVEDP is decreased; ventricular contractility is improved.**	CO and LVEDP are within acceptable limits; fatigue, dyspnea, and angina are relieved. LVEDP is decreased; stroke volume is improved; patient loses weight; dyspnea and SOB are relieved.

→ ⟩ ⟩ ⟩

PATIENT OUTCOME	DATA INDICATING THAT OUTCOME IS REACHED
Patient exhibits cardiac tolerance to ADLs and to increasing levels of activity.	Patient is normotensive. HR is within 10-20 bpm of resting rate. Patient denies symptoms of activity intolerance.
Patient copes effectively with diagnosis.	Patient verbalizes less threatening appraisal of situation and verbalizes feelings openly. Patient is able to identify different measures to use in dealing with threatening events; appears comfortable.
Patient's knowledge level is increased.	Patient verbalizes signs and symptoms to report to physician and reports appropriate changes in life-style.

PATIENT TEACHING

1. Describe the nature and type of cardiomyopathy.
2. Explain the limitations of the disease on life-style and the prognosis.
3. Explain the signs and symptoms to report to the physician.
4. Describe activity allowances and limitations. Explain the importance of avoiding isometric exercises; of resting when feeling tired; need to rest before and after heavy tasks; rest after meals; and need to avoid extreme temperatures. For patients with HCM, explain importance of avoiding all isometric or strenuous exercises and competitive sports. Examples include jogging, football, and soccer.
5. Explain dietary and fluid restrictions.
6. Explain the name, purpose, dosage, and side effects of prescribed medications; warn against the effects of abruptly stopping propranolol.
7. Explain the need for daily weights when ordered and to report increase of more than 2 pounds in 24-hour period.
8. Provide opportunity for family members to learn CPR.
9. Review importance of follow-up appointments.

Congestive Heart Failure

Congestive heart failure is a complex clinical syndrome that results from the heart's inability to increase cardiac output sufficiently to meet the body's metabolic demands.

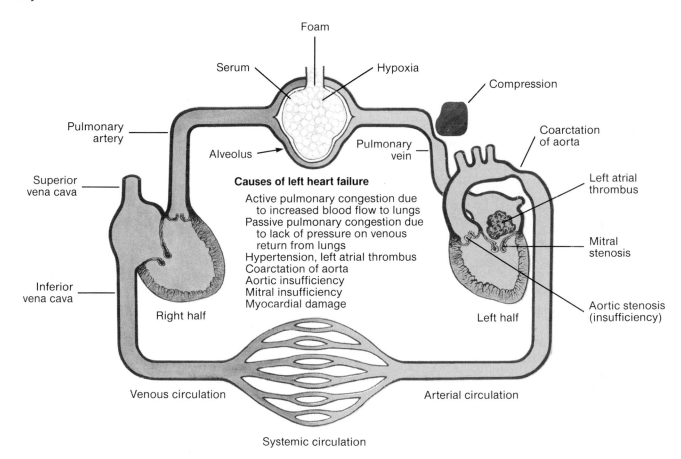

Causes of left heart failure

Active pulmonary congestion due to increased blood flow to lungs
Passive pulmonary congestion due to lack of pressure on venous return from lungs
Hypertension, left atrial thrombus
Coarctation of aorta
Aortic insufficiency
Mitral insufficiency
Myocardial damage

EPIDEMIOLOGY

Congestive heart failure (CHF) occurs as a result of damage to the myocardium. It is estimated that as many as 2 million Americans suffer from CHF and that up to 29,000 die annually from this chronic disorder.[2]

ETIOLOGY

The underlying causes of heart failure vary, but ultimately, the disorder results in the heart's inability to act as an effective pump.

Decreased myocardial contractility can result from a primary disorder or from conditions that place an excessive volume or pressure workload on the heart.

There are a number of conditions that cause pri-mary myocardial disorders and disorders that increase the heart's workload.

In addition, there are filling disorders that interfere with the heart's ability to pump blood effectively and cause a drop in cardiac output. Examples are cardiac tamponade and restrictive percarditis.

Persistent tachyarrhythmias also can reduce ventricular filling time, and marked bradyarrhythmias significantly reduce cardiac output because the ventricles cannot augment the stroke volume.

Loss of coordinated atrial contraction, as occurs in atrial fibrillation, can decrease cardiac output, presumably because of loss and the atrial "booster pump" that contributes to normal ventricular filling.

DISORDERS/CONDITIONS THAT CAN LEAD TO CONGESTIVE HEART FAILURE

Causes of decreased myocardial contractility

Coronary artery disease
Myocarditis
Cardiomyopathies
  Congestive
  Restrictive
  Hypertrophic
Infiltrative diseases
  Amyloidosis
  Tumors
  Sarcoidosis
Collagen-vascular diseases
  Systemic lupus erythematosus
  Scleroderma
Iatrogenic factors
  Drugs such as β-blockers; calcium antagonists

Causes of increased myocardial workload

Hypertension
Pulmonary hypertension
Valvular heart disease
  Aortic or pulmonic stenosis
  Mitral, tricuspid, or aortic insufficiency
Hypertrophic cardiomyopathy
Intracardiac shunting
High-output states
  Anemia
  Hyperthyroidism
  Beri-beri
  Arteriovenous fistula

PATHOPHYSIOLOGY

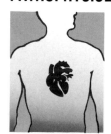

Despite the cause, the primary dysfunction in CHF remains the same: the inability of the heart to function as a pump. However, changes in the basic physiologic mechanisms of preload, afterload, and stroke volume contribute to the pathophysiologic state of heart failure.

As a result of impaired cardiac function, failure to empty venous reservoirs and reduced delivery of blood into the arterial circulation lead to increased ventricular pressures, elevated systemic and pulmonary pressures, and decreased cardiac output. Furthermore, a series of compensatory mechanisms are activated.

Activation of the sympathetic nervous system. Increased sympathetic activity represents the earliest response to decreased cardiac output and blood pressure. Stimulation of beta-adrenergic receptors results in an increase in the heart rate, stroke volume, and cardiac output. Sympathetic stimulation acts on peripheral vascular resistance. This increases venous tone by increasing systemic vascular resistance to improve venous return, which enhances ventricular filling.

Renal compensation is another mechanism activated by the drop in cardiac output and perfusion pressure. Sympathetic activity restricts renal blood flow. This in turn reduces glomerular filtration rate and triggers the renin-angiotension mechanism, leading to increased aldosterone production and tubular resorption of salt and water. **Ventricular hypertrophy** occurs in response to increased pressure workloads by increasing the wall thickness of the ventricles. The muscle mass increases in a concentric manner, with little or no change in chamber size. Clinical manifestations of heart failure can be divided into left- and right-sided failure; they can occur independently or in combination.

Left-Sided Heart Failure

Any sustained elevation in left ventricular end-diastolic pressure (LVEDP) increases left atrial pressure, which is transmitted to the pulmonary vascular bed. Clinically, this is reflected by an increase in pulmonary capillary wedge pressure (PCWP). Should this pressure exceed the colloid osmotic pressure of the pulmonary capillaries (30 mm Hg), fluid will leak into the pulmonary interstitial spaces (Figures 4-23 and 4-24). This leads to hypoxia resulting from poor oxygen exchange and clinically to dyspnea, cough orthopnea, and paroxysmal nocturnal dyspnea.

Right-Sided Heart Failure

Persistent elevation of LVEDP eventually leads to right-sided failure characterized by venous congestion in the systemic circulation. Right-sided heart failure may also occur as a primary disorder of the right ventricle as seen in tricuspid regurgitation, in right ventricular infarction, or as a result of pulmonary disease such as cor pulmonale. Clinically, distended neck veins, hepatomegaly, and dependent edema occur.

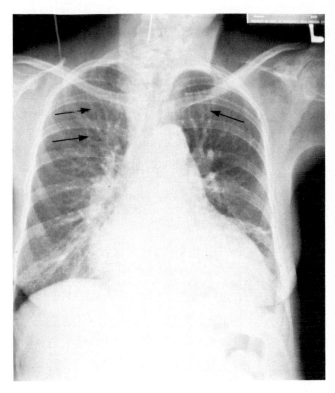

FIGURE 4-23
Pulmonary congestion. Arrows indicate upper lobe distention.
No enlarged cardiac silhouette.

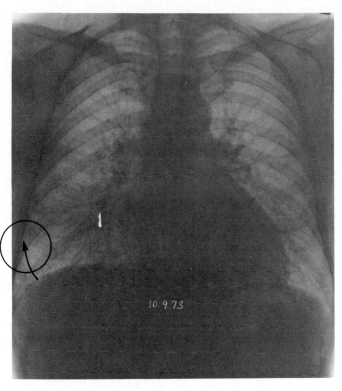

FIGURE 4-24
Interstitial edema. Hilar areas are blurred and hazy. Kerley-B
lines are indicated by arrows. Cardiac silhouette is enlarged.

DIAGNOSTIC STUDIES AND FINDINGS

Diagnostic test	Findings
Laboratory tests	
Electrolytes	Hyponatremia (dilutional) owing to water retention; urinary sodium loss in response to diuretics; hypokalemia as consequence of excessive use of diuretics or as secondary manifestation of aldosteronism; hypochloremia as result of diuretic therapy; metabolic acidosis or alkalosis
Blood chemistry	BUN, creatinine rise with decreased glomerular filtration; liver function values (SGOT, bilirubin, alkaline phosphatase) mildly increased; prothrombin time prolonged; glucose level elevated
Arterial blood gases	Hypoxemia; decreased oxygen saturation; (early) mild respiratory alkalosis; (late) hypercarbia, hypoxia
Urine studies	Urine output decreased; metabolic acidosis or alkalosis; specific gravity > 1.010 (with excessive fluid intake); < 1.035 (with decreased fluid intake); proteinuria; glucosuria
Pulmonary function tests	Reduced vital capacity; reduced total lung capacity; increased residual volume

Diagnostic study	Findings
Chest x-ray (Figures 4-23 and 4-24)	Increased pulmonary congestion: redistribution of pulmonary blood flow, interstitial edema (intraseptal edema—Kerley-B lines; perivascular edema), alveolar edema, pleural effusion; (early) little or no change in size or contour of cardiac silhouette; (late) increased cardiothoracic ratio
ECG	LV hypertrophy, RV hypertrophy, atrial hypertrophy, tachycardia, dysrhythmias
Radionuclide angiography (scintigraphy)	Estimates wall motion and shows areas of decreased myocardial perfusion. LV ejection fraction of < 30 mm is prognostic of high mortality
Echocardiogram	LV failure: increased LVEDP (> 5.6 cm), decreased wall motion
Hemodynamic monitoring (right heart catheterization)	LV failure: elevated PCWP and pulmonary artery diastolic pressure (PADP), decreased CO, decreased ejection fractions; RV failure: elevated PAP, RV pressure, and right atrial pressure (RAP)

MEDICAL MANAGEMENT

GENERAL MANAGEMENT

Physical activity: Bed rest with head of bed elevated to 45° to reduce myocardial oxygen demand and decrease circulating volume returning to heart.

Diet: Sodium restricted diet: 4 g diet means "No added salt"; 2 g diet eliminates all salt from cooking. Weigh daily to monitor fluid retention.

Oxygen therapy: Initiated if patient is hypoxic.

Other: Rotating tourniquets may be used for rapid reduction of circulating blood volume.

Hemodynamic monitoring (PAP, PCWP, SVR, CO/CI): Direct means of assessing hemodynamic status of heart and effectiveness of treatment; also assists in directing therapy.

Cardiac monitoring: Used to assess for drug-induced dysrhythmias and for dysrhythmias induced by an underlying disorder.

Intra-aortic balloon pump (IABP): Counterpulsation device that assists failing heart by decreasing afterload and increasing coronary artery perfusion.

Ventricular assist devices (VAD) (Right or left): Mechanical device that decreases the work of the myocardium while maintaining systemic pressure. Positioned outside the body or implanted into the abdomen, VAD works as an artificial pump to maintain circulation so the heart can rest and recover.

MEDICAL MANAGEMENT—cont'd

DRUG THERAPY

Diuretics: Furosemide (Lasix); Ethacrynic acid (Edecrin); Thiazides

Vasodilators

Nitrates: Nitroprusside sodium (Nipride); Isosorbide dinitrate (Isordil); Nifedipine (Procardia, Adalat)

Antihypertensives (for vasodilator effect):   Hydralazine (Apresoline)

Beta-adrenergic blocking agents: Prazosin (Minipress); Phentolamine (Regitine)

Angiotensin-converting enzyme (ACE) inhibitors: Captopril (Capoten)

Morphine sulfate

Inotropic agents:
   Cardiac glycosides—Digitalis*
   Adrenergic drugs—Dopamine (Intropin)
   Dobutamine (Dobutrex); Milrinone (Amrinone)

SURGERY

Directed by underlying condition; mortality is greater among patients with LV dysfunction.
Cardiac transplantation may be considered.

*NOTE: Commonly used but use is limited because toxic effects occur when blood levels exceed 2 ng/ml—more likely in patients who are small, elderly, or who have chronic obstructive pulmonary disease.

1 ASSESS

ASSESSMENT	OBSERVATIONS	
	LEFT-SIDED FAILURE	RIGHT-SIDED FAILURE
General complaints	Dyspnea, orthopnea, PND, fatigue, restlessness, insomnia, anorexia	Fatigue, anorexia, nausea, vomiting
Skin	Pallor, diaphoresis	Diaphoresis
Cardiovascular system	Left ventricular S_3 Systolic murmur at apex Precordial movement—displaced apical impulse and palpable thrills Tachycardia; pulsus alternans	Right ventricular S_3 (heart beat at lower LSB) Systolic murmur Precordial movement—RV impulse along LSB or xiphoid Hepatojugular reflex Elevated JVP (rise in "a" and "v" waves)

→ › ›

	OBSERVATIONS	
ASSESSMENT	LEFT-SIDED FAILURE	RIGHT-SIDED FAILURE
Hemodynamic parameters	Increased PCWP, PAP	Increased RAP
Pulmonary system	Crackles Rapid labored respiration Cough Frothy or blood-tinged sputum	
Gastrointestinal system		Weight gain Abdominal distention RUQ pain, Ascites Hepatomegaly Splenomegaly
Peripheral vascular system		Dilation of peripheral veins Edema (firm, pitting) in peripheral extremities, sacrum, and genitalia

2 DIAGNOSE

NURSING DIAGNOSIS	SUBJECTIVE FINDINGS	OBJECTIVE FINDINGS
Decreased cardiac output related to mechanical factors (preload, afterload, contractility)	Complains of fatigue, weakness, effort intolerance, breathlessness, and altered mental status	Tachycardia, pulsus alternans, weak thready pulse, decreased peripheral pulses, hypotension, narrowed pulse pressure, pallor, diaphoresis, cool skin, cyanosis, decreased urine output (<30 ml/h) Increased PCWP, SVR; decreased CO/CI Breath sounds: crackles, wheezes
Fluid volume excess related to increased levels of aldosterone, sodium retention, and antidiuretic hormone (ADH) secondary to reduced glomerular filtration rate	Patient complains of SOB, weight gain	Weight gain, peripheral edema, anasarca Breath sounds: crackles, wheezes Tachypnea, jugular venous distention, Positive hepatojugular reflux Changes in mental status Heart sounds: S_3

NURSING DIAGNOSIS	SUBJECTIVE FINDINGS	OBJECTIVE FINDINGS
Impaired gas exchange related to alveolar-capillary membrane changes due to increased pulmonary capillary pressure	Patient complains of SOB, DOE, hoarseness Cough: moist Apprehension	Restlessness, confusion Orthopnea, tachypnea: shallow Breath sounds: crackles in independent parts of lung or extending upward toward apex Pallor, diaphoresis, cyanosis Sputum is pink, frothy Blood gases: hypocapnea ($\downarrow$ Pa_{CO_2}), hypoxia ($\downarrow$ Pa_{O_2}), respiratory alkalosis Chest x-ray: Bilateral interstitial and/or alveolar infiltrates, Kerley-B lines PCWP: 14-20 mm Hg—mild 25-30 mm Hg—severe
Activity intolerance related to weakness secondary to decreased CO	Patient complains of progressive decrease in ability to perform ADLs Fatigue, generalized weakness	Response to activity: exertional dyspnea, tachypnea, tachycardia, irregular heart rate, hypotension ECG: dysrhythmias during or following activities
Altered nutrition: less than body requirements related to impaired absorption of nutrients due to decreased CO	Patient complains of anorexia, nausea, increased fatigue, muscle weakness	Dry body weight <20% of ideal weight for age, height, and body size; decreased triceps skinfold measurements; wasted appearance Serum albumin: <3.5 mg/dl Transferrin level: <200 m/dl Lymphocyte count: <20% of WBC Mouth: stomatitis; tongue swollen, beefy red; gums spongy, bleed easily Skeletal: ribs, scapula, legs are thin, despite a swollen or enlarged abdomen
Impaired skin integrity related to impaired circulation and metabolic state	Patient complains of pain or discomfort over pressure areas	Skin (dependent areas and bony prominences): edema, redness, irritation, excoriation

Other related nursing diagnoses

Ineffective individual coping and **ineffective family coping** related to changes in self-concept, role performance, or powerlessness
Self-care deficit related to debilitated state
Noncompliance (medications, diet therapy) related to ineffective coping

3 PLAN

Patient goals

1. Patient will demonstrate improved cardiac output.
2. Patient will achieve a normovolemic balance.
3. Patient will demonstrate improved gas exchange.
4. Patient will demonstrate improved tolerance to increased levels of activity.
5. Patient will achieve and maintain adequate nutritional intake.
6. Patient will maintain skin integrity.
7. Patient will demonstrate increased level of knowledge.

→ > >

4 IMPLEMENT

NURSING DIAGNOSIS	NURSING INTERVENTIONS	RATIONALE
Decreased cardiac output related to mechanical factors (preload, afterload, contractility)	Assess and monitor BP, apical pulse, HR and respirations, heart and lung sounds, level of consciousness q 4 h or as needed.	To detect early signs and symptoms of decreased CO, and/or to detect signs of disease progression or improvement.
	Maintain bed rest as indicated by condition; elevate head of bed to 30°-60°, have patient lean forward on padded over-bed table; administer oxygen as ordered.	To conserve energy and decrease cardiac workload by decreasing oxygen demand; to facilitate ventilation and decrease workload of breathing.
	Monitor hemodynamic parameters: BP, arterial pressures, PAP, PCWP, CO/CI, SVR.	To evaluate preload and afterload parameters and/or to assess response to therapy.
	Administer drug therapy as ordered— vasodilators, inotropic agents, angiotensin inhibitors. Monitor for signs of drug toxicity.	Vasodilators decrease preload and afterload, inotropic agents improve myocardial contractility, and angiotensin inhibitors decrease SVR.
	Restrict activities as indicated by condition; implement measures that promote rest, such as spacing procedures and treatments so that patient can rest between activities.	To avoid fatigue, which increases oxygen demand.
Fluid volume excess related to increased levels of aldosterone, sodium retention, and antidiuretic hormone secondary to reduce renal blood flow	Assess and monitor the following: Increase or decrease in jugular venous distention; intake and output—report output of <30 ml/h or intake > output on daily basis. Auscultate heart (S_3, S_4) and lung sounds q 4-8 h. Weigh patient daily; report increase >1-2 kg/day (2.2 lbs).	To detect signs of fluid retention, increased congestion, and/or response to therapy. Daily weight fluctuations are often due to water loss or gain. One kg of body weight reflects one L of fluid, indicating need for additional diuretics.
	Maintain patient on IV.	To access vein for emergency drug administration.
	Administer medications as ordered: Rapid-acting diuretics Positive inotropic and arterial dilators	Diuretics decrease circulating volume; inotropic agents improve renal blood flow.
	Restrict dietary sodium intake and fluid intake.	To control sodium resorption and fluid retention due to excessive aldosterone secretion.
	Monitor electrolytes daily, especially sodium and potassium.	Low serum sodium needs to be evaluated to determine if hyponatremia is dilutional due to excessive water retention, thus masking real total body excess of sodium vs true low sodium concentration. Because potassium is lost with loop diuretics, hypokalemia may occur, resulting in ventricular ectopy, particularly if patient is also on digitalis.

NURSING DIAGNOSIS	NURSING INTERVENTIONS	RATIONALE
Impaired gas exchange related to alveolar-capillary membrane changes due to increased pulmonary capillary pressure	Assess and monitor for changes in respiratory function.	To detect signs and symptoms of impaired ventilation and perfusion.
	Monitor serial arterial blood gases.	To identify hypoxemia, hypercapnia, and to determine need for assisted ventilation.
	Auscultate lung sounds q 4 h.	To detect increases in congestion and determine adequacy of ventilatory effort.
	Monitor chest x-rays.	To identify changes reflecting increased or resolution of pulmonary congestion.
	Monitor hemodynamic parameters: PAP, PCWP as indicated.	Pressure values are indicators of degree of pulmonary congestion.
	Elevate head of bed; have patient lead forward on padded over-bed table; reposition q 2-4 h as indicated by condition.	To decrease work of breathing and enhance ventilation and gas exchange particularly to lower lung area.
	Administer oxygen therapy as ordered, via nasal prongs, mask, or positive-pressure device. Prepare for intubation and assisted mechanical ventilation if required.	To increase arterial oxygenation (Pa_{O_2}); to correct hypoxemia and hypercapnia.
	Provide humidified inspired air as ordered.	To liquefy secretions.
	Instruct patient to cough and deep breathe.	To facilitate ventilation and remove pulmonary secretions.
	Administer medications as ordered: Morphine, rapid-acting diuretics	Morphine decreases pulmonary vascular congestion due to transient arterial or venous dilation and decreases anxiety. Diuretics decrease pulmonary congestion by reducing circulating blood volume.
	Instruct patient to avoid smoking or use of tobacco products.	Nicotine is a cardiac stimulant, which causes vasoconstriction and reduces oxygen availability.
	Provide brief explanations for all treatments and procedures.	To prevent hyperventilation resulting from fear or anxiety.
Activity intolerance related to weakness secondary to decreased CO	Assess and monitor for signs of activity intolerance.	In the setting of compromised myocardium, the heart is unable to effectively increase stroke volume in response to increased demands, which contributes to increased weakness and fatigue.
	Check BP, HR, and respiration before and after activity.	Orthostatic hypotension can result from prolonged period of bedrest.
	Maintain on bed rest or on chair-rest with feet elevated as indicated.	Patient may find confinement to bed rest more fatiguing.

➔ ❯ ❯

NURSING DIAGNOSIS	NURSING INTERVENTIONS	RATIONALE
	Identify factors known to cause fatigue, restrict and/or limit as indicated, e.g., number of visitors and their length of stay.	To promote energy conservation.
	Space treatments and procedures to allow for periods of uninterrupted rest; provide periods of rest throughout day and evening.	To ensure periods of complete rest.

	Implement measures that will improve activity tolerance by minimizing fatigue:
	  Bathing—shower with chair vs self-bath
	  Toileting—bedside commode vs bedpan or urinal
	  Up in chair with legs elevated vs complete bedrest
		To limit or reduce energy expenditure.

	Increase activity level as indicated by condition; assess activity tolerance and activity progression.	To evaluate improved myocardial performance.
Altered nutrition: less than body requirements related to impaired absorption of nutrients due to decreased CO	Observe patient daily for signs of malnutrition and cardiac cachexia.	Nutritional deficits occur as result of (1) body's inability to absorb nutrients because of poor tissue perfusion, and (2) hypermetabolic state that occurs in heart failure—patient's intake and malabsorption are unable to meet increased demand.
	Evaluate laboratory data.	Malnutrition and protein depletion are reflected as low levels of serum transferrin and lymphocytes.
	Determine patient's baseline weight. Weigh daily: upon rising, after voiding, with same clothing.	To assess actual weight loss and to obtain consistent and accurate body weight, which will assist in determining caloric needs.
	Maintain diet as ordered; consult with dietitian as indicated.	To ensure that diet will meet required caloric needs.
	Supplement meals with high caloric feedings.	To maintain minimum required caloric intake.
	Carry out measures to improve appetite.	Controlling/promoting environment and psychosocial factors enhances appetite.
	Offer small frequent meals.	Enlarged liver, ascites, GI hypomotility, and delayed gastric emptying can contribute to feeling of fullness as well as nausea and vomiting.
	Permit patient to choose foods. Where possible, encourage family to bring food from home and assist with feedings.	Psychosocial support is enhanced by encouraged participation in meals and by providing involvement by support systems.

NURSING DIAGNOSIS	NURSING INTERVENTIONS	RATIONALE
	Remove unsightful and odorous items from room during mealtime.	To reduce noxious stimuli, which may contribute to nausea.
	Arrange medication schedule so it does not interfere with meals.	Side effects of certain medications may contribute to loss of appetite, e.g., bitter taste of medication, dry mouth.
	Administer antiemetics/analgesics before meals.	To ensure patient comfort and improve appetite.
Impaired skin integrity related to impaired circulation and metabolic state	Assess skin integrity daily, noting color, texture, and temperature.	Chronic malnutrition state interferes with normal tissue integrity and wound healing, which results in loss of subcutaneous tissue and muscle mass.
	Initiate measures to maintain skin integrity. If *on bed rest:* turn and reposition q 2-4 h; use all 4 sides. Use pull sheet to lift or move patient. Keep linens clean and wrinkle free. Provide alternative preventive measures for patients on prolonged bedrest: air pressure beds, alternating pressure mattresses, sheepskin, heel guards.	To relieve pressure areas and to improve circulation and joint mobility. To prevent friction and injury to epidermis as patient slides up in bed. To prevent skin breakdown and enhance circulation.
	Encourage ambulation; have patient sit in chair limiting time to <2 h. Administer skin care daily; massage bony and/or pressure areas. NOTE: To avoid skin excoriations, do not massage reddened areas.	To promote circulation to all body parts. To increase tissue perfusion to affected areas.
	Keep skin clean and dry.	Moisture contributes to skin breakdown and infection.
	Initiate decubitus care at first signs of breakdown or ulceration.	Decubitus development is a rapid process.
Knowledge deficit	See Patient Teaching.	

5 EVALUATE

PATIENT OUTCOME	DATA INDICATING THAT OUTCOME IS REACHED
Ventricular function is improved.	HR and PCWP are decreased. CO is increased. Mental status is improved. Urine output is increased.
Fluid overload is decreased.	Patient verbalizes. He is able to perform ADLs without difficulties; ECG, BP, HR and respiratory rate within acceptable limits (HR within 20 bpm of resting rate) during activity.
Gas exchange is improved.	Lung sounds are clear. Anxiety level is diminished. Orthopnea and dyspnea are reduced. Hypoxemia and hypercarbia are absent. Respirations are improved.
Activity level is improved.	Patient verbalizes. He is able to perform ADL without difficulties; ECG, BP, HR and respiratory rate within acceptable limits (HR within 20 bpm of resting rate) during activity.

PATIENT OUTCOME	DATA INDICATING THAT OUTCOME IS REACHED
Nutritional status is improved.	Dry body weight normal or improved for age and body build. Improved appetite, good skin turgor, increased muscle mass, and improved energy.
Skin integrity is improved and/or maintained.	Skin: intact, warm, dry, signs of healing over areas of breakdown.
Patient's knowledge level is increased.	Patient verbalizes knowledge regarding importance of daily weight, taking prescribed medication, activity allowances and limitations, and dietary restrictions.

PATIENT TEACHING

Instruction is directed toward long-term maintenance of the therapeutic program.

1. Describe the disease process, the underlying cause, and any precipitating factors.
2. Instruct the patient to report symptoms of fluid retention and/or failure to physician: weight gain of >2 lb in 24 h, DOE, PND, and effort intolerance.
3. Instruct the patient to limit the intake of salt in diet and avoid foods that have a high sodium content, such as most canned foods, luncheon meats, "fast-foods" (i.e. hamburgers) cheeses; instruct the patient to read labels for sodium content before buying.

Provide information about alternative ways to season food. Refer to dietitian as necessary.

4. Instruct the patient to pace activities to avoid over-exertion and fatigue—to slowly increase and pace activities, to rest between periods of activity, and to use energy-saving techniques (e.g. sitting to brush hair and to prepare foods, and using a shower chair).
5. Teach the patient to weigh daily in the morning before the first meal with the same scale and wearing the same clothing, and to report weight gain of >2 lb in 24 h.
6. Teach the patient the name and method of administration of drugs and their potential side effects.

Shock

Shock is an abnormal physiologic state that is the first phase of the body's alarm reaction to an insult or injury that progresses to multiple organ system failure.

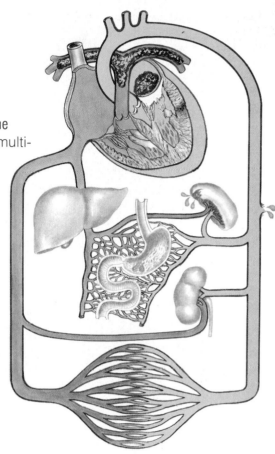

Primary insufficiency of cardiac output

A. Infarction
Myocarditis
Rupture of valve cusps
Rupture of chordae tendineae

B. Pericardial tamponade
Embolism
Obstruction by thrombus
Tachycardias
Dysrhythmias (severe)

Hypovolemia

A. Hemorrhagic loss of blood
Loss of plasma
Burns
Dehydration
Heat exhaustion

B. Severe infection
Anaphylaxis
Pain
Heat stroke

Most commonly shock occurs as an extreme pathophysiologic syndrome associated with abnormal cellular metabolism, which in most cases is due to inadequate tissue perfusion. If shock is untreated, progressive circulatory collapse and impaired cellular metabolism develop, leading eventually to death.

PATHOPHYSIOLOGY

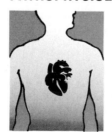

Various methods of identifying or classifying shock have been used. The following four categories based on etiology are commonly used in the clinical setting. These categories are (1) **hypovolemic** (including hemorrhage and dehydration); (2) **vasogenic,** including sepsis, anaphylaxis, and deep anesthesia effects; (3) **Cardiogenic,** including acute myocardial infarction and other cardiac-related etiologies; and (4) **Neurogenic.**

Hypovolemic Shock

Hypovolemic, or "cold", shock results from a decrease in intravascular volume and generally occurs when there is an associated deficit of at least 15% to 20% of the total blood volume. Hypovolemia is the most common cause of hypotension in critically ill patients, particularly in the postoperative phase.

Hypovolemic shock may be caused by excessive loss of plasma volume as occurs in burns or pancreatitis when extracellular fluid is sequestered in injured or inflamed tissue cells. Severe dehydration and hypovolemia may also be induced by diabetic ketoacidosis, excessive vomiting, or diarrhea. The most common cause of hypovolemic shock, however, is excessive loss of blood through trauma of a major blood vessel or vascular organ such as the kidney, spleen, or liver; through injury or disease of the gastrointestinal system such as rupture of esophageal varices; or through defects in vascular structures that lead to rupture as with aneurysms.

The severity of hypovolemic shock is related to the amount and rate of volume loss. If volume is replaced quickly, the shock state can be easily reversed, but if low aortic pressures persist longer than 60 minutes, the process may be irreversible.

The major hemodynamic changes initially associated with uncompensated fluid loss are low cardiac output, increased systemic vascular resistance, and decreased central venous pressure. Clinically the patient presents the classic symptoms of shock: cool clammy skin, increased heart and respiratory rates, and decreased urine output owing to compensatory vasoconstriction. The blood pressure may be normal or low, particularly in the early phase of "cold shock."

Vasogenic Shock

Unlike hypovolemic shock, which leads to vasoconstriction, vasogenic shock results in massive vasodilation from an increase in total vascular capacity. Circulating volume is lost because of venous pooling, increased capillary permeability, and third spacing of fluid. If intravascular volume is not replaced, hypovolemia will occur. Whereas a patient with hypovolemia has cold extremities as a result of vasoconstriction, a patient with vasogenic shock has warm extremities, giving rise to the term "warm shock." Warm shock is present in 30% to 50% of patients in the early phase of septic shock.

The most common form of vasogenic shock is sepsis, but it may also occur as a result of other factors, including anaphylactic reactions from drugs, insect stings, and food allergies.

Septic shock is commonly related to the release of bacterial endotoxins following a gram-negative bacterial infection. The organisms most frequently found in septic shock are the gram-negative bacteria *Escherichia coli, Klebsiella, Enterobacter, Pseudomonas, Serratia, Proteus,* and *Bacteroides fragilis;* the gram-positive bacteria *Staphylococcus, Pneumococcus,* and *alpha-* or *beta-Streptococcus;* and the fungus *Candida.* Many are part of the natural body flora or are common in the hospital environment. The microbes associated with the highest mortality are *Proteus, Pseudomonas, Candida,* and *B. fragilis.* Although patients in critical care units are the most vulnerable to hospital-acquired infections, a large subset of patients in general hospital units is also vulnerable. Patients particularly susceptible to septic shock are the elderly, immunosuppressed patients, patients who have indwelling catheters (urinary, intravenous, or intracardiac) or urinary tract infection, and patients who have undergone manipulative instrumentation or gastrointestinal or genitourinary surgical procedures.

Although deaths from septic shock have decreased since the 1960s, the mortality continues to be as high as 50%. This is due to several factors, the most striking of which are the changing pattern of microbial resistance to antimicrobial agents[15, 60] and the rapidly changing microbial profile.

Although the exact mechanism by which toxins produce septic shock is unclear, certain hemodynamic changes have been recognized. In early phases a hyperdynamic state exists in which the cardiac output, stroke volume, and heart rate are increased and the systemic vascular resistance and central venous pressure are decreased. The patient appears warm, dry, and flushed because of generalized vasodilation and venous pooling. This hyperdynamic state is probably due to the effects of various vasoactive substances released by the exotoxins or from the injured or infected tissue.

The circulatory changes combined with the decreased systemic vascular resistance may stimulate sympathetic response, causing the increased heart rate and maintenance of normal blood pressure that occurs during this "warm" shock phase.

If hyperdynamic shock is allowed to persist, the continued increase in capillary leaking will potentiate hypovolemia to the point that the process will convert to a hypodynamic phase known as the "cold" phase of septic shock. In this state the systemic vascular resistance increases, cardiac output drops, and the patient appears cold, pale, and clammy. The cause of this change is related to ineffective circulating blood volume, sympathetic vasoconstriction, and pump failure.[60]

In **anaphylactic reactions** from drugs, insect stings, or food allergies, the mechanism involved is an antibody-antigen interaction that provokes the release of chemical mediators such as histamine. These mediators act primarily on the vascular membranes and smooth muscles. Histamine release causes veins and arterioles to dilate, decreasing cardiac output and arterial pressure. In addition, histamine increases capillary permeability, causing fluid to escape from the intravascular compartment into the interstitial space. The result is volume depletion; however, while plasma water is removed from the capillaries, the red cells remain and the hemoglobin levels and hematocrit values rise. The immediate clinical reactions in anaphylaxis are pharyngeal and laryngeal edema, probably stemming from effects of histamines, and bronchoconstriction with the immediate threat of death from asphyxiation.

Deep anesthesia can cause severe depression of the vasomotor centers of the brain, which may result in vasomotor collapse and venous pooling. These in turn decrease venous return to the heart and diminish cardiac output.

Cardiogenic Shock

Cardiogenic shock occurs when the heart cannot maintain an adequate cardiac output to meet the body's metabolic demands.

The most common cause of cardiogenic shock is myocardial infarction, but it may be the result of a variety of cardiac disorders: acute myocardial infarction, end-stage cardiomyopathy (congestive, hypertrophic, or restrictive), valvular heart disease, cardiopulmonary bypass, and cardiac tamponade. The cardinal feature of cardiogenic shock is inadequate tissue perfusion and oxygen delivery resulting from a severely impaired ventricle.

Despite advances in pharmacology and hemodynamic monitoring, the incidence of cardiogenic shock resulting from myocardial infarction remains at 10% to 15%, with a mortality greater than 60%. Since the prognosis depends largely on the extent of myocardial damage, current therapies focus on early intervention to reduce ischemia and limit permanent myocardial damage.[13]

In patients with myocardial infarction, shock develops as a result of abnormal reflexes arising from the ischemic myocardium. The consequent inability to increase systemic vascular resistance makes it difficult to maintain an adequate arterial pressure. This leads to hypoperfusion of an already ischemic myocardium, producing further damage and further insufficiency of the pumping action of the left ventricle. Failure of the left ventricle to generate sufficient energy to pump blood into the systemic circulation further contributes to decreased coronary perfusion and decreased myocardial oxygen supply.

Cardiogenic shock has been correlated with destruction of 40% or more of left ventricular muscle mass. The mechanism of cardiogenic shock is complex, with a vicious cycle of metabolic and hemodynamic changes that lead rapidly to further deterioration of cardiac function.[60] If left untreated, the reduction in tissue blood flow and oxygen delivery to the myocardium results in progressive circulatory collapse, impaired cellular metabolism, and eventual death.

The basic pathophysiologic defect associated with severe myocardial ischemia or necrosis is severely depressed ventricular function, which results in reduced cardiac output and inadequate tissue perfusion. The magnitude of impairment in ventricular function is related to total myocardial damage and the balance between oxygen supply and demand.

Neurogenic Shock

Neurogenic shock is produced by damage to or pharmacologic block of the vasomotor center of the medulla, resulting in vasodilation and increases in the vascular space. This leads to a relative hypovolemia brought on by a decrease in systemic vascular resistance, with peripheral pooling and a decrease in venous return. The result is a drop in cardiac output leading to tissue hypoperfusion.

Neurogenic shock most commonly results from spinal anesthesia or upper spinal cord injury.

Compensatory Mechanisms of Shock

A number of compensatory mechanisms are activated to maintain cardiovascular dynamics when arterial pressure and tissue perfusion are reduced. These compensatory mechanisms are mediated by the sympathetic nervous system and the release of endogenous vasoconstrictor and hormonal substances.[38,131]

Baroreceptors. A reduction in mean and arterial pressure and pulse pressure is sensed by baroreceptors in the carotid sinus and aortic arch, and they produce a generalized sympathetic stimulation with secretion of epinephrine and norepinephrine. The result is increases in peripheral vascular resistance, arterial pressure, and myocardial contractility.

Fluid shifts. The major endogenous vasoactive substances released during shock are catecholamines and vasopressin, which augment sympathetic activity when activated further. The release of these vasoactive substances also causes a reduction in vascular capacitance, which facilitates the osmotic movement of interstitial fluid into the vascular compartments to restore blood volume.

Renin-angiotensin-aldosterone system. When renal ischemia occurs, the renin-angiotensin-aldosterone system is activated to help maintain blood pressure and intravascular volume. The reduction of renal perfusion pressure results in release of renin, which in time is converted to angiotensin II, a powerful vasoconstrictor. Angiotensin II stimulates the release of aldosterone, which enhances sodium and water resorption by the renal tubules to help maintain intravascular volume.

Antidiuretic hormone. The release of antidiuretic hormone (ADH) from the posterior pituitary gland in response to hypotension is another hormonal system that plays a role in volume regulation during circulatory shock. ADH enhances resorption of sodium and water by increasing permeability of the renal tubules.

Progressive Shock

If the compensatory mechanisms are insufficient to restore effective perfusion to vital organs, circulatory function deteriorates further, perpetuating a cycle of progressive, irreversible changes that decrease cardiac output.

Cellular deterioration. As shock becomes severe, local changes in cellular metabolism occur. Prolonged tissue ischemia results in incomplete oxidation at the cellular level, diminishing mitochondrial activity. Cellular adenosine triphosphate (ATP) stores consequently begin to be used, and the cells resort to anaerobic metabolism of glucose to provide energy. This anaerobic process of glycolysis leads to the production of lactic acid, which builds up in the blood. The effects of an acidic pH include depressed myocardial function and a decreased vascular response to epinephrine and nor-epinephrine, thus potentiating the vasomotor collapse seen late in shock.[13,38]

Another significant cellular change resulting from continued cellular ischemia is the release of vasoactive metabolites into the systemic circulation. Substances such as bradykinin, histamine, serotonin, and pros-taglandins, along with decreased vascular tone, lead to increases in venous pooling and capillary permeability. Excessive vasodilation then decreases venous return and cardiac filling. The increased permeability of the capillaries allows large quantities of fluid to escape into the interstitial spaces.

Organ and Tissue Changes

As the shock syndrome becomes severe, generalized organ deterioration begins.

Renal function. Although diminished renal perfusion activates certain compensatory mechanisms, in the early phase of shock prolonged decreased renal blood flow leads to renal ischemia and acute tubular necrosis. Clinically this is evidenced by fluid, electrolyte, and metabolic disturbances.

Pulmonary function. Ischemia to the pulmonary circulation in the early phases of shock can sufficiently damage pulmonary function to cause adult respiratory distress syndrome. Damage to the pulmonary capillary endothelial cells causes increased capillary permeability, which leads to interstitial and alveolar edema that impairs gas exchange. The resulting hypoxemia and respiratory acidosis further reduce tissue oxygen delivery and organ function.

Gastrointestinal function. Ischemic damage to the gastrointestinal tract causes a loss of the protective mucosal covering in the intestine. This can lead to intestinal damage and necrosis by digestive enzymes. It may also account for the release of bacteria and bacterial toxins into the bloodstream, causing sepsis and further circulatory dysfunction.

The reticuloendothelial system may also be damaged during shock, impairing the patient's ability to withstand infection.

Intravascular clotting. As the products of cellular deterioration begin to accumulate in the capillaries and vascular dilation occurs, blood flow becomes extremely sluggish. The stagnation, along with local chemical changes in the capillaries, leads to blood aggregation and intravascular clotting. The formation of microemboli enhances tissue ischemia by further decreasing blood flow through the capillaries. This hypercoagulability response may occur as an early compensatory mechanism, particularly with hemorrhage. In the late stages of shock, however, a reversal in coagulation occurs, leading to a hypocoagulability state. This results from loss in clotting factors through bleeding or decreased production owing to poor tissue perfusion. It may also be the result of a consumption of clotting factors that is seen in disseminated intravascular coagulation.

Myocardial depression. Except in cardiogenic shock, the major cardiac effects of shock occur in the late stage and are by far the most important factor in the progressive deterioration caused by shock. As arterial pressure continues to drop, so does coronary blood flow. This leads to depressed myocardial function and a further reduction of cardiac output. Myocardial contractility is depressed further by the combined effects of toxins, acidosis, and tissue hypoxia that result from cellular deterioration. Thus circulatory failure is a syndrome that involves all systems, and it is usually the deterioration of heart function that makes shock irreversible.

COMPLICATIONS

Myocardial failure
Adult respiratory distress syndrome (ARDS)
Gastrointestinal bleeding
Disseminated   intravascular   coagulation
  (DIC)
Hepatic failure
Kidney failure

DIAGNOSTIC STUDIES AND FINDINGS

Diagnostic test	Findings
Hematocrit	Decreased, however in hypovolemia may be increased due to intravascular fluid shift
Hemoglobin	Decreased in hemorrhage
White blood count (WBC) with differential	Leukopenia in gram-negative sepsis; leukocytosis with increased neutrophils in all forms of shock
Erythrocyte sedimentation rate (ESR)	Increased in response to tissue injury
Cultures (blood [obtain two to four cultures from different sites] urine, sputum)	Positive growth of an organism in septic shock
Serum electrolytes	
Sodium	Increased during diuretic phase of acute tubular necrosis; decreased with administration of hypotonic fluid following fluid loss
Potassium	Increased with cellular death during oliguric phase, in acidosis, and after transfusion reactions
Serum chemistry	
BUN, creatinine	Increased, reflecting impaired renal function
Lactate levels	Increased
Glucose levels	Increased in early shock, reflecting release of liver glycogen stores in response to catecholamines
Coagulation studies	
Prothrombin time (PT)	Prolonged
Partial thromboplastin time (PTT)	Prolonged
Platelets, fibrinogen levels	Decreased
Fibrinogen degradation levels (FDL)	Increased as clotting factors are consumed
Fibrinogen	Decreased due to clotting in capillaries
Arterial blood gases	Hypoxemia ($Pao_2 < 80$ mm Hg); respiratory alkalosis ($Paco_2 < 35$ mm Hg) due to impaired alveolar oxygen diffusion; metabolic acidosis (pH < 7.35) due to rising lactic and pyruvic acid levels from anaerobic metabolism
Urine studies	
Specific gravity	Increased in response to action of ADH and during oliguric phase
Osmolality	High during oliguric phase
Sodium	Decreased
Sugar and acetone	Increased
ECG (12-lead and continuous monitoring)	Heart rate; tachycardia, dysrhythmia; ischemic changes
Chest roentgenogram	Early: normal
	Late: shows progressive signs of pulmonary congestion
Hemodynamic monitoring (PAP, PCWP, CO	Provides information regarding serial changes in LV function in response to specific treatments, e.g., fluid replacement

MEDICAL MANAGEMENT

GENERAL MANAGEMENT

Fluid-volume regulation: Except with patients in cardiogenic shock, restoration of intravascular volume is the most significant therapeutic intervention, particularly in the early phases of therapy.

Volume replacement should be initiated rapidly with 3-5 L of saline or other volume expanders over a 30-60-min period. Ringer's lactate provides effective intravascular expansion and is the usual fluid of choice; however, a buffered solution with lactate may be used for severe shock.

Regulation of fluids should be based on hemodynamic response to the rapid fluid infusion. Careful monitoring of MAP, PCWP or CVP, and urine output is used to guide fluid replacement.

Blood plasma expanders should be given after the initial volume deficit is corrected. In cases of massive hemorrhage, replacement should be with whole blood if the hematocrit value <30%. If the hematocrit value >30%, plasma expanders may be given. Packed cells are used if the RAP or PCWP is elevated and in cases such as cardiogenic shock, in which myocardial dysfunction limits the amount and speed of fluid replacement.

In a patient in shock after acute MI, volume deficits may occur and fluid replacement may be necessary to restore a depressed CO to normal. Continuous monitoring of PCWP is the most precise method of determining volume deficits. If PCWP <15-18 mm Hg, fluid replacement may be given to increase CO (Starling's law). The PCWP should be kept <18 mm Hg to avoid pulmonary congestion.

If the PCWP of a patient in shock is elevated, fluid replacement is contraindicated and diuretics may be necessary to return the PCWP to therapeutic range. Diuretics are generally given only to patients in cardiogenic shock with an elevated PCWP. They reduce preload through their effect on venous capacitance and decrease total circulating fluid.

Oxygenation: Ventilation/perfusion ratios should be determined early to ensure adequate ventilation. Oxygen exchange may be impaired in patients with shock, especially if CO is decreased. Oxygen therapy should be given from the onset of treatment to maintain an arterial Po_2 of at least 80 mm Hg. Intubation may be indicated if arterial blood gas assays show worsening hypoxemia despite high oxygen concentrations. The indications for mechanical ventilation are a Pao_2 <50 mm Hg while the patient is receiving oxygen concentrations of 50%, a vital capacity <15 ml/kg body weight, a Pco_2 >45 mm Hg, and an arterial pH <7.25.

Hemodynamic monitoring: For diagnostic information and evaluation of ongoing therapy, arterial pressures, PAP, and PCWP should be monitored initially every 5-10 min. A CI of <2 L/min reflects a shock state.

Acid-base balance: Frequent monitoring of acid-base balance is necessary to avert profound acidosis. Intravenous administration of sodium bicarbonate may be necessary to maintain or correct the pH to 7.35.

Renal function: Hourly urine output measurements with frequent checks are necessary to determine adequate kidney perfusion. Urine output <30 ml/h reflects inadequate renal perfusion. Elevated serum BUN and creatinine levels reflect renal dysfunction.

Nutrition: Shock patients should receive nothing by mouth, but care must be taken to provide nutrition, preferably with hyperalimentation, owing to altered liver function, which contributes to the depleted nutritional stores created by shock state.

Activity: Efforts should be made to minimize energy expenditure. The patient should be maintained on complete bed rest in a supine position, with legs elevated to 45°.

ADJUNCTIVE THERAPY

Intraaortic balloon pump (IABP):   Counterpulsation is the most frequently used method of mechanically assisting circulation to prevent cardiovascular collapse. Counterpulsation augments aortic pressure during diastole with subsequent reduction of afterload, thus effectively reducing the work of the myocardium and improving coronary blood flow.

MEDICAL MANAGEMENT—cont'd

A catheter with a 10-50 cc balloon is inserted into the femoral artery and positioned in the thoracic aorta just distal to the left subclavian artery. With the ECG used for synchronization, the balloon is inflated during diastole and deflated during systole.

Ventricular assist devices (VAD): Ventricular assist devices perform the work of the failing ventricle. VADs approximate normal hemodynamic parameters, supporting circulation for several days.

DRUG THERAPY

Maintenance of adequate hemodynamic state: In shock, myocardial dysfunction develops as a result of workload, limited coronary blood flow, and decreased myocardial oxygenation. Sympathomimetic agents are used to maintain an adequate hemodynamic state. The effects of these agents are mediated through the action of alpha- and beta-adrenergic receptors. Alpha-receptors located in the smooth muscle of the vascular bed cause vasoconstriction, thereby increasing peripheral resistance and venous return. By contrast, $beta_1$-receptors are located in the myocardium, arteries, and lungs. Myocardial beta-receptors act to increase HR and contractility, whereas activation of $beta_2$-receptors causes vasodilation.

The various adrenergic drugs differ with respect to their relative alpha (peripheral) and beta (peripheral, myocardial) effects. The rationale for selecting any drug depends on the specific vascular bed on which the drug acts and the desired cardiovascular effect. In cardiogenic shock, for example, drugs with positive inotropic and vasoconstrictor properties are used to increase CO by augmenting myocardial contractility and to improve blood flow to vital organs by increasing total vascular resistance. Dopamine, norepinephrine, and epinephrine, which have both constrictor and inotropic properties, are commonly used in treatment of cardiogenic shock.

The following agents are most commonly used in the treatment of patients with shock.

Adrenergic drugs: Dopamine (Intropin) is one of the most widely used drugs in the treatment of shock. Its effects depend on the dose used. In low doses (2-5 µg/kg/min) it produces dilation of renal, mesenteric, coronary, and cerebral blood vessels. In higher doses (6-15 µg/kg/min) it improves CO by increasing contractility (beta effect) but has no effect on BP. At therapeutic levels (10-15 µg/kg/min) dopamine increases CO and BP with little change or reduction in PVR. The increase in BP is due primarily to an enhanced CO. In addition, the vasodilator effect on renal blood vessels increases renal blood flow, which improves urine output. In very high doses (>20 µg/kg/min) dopamine causes generalized vasocon-striction (alpha effect), which opposes the desired vasodilator effect obtained with lower doses. Infusions should be started with low doses (3-5 µg/kg/min), increasing slowly until optimum arterial pressure is achieved.

Dobutamine (Dobutrex) is used primarily for the inotropic effect. It stimulates $beta_1$-receptors to increase myocardial contractility and stroke volume, resulting in improved CO. Since dobutamine has minimal $beta_2$ and alpha effects, it produces little change in BP and HR; however, systolic blood pressure may be increased because of increased CO. Coronary blood flow and MV_{O_2} are also increased because of increased myocardial contractility. Infusions begin at 2-4 µg/kg/min, with therapeutic doses between 2.5 and 10 µg/kg/min.

Epinephrine is a potent beta- and alpha-catecholamine and causes vasoconstriction of the splanchnic and renal beds. Although it does increase CO, its effects on PVR do not favor redistribution of blood flow to vital organs. It is also considered less advantageous than other adrenergic drugs because it increases automaticity, which can initiate serious dysrhythmias.

Norepinephrine has both alpha and beta actions. It increases myocardial contractility by stimulating $beta_1$-receptors and causes arteriovenous constriction by stimulating alpha-receptors. Thus norepinephrine increases systemic arterial pressure by increasing the cardiac output and peripheral vascular resistance. Once again the actual hemodynamic effects depend on the dose employed. With small doses a beta effect predominates, causing slight increases in BP and CO. With very high doses norepinephrine produces significant vasoconstriction, causing an increased SVR and BP. However, the CO may fall despite the positive inotropic effect. The usual starting dose is 2-8 µg/min. Norepinephrine should be administered through an indwelling catheter placed in a large vein, since it is known to cause tissue necrosis with extravasation. The disadvantage of this drug is its vasoconstricting effect on the kidneys, which can result in impaired renal perfusion and oliguria.

MEDICAL MANAGEMENT—cont'd

Isoproterenol (Isuprel) acts as a peripheral dilator through $beta_2$ stimulation. More important is the $beta_1$ effect, which augments myocardial contractility and HR, thereby improving CO. However, it may cause a substantial increase in myocardial oxygen demand, which can exacerbate myocardial ischemia in a patient with cardiogenic shock.

Cardiac glycosides: The role of digitalis in the treatment of shock is now being questioned. It has been noted that inotropic drugs such as digoxin become less effective as the degree of LV failure increases. As an inotropic agent for treatment of severe or cardiogenic shock, digitalis is relatively weak when compared with the sympathomimetic drugs. In addition, it could be hemodynamically detrimental because of the increased MVo_2 produced by the increased contractility, as well as by the decrease in afterload associated with it. Furthermore, because of the impaired renal function, acidosis, and hypoxia occurring in shock states, the patient is predisposed to digitalis-induced dysrhythmias.[38]

Vasodilators: Vasodilator therapy is generally limited to patients with failing ventricular function; its usefulness in the routine treatment of cardiogenic shock is still a subject of debate. However, it may be useful in treating patients with severe hypotension whose severe vasoconstriction continues despite volume replacement. Excessive vasoconstriction, which occurs initially as a compensatory response to hypoperfusion, can reduce blood flow and oxygen delivery, and can cause such a loss of intravascular volume that it leads to further reduction of CO. The rationale for using vasodilator therapy in shock is to break this progressive positive-feedback cycle.

Vasodilators improve LV function by decreasing myocardial oxygen demand through the reduction of preload and afterload. These drugs have no direct inotropic action on the heart. The increased cardiac output produced by vasodilators is caused by the changes in preload and afterload.

Arterial vasodilators are used to decrease PVR, which then decreases resistance to LV ejection and therefore afterload. Venodilators are used to increase venous capacitance, causing a decrease in venous return that will decrease PCWP and preload.

The potential role of vasodilator therapy in treating cardiogenic shock merits further study. Although inappropriate as a single form of therapy, the use of vasodilators combined with external counterpulsation and other inotropic agents appears to be effective in providing efficient ventricular function. Nitroprusside and phentolamine are the vasodilator agents most commonly used in the treatment of cardiogenic shock.

Antihypertensive agents: Nitroprusside (Nipride, Nitropress) causes both arterial and venous dilation, thereby decreasing venous return and LV filling (decreased preload), as well as resistance to LV ejection (decreased afterload). The drug is administered intravenously with an initial dose of 0.5-10 $\mu g/kg/min$, which is increased in increments of 5-10 $\mu g/kg/min$ every 5 min or until there is an improvement in hemodynamics. Fluid replacement may be required if filling pressures drop excessively. Fluid volumes should be determined before administration of these agents. In hypovolemic patients, massive vasodilation will only worsen the clinical picture by further decreasing venous return.

Alpha-adrenergic blocking agents: Phentolamine mesylate (Regitine) inhibits vasoconstriction by blocking alpha-adrenergic receptors. It lowers arterial pressure, thereby decreasing afterload. The drug is given intravenously at a dosage of 0.1-2 mg/min.

1 ASSESS

ASSESSMENT	OBSERVATIONS		
	HYPOVOLEMIC SHOCK	CARDIOGENIC SHOCK	VASOGENIC SHOCK
General complaints	Anxiety, restlessness	Anxiety, restlessness	Anxiety, restlessness
Level of consciousness	Lethargy; confused, stupor, coma	Lethargy, confused, coma	Lethargy, stupor, coma
Temperature	Increased or decreased	Increased	Increased or decreased
Cardiovascular system			
Heart rate, rhythm **Heart sounds** **Blood pressure**	Increased, pulse thready	Increased, pulse thready S_3, S_4	Increased, pulse thready
Early	Pulse pressure decreased; diastolic pressure increased	Pulse pressure decreased; diastolic pressure increased	Normal; pulse pressure decreased
Late	Systolic pressure decreased	Systolic pressure decreased	Systolic pressure decreased
Skin	Cool, moist, clammy, pale	Cool, moist, clammy, pale, cyanosis	Early: warm, dry Late: cool, moist, clammy; color—pale, cyanosis
Capillary refill time	Decreased	Decreased	Decreased
Peripheral pulses	Absent or diminished	Absent or diminished	Absent or diminished (late)
JVP	Absent or flat	Elevated	
Respiratory system			
Respiratory rate	Increased hyperventilation	Increased Late: Cheyne-Stokes respirations; apnea	Increased Late: Cheyne-Stokes respirations
Breath sounds	Early: clear; late: crackles	Crackles	Crackles
Renal system	Decreased (<20 ml/mm); anuria	Decreased (<20 ml/mm); anuria	Decreased (<20 ml/mm); anuria
Gastrointestinal system	Hemorrhage: guaiac positive stools; nausea, hypoactive bowel sounds	Nausea, hypoactive bowel sounds	Nausea; hypoactive bowel sounds

→ ⟩ ⟩

ASSESSMENT	OBSERVATIONS		
	HYPOVOLEMIC SHOCK	CARDIOGENIC SHOCK	VASOGENIC SHOCK
Neuromuscular system	Muscle aching; diminished deep tendon reflex responses	Muscle aching; diminished deep tendon reflex responses	Muscle aching; diminished deep tendon reflex responses
Hemodynamic findings			
RAP	Decreased	Normal or increased	Decreased
PCWP	Decreased	Increased	Decreased
SVR	Increased	Increased	Decreased
CO	Decreased	Decreased	Early: increased; late: decreased
CI	No change	Decreased	Early: increased or decreased; late: decreased
SV_{O_2}	Low	Increased	Low

2   DIAGNOSE

NURSING DIAGNOSIS	SUBJECTIVE FINDINGS	OBJECTIVE FINDINGS
Altered tissue perfusion (cerebral, cardiopulmonary, renal, and peripheral) related to decreased CO	Complains of restlessness, thirst	Cerebral: changes in mentation/sensorium; confusion, somnolence Cardiopulmonary: hypotension, decreased pulse pressure, tachycardia Renal: decreased urine output, decreased specific gravity, elevated BUN, and creatinine clearance Peripheral: poorly palpable peripheral pulses; skin cool, clammy, and pale, blanching of nail beds
Decreased cardiac output related to mechanical factors (preload, afterload, contractility)	Complains of fatigue, chest pain	Skin pallor, cyanosis, diaphoresis, oliguria, anuria, hypotension, tachycardia, jugular venous distension, decreased peripheral pulses
Fluid volume deficit related to hemorrhage, fluid loss	Complains of thirst, apprehensiveness	Apathy, poor skin turgor, dry mucous membranes, decreased systolic BP, decreased urine output (< 0.5 ml/kg/h), increased specific gravity, decreased urine sodium, tachycardia, flat neck veins, decreased JVP, decreased RAP, PCWP, CO, or CVP

NURSING DIAGNOSIS	SUBJECTIVE FINDINGS	OBJECTIVE FINDINGS
Impaired gas exchange related to increased pulmonary capillary permeability	Complains of apprehensiveness, anxiety, dyspnea	Restlessness, confusion progressing to somnolence; diaphoretic; tachypnea: rate > 20 breaths/min Skin: pale to cyanosis Breath sounds: crackles, rhonchi; diminished breath sounds Arterial blood gases: Pao_2— < 80 mm Hg pH: < 7.35 PCo_2: < 35 mm Hg
Anxiety related to actual and perceived threat to biologic integrity	Verbalizes fear, apprehension	Restlessness, poor eye contact, extraneous movements, anxiety, facial tension, diaphoresis, tachycardia, hyperventilation
Altered nutrition: less than body requirements related to depleted glycogen stores	Complains of nausea, anorexia, weakness, altered taste sensation	Vomiting, decreased body weight $\geq$ 10% to 20% under ideal body weight; weakness of muscles required for swallowing or chewing Caloric intake inadequate to meet metabolic needs Malnutrition: decreased BUN, serum albumin, protein, Hgb, lymphocyte and transferrin levels Decreased triceps skinfold measurement; stomatitis
Potential for infection related to sepsis and impaired immune response	Verbalizes feeling warm, uncomfortable, achy	Elevated temperature; tachycardia; positive cultures: blood, urine secretions, or wound drainage WBC: leukocytosis Bacterial: increased neutrophils (bands) Viral: increased lymphocytes; increased ESR Serum glucose: increased
Impaired skin integrity related to mechanical factors (pressure, irritation) internal factors, altered nutritional state, altered metabolic state, altered circulation	Patient complains of soreness, pressure, pain, altered sensation	Evidence of irritation; erythema; warm to touch; swelling; evidence of breakdown; broken skin; blisters

3 PLAN

Patient goals

1. The patient will demonstrate improved tissue perfusion and cellular oxygenation.
2. The patient will demonstrate improved cardiac output.
3. The patient will demonstrate stable fluid balance.
4. The patient will demonstrate improved ventilation and adequate oxygenation.
5. The patient will demonstrate reduction in anxiety state.
6. The patient will maintain adequate nutritional state.
7. The patient will be free of signs and symptoms of infection.
8. The patient will maintain skin integrity.

4 IMPLEMENT

NURSING DIAGNOSIS	NURSING INTERVENTIONS	RATIONALE
Altered cerebral, cardiopulmonary, renal, and peripheral tissue perfusion related to decreased CO	Assess for signs, symptoms indicative of altered tissue perfusion.	Early compensatory mechanisms, such as fluid shift, sympathetic stimulation, contribute to maintaining adequate tissue perfusion; however, as shock state progresses, vital functions begin to rapidly deteriorate.
	Maintain complete bedrest in flat position; keep warm.	To minimize metabolic needs and facilitate circulation.
	Perform neurologic checks observing for signs of altered sensorium.	Altered sensorium reflects inadequate cerebral blood flow and change in systemic perfusion.
	Measure intake and output q 1-2 h or as indicated; report output < 30 ml/h	To evaluate kidney function and body volume.
	Check BP, peripheral pulses q 1-2 h as ordered. Administer parenteral therapy as ordered: using PAP, PCWP to monitor response.	To assess for signs of vasoconstriction and tissue perfusion.
Decreased cardiac output related to mechanical factors (preload, afterload, contractility)	Assess and monitor for signs and symptoms indicative of decreased CO; report subtle and rapid changes to physician; determine if shock state is caused by hopovolemia vs that caused by LV dysfunction.	Survival depends on careful assessment of signs and contributing failures; assists in the prevention and/or restoration of ventricular function.
	Maintain bed rest, position patient in supine position with head and shoulders only slightly more elevated than chest, with legs elevated 45° (in absence of head injury).	To promote energy, increase venous return from lower extremities, and avoid decrease in BP.
	Check body temperature as indicated; administer antipyretics as ordered.	Elevated temperature increases cardiac work and myocardial oxygen demand.

NURSING DIAGNOSIS	NURSING INTERVENTIONS	RATIONALE
	Monitor hemodynamic parameters as ordered: MAP; PAP, PCWP.	Evaluate patient's clinical status and/or response to therapy. Decrease in aortic pressure and increase in LVEDP can lead to hypoperfusion of coronary arteries, which results in myocardial ischemia.
	Measure and calculate CO and CI.	To evaluate cardiac function, CI is more specific determinant of CO because it compares individual differences of CO in relation to body size.
	Calculate SVR as ordered.	To determine LV afterload.
	Frequently assess cardiovascular response to drug therapy; adjust flow/dosage according to BP, HR response	To evaluate for signs of improved myocardial function; to identify early signs of toxic effects of agents.
	Administer drugs as ordered: sympathomimetic and vasodilator drugs.	To increase myocardial contractility and reduce afterload.
	Administer plasma volume expanders as ordered; adjust flow rate according to PAP, PCWP readings.	To maintain adequate circulating volume; if problem related to hypovolemia, will need to initiate fluid challenges as ordered.
	Monitor intra-aortic balloon pump as indicated, assessing cardiac response.	To augment circulating blood volume and diminish oxygen demand by decreasing afterload and increasing coronary artery perfusion, resulting in improved stroke volume and CO.
	Place on cardiac monitor; observe for cardiac dysrhythmias and initiate antiarrhythmic therapy as indicated.	Cardiac dysrhythmias may result from depressed myocardial contractility and decreased coronary perfusion or may reflect side effects of medication, electrolyte imbalance.
	Restrict and plan activities as indicated; provide rest between procedures.	To decrease metabolic and oxygen demands.
	Measure intake and output q 1-2 h; monitor indices of renal function: BUN, creatinine.	To assess for signs of continued depressed CO and presence of hypovolemia.
Fluid volume deficit related to hemorrhage, fluid loss	Assess for signs and symptoms of fluid volume deficit.	Inadequate circulating volume may result from fluid regulating mechanisms, which respond to conserve and restore plasma volume. The capillary-fluid shift mechanisms increase intravascular volume by moving fluid from tissues into capillaries.
	Monitor BP, pulse, and respirations q 15 min during acute phase, increasing to q 2 h as condition stabilizes.	To determine stabilization vs progressive deterioration; may be used as early indicator that more fluids are required.

→ > >

NURSING DIAGNOSIS	NURSING INTERVENTIONS	RATIONALE
	Administer fluids as ordered: plasma volume expanders, saline solutions, and dextran.	To restore blood volume.
	Monitor hemodynamic parameters: RA, CVP, PCWP, PAP.	To accurately monitor response to fluid replacement therapy; to monitor that shock state is due to decreased circulating volume and not to heart failure.
	Maintain accurate intake and output q 1 h as indicated.	To assess kidney function as well as circulating fluid volume; need to monitor kidney function to avoid fluid overload.
	Monitor specific gravity q 1 h while patient remains unstable, then q 4-8 h.	To evaluate need for further fluids or need of diuretic; an increase in specific gravity indicates kidney is attempting to retain fluid and sodium.
	Monitor serum and urine sodium laboratory values.	Hyponatremia reflects dilutional effect of fluid excess. Decreased urine sodium with an increased specific gravity reflects kidney's attempt to retain fluid and sodium.
	Monitor serum potassium laboratory values.	Hyperkalemia: potassium excess as result of decreased kidney function. Hypokalemia: may reflect loss of potassium in association with acidosis.
	Monitor chemistries.	BUN, creatinine: reflect kidney function. Hct, HgB: reflect fluid status; can influence oxygen-carrying capacity.

	Monitor ABG.	To monitor acid-base balance:
		  pH < 7.35: intracellular acidosis
		  HCO_3^-: metabolic acidosis
		  $Pa_{CO_2} < -35$: compensatory alkalosis

	Evaluate for hidden fluid loss.	Internal fluid loss into body spaces can occur (e.g., gastrointestinal bleeding, peritoneal bleeding, hemothorax).
	Maintain bed rest in supine position. For hypovolemic shock in absence of head trauma, elevate feet and legs 6 to 8 in.	To increase venous return.
Impaired gas exchange related to increased pulmonary capillary permeability	Assess for alterations in respiratory function.	To assess adequacy of blood oxygenation and determine need of endotracheal intubation. Mechanical ventilation is required if hypoxemia and hypercapnia cannot be corrected.

NURSING DIAGNOSIS	NURSING INTERVENTIONS	RATIONALE
	Monitor serial ABG.	An increased alveolar-arterial (A-a) gradient suggests decreased oxygen lung perfusion and impending respiratory failure.
	Monitor mixed SVO_2 if PA catheter in place; report if $SVO_2 < 60\%$.	SVO_2 drops when CO decreases; reflects decrease in tissue perfusion.
	Auscultate lung sounds q 1-2 h.	To detect adventitious sounds (crackles, wheezes, rhonchi), which indicate pulmonary congestion, or diminished sounds, reflecting atelectasis.
	Monitor respiratory pattern, noting rate, rhythm, and use of accessory muscles.	Tachypnea may reflect compensatory respiratory alkalosis, hypoxemia, pulmonary edema, atelectasis.
	Assess mental status.	Alteration in level of awareness may reflect cerebral perfusion problems.
	Assess skin color.	Central cyanosis generally reflects hypoxemia.
	Administer oxygen as ordered, via mask or through endotracheal tube; prepare for intubation and assisted ventilation as indicated.	To ensure oxygen delivery and optimal gas exchange ($PaO_2 = 80\text{-}100$ mm Hg).
	Review serial chest roentgenograms as ordered.	To assess for signs of increased congestion, atelectasis.
	Maintain patent airway; suction as indicated.	To clear airway and improve oxygen delivery.
	Maintain patient on bed rest.	To decrease oxygen demand and oxygen consumption.
Anxiety related to actual or potential biologic integrity	Assess for signs and symptoms of fear and anxiety; determine if appropriate or inappropriate.	A moderate degree of situational anxiety is appropriate; severe anxiety or panic leads to sympathetic arousal, causing increased metabolic expenditure.
	Determine patient's source of fear and anxiety.	To determine patient's perception of situation; to correct any misconceptions; and to assist patient to deal with feelings.
	Explain all procedures and treatment, offering brief explanations.	To minimize feelings of uncertainty and total loss of control.
	Anticipate needs.	To minimize expenditure of energy.
	Stay with patient to offer reassurance; use calm, soft voice.	Provides a sense of security that he/she is not alone.

NURSING DIAGNOSIS	NURSING INTERVENTIONS	RATIONALE
	Allow family members to visit or remain with patient if possible.	Presence of a familiar and supportive person may help to minimize anxiety by providing comfort and reassurance.
	Initiate comfort measures such as quiet, restful environment.	To minimize internal and external arousal.
	Encourage expressions of feelings, such as crying.	To release feelings of tension and stress.
Altered nutrition: less than body requirements related to depleted glycogen stores	Document weight upon admission.	To establish baseline and evaluate actual weight loss.
	Assess signs of early malnutrition; monitor laboratory values daily.	Important to assess early in order to maintain optimal nutritional support.
	Weigh daily at same time of day, using same scale and same amount of clothing.	To ensure accurate weight measurement.
	Monitor daily amount of food and liquid intake; assist with feedings as indicated.	To determine need for supplemental or parenteral feedings.
	Begin tube feedings, intralipids, and/or hyperalimentation as ordered.	To improve and maintain nutritional status.
Potential for infection related to sepsis and impaired immune response.	Assess for signs and symptoms of systemic infection.	To identify developing sepsis.
	Identify and monitor potential sites of infection: IV and pressure catheters, wounds, and sutures.	To detect signs of developing localized infections; due to impaired immune response, patient is at risk for developing nosocomial infections.
	Change line tubing and wound dressings daily using strict asepsis.	To minimize potential for bacterial and nosocomial infections.
Impaired skin integrity related to mechanical factors and internal factors	Assess and monitor skin integrity q 4-8 h; perform skin care q 1-2 h, carefully observing bony prominences for pressure points and evidence of breakdown.	To detect early signs of irritation to initiate preventive care and avoid progressive skin breakdown and infection.
	Provide convoluted foam mattress, sheepskin mattress, or air-pressure mattress as ordered.	To minimize skin pressure.
	Turn patient q 1-2 h as condition permits.	Decubitus ulcer formation is based on time and pressure relationship, therefore need to alternate body positions frequently.
	Begin passive range of motion exercises as condition permits.	To avoid muscle contractions.

NURSING DIAGNOSIS	NURSING INTERVENTIONS	RATIONALE
	Initiate an aggressive therapeutic plan at early signs of skin irritation or breakdown: regular cleansing of area; massage *around* affected area—do not massage reddened or irritated site.	To prevent further breakdown and possible infection. To improve circulation.

5 EVALUATE

PATIENT OUTCOME	DATA INDICATING THAT OUTCOME IS REACHED
Tissue perfusion is improved.	Patient is alert and oriented, is normotensive; urine output is normal, skin warm and dry; peripheral pulses >2+.
Cardiac output is improved.	Patient is normotensive; CO is 4-5 L/min; PCWP is 10-15 mm Hg; skin is warm and dry; patient is resting quietly.
Fluid volume is restored.	Patient is normotensive; PCWP is 10-15 mm Hg; urine output is increased; P_{CO_2} is 35 to 45 mm Hg; pH is 7.35 to 7.45.
Gas exchange is improved.	Pa_{O_2} is 80-100 mm Hg; P_{CO_2} is 35-45 mm Hg; lungs are clear; patient verbalizes breathing easier.
Anxiety is decreased.	Patient verbalizes fears and asks questions; patient appears relaxed and is resting quietly.
Nutritional status is maintained or improved.	Weight remains stable or increases. Albumin, transferrins within normal limits; nitrogen balance is maintained; patient is eating.
There is no infection.	Patient is afebrile; WBC, glucose within normal limits; cultures are negative.
Skin integrity is maintained or improved.	Skin and tissue are intact, without evidence of irritation or breakdown.

PATIENT TEACHING

1. Explain all procedures and treatments as they occur. Refer to primary disorder for specific teaching protocol.

Hypertension

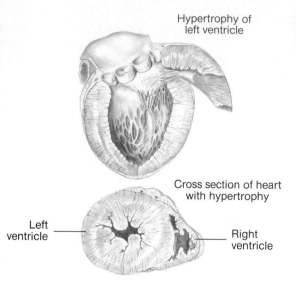

Hypertrophy of
left ventricle

Cross section of heart
with hypertrophy

Left
ventricle

Right
ventricle

Hypertension

Hypertension is an intermittent or sustained elevation in systolic or diastolic blood pressure. It is a major cause of cerebrovascular accident (stroke), cardiac disease, and renal failure.

Hypertension may be defined as a blood pressure greater than 160/90 mm Hg. Persons with blood pressures less than 140/80 mm Hg are normotensive. Table 4-2 defines further categories of hypertension.[76] Although there is no way of predicting in whom high blood pressure will develop, hypertension can be detected easily. Therefore, the major emphasis in the control of hypertension should be on early detection and effective treatment.

EPIDEMIOLOGY

Based on data from the Joint National Committee Report on Detection, Evaluation, and Treatment of High Blood Pressure, it is estimated that 60 million Americans are diagnosed with hypertension, and an additional 25 million have border-line hypertension.[167] Half of those affected are unaware of their hypertension.

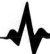

Table 4-2

CLASSIFICATION OF HIGH BLOOD PRESSURE*

Category	Range (mm Hg)
Normal BP	< 140/80
Borderline	140 to 159/85 to 89
Isolated systolic hypertension	≥ 160
Mild hypertension	90 to 104 (diastolic BP)
Moderate hypertension	105 to 114 (diastolic BP)
Severe hypertension	115 or greater (diastolic BP)

*Represents the average of two or more measurements taken on two separate occasions.
SOURCE: 1984 Report of Joint National Committee on Detection, Evaluation, and Treatment of High Blood Pressure.

ETIOLOGY

Primary (essential) hypertension, the most common form of hypertension, accounts for 90% of all clinical cases of hypertension. However, the exact causes remain unclear. There are several theories to explain the mechanisms involved. Some include:

Neural theory—an abnormal condition in which excessive neurohumoral stimulation results in increased muscle tone.

Sympathetic nervous system activation—increased CNS activity could raise blood pressure by increasing renin via the release of catecholamines, or by causing veno-arterial constriction.

Renin-angiotension-aldosterone system—stimulation and production of high plasma levels of renin (an enzyme produced by juxtaglomerular cells) results in the production of angiotension I and II, which are vasoconstricting substances. Angiotension II leads to venoarterial constriction, which stimulates aldosterone, resulting in retention of salt and water (Figure 4-25).

Vasodepressor—decreased concentration of vasodilatating substances, e.g., prostaglandins and kinins.

While an exact cause is not known, several factors have been identified as contributing to the development of hypertension.

Secondary hypertension refers to elevated blood pressure that is related to some underlying condition. The most common causes of secondary hypertension are renal failure, renovascular disease, and use of oral contraceptives in women. Other conditions that may lead to secondary hypertension include renal parenchymal disorders, renal artery disease, endocrine and metabolic disorders, CNS disorders, and coarctation of the aorta.

Age, family history. While absolute figures are not clear, there is evidence to suggest that between from

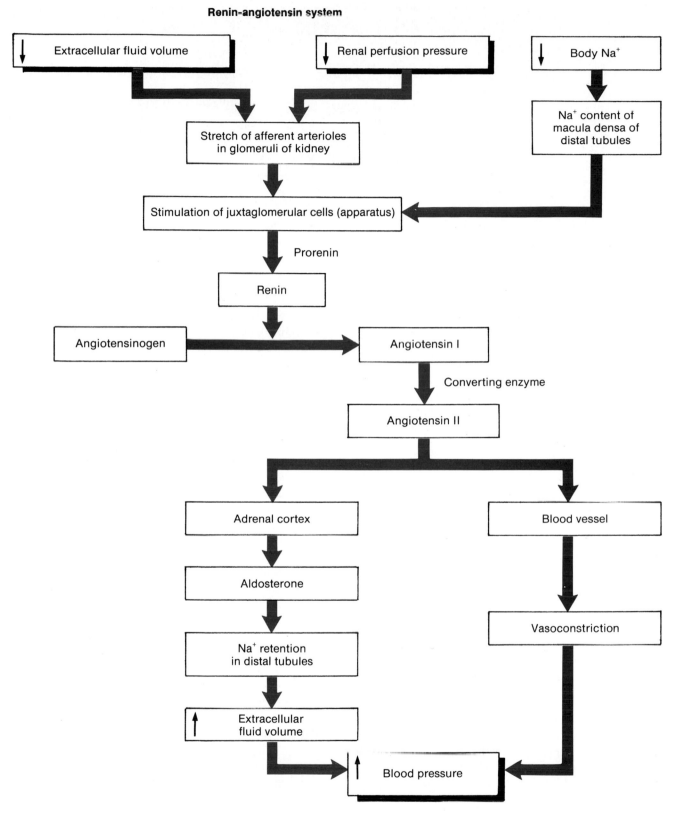

FIGURE 4-25
Complex relationship between extracellular fluid volume and pressure as medicated by renal hormonal mechanisms. These involve production of renin and angiotensin.

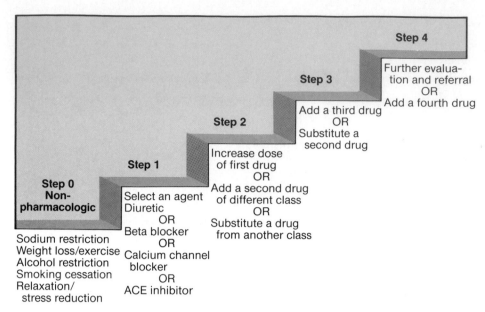

Step 4
Further evalua-
tion and referral
OR
Add a fourth drug

Step 3
Add a third drug
OR
Substitute a
second drug

Step 2
Increase dose
of first drug
OR
Add a second drug
of different class
OR
Substitute a drug
from another class

Step 1
Select an agent
Diuretic
OR
Beta blocker
OR
Calcium channel
blocker
OR
ACE inhibitor

Step 0
Non-
pharmacologic
Sodium restriction
Weight loss/exercise
Alcohol restriction
Smoking cessation
Relaxation/
stress reduction

2% to 12% of our young population has high blood pressure. The risk for developing primary hypertension is higher if one (28%) or both (41%) parents are hypertensive.[2,76] In the elderly, high blood pressure is the major cardiovascular risk factor. Reported prevalence rates indicate that 20% of the total elderly population have isolated systemic hypertension (systolic pressure > 160 mm Hg) or mild diastolic hypertension (≥ 90 mm Hg).[148]

Race, sex. Prevalence rates for hypertension vary widely with race and sex. In the United States, hypertension among black Americans is 38.2% as compared with 28.8% among whites. In addition, hypertension is more severe with greater risk of target organ damage for blacks than for whites. Among sexes, males have a higher prevalence rate than females, but the rate in females rises if she uses oral contraceptives, is overweight, or has a family history of high blood pressure.

In addition to these unavoidable factors, obesity, cigarette smoking, stress, and a high dietary intake of salt and saturated fats may contribute to the development of hypertension.

PATHOPHYSIOLOGY

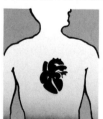

Accelerated (malignant) hypertension is a state in which the blood pressure is extremely high (diastolic pressure greater than 120 mm Hg). It is accompanied by acute hypertensive retinopathy, nephrosclerosis, and encephalopathy.

The pathogenesis of hypertension is complex because various homeostatic mechanisms contribute to the maintenance of normal arterial pressure.

Cardiac output (stroke volume × heart rate) and pe-

ripheral vascular resistance are the hemodynamic determinants of arterial pressure. Increases in blood volume (high-output states), heart rate, or arterial vasoconstriction that causes an increase in peripheral resistance can lead to a hypertensive state.

Stimulation of stretch receptors (baroreceptors) in the wall of the carotid sinus and the aortic arch stimulate the sympathetic nervous system, which results in increased levels of epinephrine and norepinephrine. This in turn results in an increase in cardiac output and/or systemic vascular resistance. In many hypertensive patients, the cardiac output will remain normal while total peripheral resistance is elevated. The mechanism to explain the increased systemic resistance remains unclear.

Target organ involvement. Clinically, patients with mild to moderate hypertension remain asymptomatic. However, the effect of hypertension is observed in the effect it has on various organs, including the heart and kidneys.

Cardiovascular system. Persistent hypertension leads to concentric hypertrophy of the heart. This is thought to be due to prolonged exposure to elevated peripheral resistance (afterload) and as a primary effect on heart muscle.

COMPLICATIONS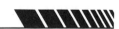

Hypertensive crisis
Coronary artery disease
Cerebrovascular disease (stroke)
Renal disease
Congestive heart failure
Peripheral vascular disease
Aortic aneurysm and dissection
Sudden death

DIAGNOSTIC STUDIES AND FINDINGS

Diagnostic test	Findings
Laboratory tests	
Urine studies including microscopic examination	Proteinuria, hematuria
Blood chemistry	BUN >20 mg/dl
	Creatinine > 1.5 mg/dl
	Potassium >5 mEq/L in renal failure; <3.5 mEq/L in primary aldosteronism and with diuretic administration
	Cholesterol and lipid levels elevated in hyperlipidemia
	Uric acid level may increase with diuretic therapy
	Calcium level may increase with diuretic therapy
Electrocardiogram (ECG)	LV hypertrophy: increased QRS voltage
	Myocardial ischemia: ST depression, T wave inversion
Chest x-ray	PA view: increased convexity of left heart border
	Increased C-T ratio
Arterial BP	Diagnosis is made on the basis of an average of two or more BP measurements taken on two or more subsequent occasions

MEDICAL MANAGEMENT

GENERAL MANAGEMENT

Stepped-Care approach in the treatment of high blood pressure is based on recommendations of the 1984 Joint National Committee on Detection, Evaluation, and Treatment of High Blood Pressures for Drug Therapy. Step 0 is nonpharmacologic therapy. If control is inadequate, then drug therapy is initiated. Step 1 begins with small doses of an agent, then increasing the dose or adding or substituting another in increasing dosages until BP control is achieved.

NONPHARMACOLOGIC THERAPY (STEP 0)

Dietary management:
   Sodium restriction—may range from mild to rigid restriction depending on degree of hypertension; recommended dietary restriction 2-6 g/day.
Alcohol—limit intake to 2 oz of alcohol per day.
Caffeine—restrict intake.
Cholesterol, lipids, saturated fats—reduce intake.

Smoking cessation

Weight control: Recommend weight loss of 5% or more in obese patient.

Exercise: Aerobic exercise appropriate for age and health status; refer to cardiac rehabilitation for prescribed exercise program; avoid isometric exercises.

Stress reduction and management

Monitoring of BP: Monitor on regular basis; frequency determined by blood pressure elevations.

DRUG THERAPY

Diuretics: Thiazides; loop diuretics; potassium-sparing diuretics

Calcium channel blockers

Adrenergic blocking agents: beta- adrenergic blocking agents; alpha- adrenergic blocking agents; adrenergic antihypertensive agents

Angiotensin-converting enzyme (ACE) inhibitors

1 ASSESS

Patients with mild to moderate hypertension are asymptomatic, and physical examination findings are usually normal, with the exception of BP (See Table 4-2)

ASSESSMENT	OBSERVATIONS
General complaints	Headaches, dizziness, fatigue, vertigo, palpitations; in severe hypertension, throbbing suboccipital headache (may be present when patient awakens in morning, disappearing spontaneously after several hours); epistaxis
BP	In both arms; sitting, standing, and supine; determined over at least two occasions; $\geq$ 160/90 mm Hg or higher
Pulse	Tachycardia; bounding; femoral delays as compared with radial or brachial pulsation
Precordium	Displaced but forceful apical impulse; ventricular heave (apical lift)
Heart sounds	Bruits over carotid and femoral areas; accentuated S_2 at base; apical systolic murmur; audible S_4; early diastolic blowing murmur (right and left sternal borders and intercostal spaces)
Optic fundi	Retinal changes: grade I—minimal arterial narrowing or irregularity; grade II—marked arteriolar narrowing and irregularity with focal tortuosity or spasm; grade III—marked arteriolar narrowing and irregularity with generalized tortuosity, flame-shaped hemorrhages, cotton-wool exudates; grade IV—same as grade III plus papilledema

2 DIAGNOSE

NURSING DIAGNOSIS	SUBJECTIVE FINDINGS	OBJECTIVE FINDINGS

Altered health maintenance related to high BP	Reports lack of knowledge regarding high BP and prevention
	Reports life-style that contributes to increased risk for high BP:
	  Diet high in sodium
	  Smoking/tobacco use behavior
	  Sedentary life-style
	  High stress/tension levels
	  Failure to have BP screening if at added risk for race and family history
	  For women—use of oral contraceptives
		BP that is borderline, mild, moderate, or severe; obesity; signs and symptoms of target-organ damage

Noncompliance related to negative side effects of prescribed treatment and conflict with health motivation and sociocultural influences	Reports noncompliant behavior; statements from significant others that describe noncompliant behavior	Diagnostic or laboratory tests indicating noncompliant behavior; evidence of target organ involvement; exacerbation of symptoms; failure to keep appointments

Other related nursing diagnoses

Potential altered tissue perfusion (cerebral, renal, and peripheral vascular) related to increased peripheral vascular resistance

3   PLAN

Patient goals

1. Patient will describe health care behaviors to prevent and/or control high blood pressure.
2. Patient will demonstrate knowledge and self responsibility for maintaining a life-style that promotes blood pressure control.
3. Patient will identify reasons and/or experiences for failure to adhere to prescribed therapeutic regimen.
4. Patient demonstrates increased level of knowledge.

4   IMPLEMENT

NURSING DIAGNOSIS	NURSING INTERVENTIONS	RATIONALE
Altered health maintenance related to high BP	Assess for life-style factors that contribute to increasing risk of high BP.	Personal, social, and situational factors that influence life-style must be explored and identified to promote behavior change and acceptance of therapeutic plan.
	Assess signs and symptoms of target organ involvement.	Signs of target organ involvement suggest high BP of long standing and/or noncompliance with medical regimen.
	Identify any misconceptions in patient's knowledge base regarding disease.	Understanding of the disease and therapeutic recommendations must be clear; inaccurate perceptions lead to feelings of frustration, anger, or noncompliance.
	Obtain and record BP, involving patient with procedures and reading.	Active participation increases understanding and awareness.
	Instruct patient in antihypertensive therapy as ordered; initiate patient participation early in the administration of drug therapy, reviewing drug names, dosage, side-effects to expect and report.	Early involvement in the administration of drug therapy will permit patient to verbalize questions and concerns, which contribute to knowledge, skills, and positive attitudes toward long-term maintenance.
	Initiate health education program; encourage patient to participate in designing program; involve family or significant other (see Patient Teaching).	Behavior changes begin with clear understanding of disease process; active participation enables patient to make choices, which promotes assuming responsibility in own care.
	Provide information regarding various measures to assist in changing health behavior, e.g.: Weight—how to minimize weight gain Smoking—use of support groups, self-help books, smoking clinics Exercise—methods of integrating exercise into life-style Stress—stress relaxation classes, biofeedback, visual imagery, deep breathing	Provides patient with sense of having certain choices in the selection of strategies to modify or change behavior.

→ › ›

NURSING DIAGNOSIS	NURSING INTERVENTIONS	RATIONALE
Noncompliance related to negative side effects of prescribed treatment and conflict with health motivation or sociocultural influences	Assess data to determine that reported behavior is noncompliant and not due to lack of understanding.	Noncompliance implies that patient has awareness skills and has verbalized intention of following therapeutic recommendations, but for various reasons has chosen not to follow treatment regimen.
	Together with patient, explore other factors that may be influencing patient's ability to adhere to therapeutic plan: financial status, age, culture, occupation.	In addition to personal factors, lack of support systems or environmental or situational barriers also can interfere with patient's desire to comply.
	Explore with patient conflicts between personal values and beliefs and recommended regimen; explore alternatives or revisions of treatment plan that are more compatible with life-style.	To provide insights into factors that are contributing to noncompliance.
	Review and outline individual behaviors that place patient at risk for cardiac event; clarify any misconceptions patient may have regarding disease state.	Acceptance of therapeutic plan is dependent on fact that patient believes he/she is vulnerable to illness or disease outcome.
	Explore alternative measures to increase compliant behaviors such as contracting, self-monitoring behavior modification, shaping behavior, support or reference groups.	Promotes sense of maintaining control in making choices.
Knowledge deficit	See Patient Teaching.	

5 EVALUATE

PATIENT OUTCOME	DATA INDICATING THAT OUTCOME IS REACHED
BP is within acceptance limits.	BP ≤ 140/80 mm Hg; patient has no complaints of headache, dizziness, etc; laboratory values are within normal limits.
Patient demonstrates knowledge and self-responsibility for controlling BP.	Patient reports taking medication, loses weight, stops smoking, participates in physical activities; patient reports periodic self-monitoring of BP.
Patient complies with therapeutic plan.	Patient discusses feelings of frustration related to taking medication, changing life-style, engages in active participation in exploring ways to accept therapeutic plan.
Patient's level of knowledge is increased.	Patient verbalizes understanding of disease process and associated risk factors; patient return demonstrates BP monitoring and reports appropriate life-style changes.

PATIENT TEACHING

1. Instruct patient and family in the following: what is blood pressure; definition of high blood pressure; factors contributing to increase, identifying which are avoidable; and the effects of high blood pressure on the heart, kidneys, and brain.
2. Instruct the patient and family in blood pressure monitoring, procedure for taking blood pressure at home, frequency of monitoring, influencing factors, interpretation of results, and actions to take if significant change occurs.
3. Explain diet therapy, including sodium, calorie, and lipid restrictions as ordered; include the rationale in explanation. Discuss the importance of restricting alcohol intake.
4. Explain the importance of weight control—that in overweight persons, losing 5 pounds will lower blood pressure.
5. Explain the importance of eliminating smoking. Refer the patient to cessation support groups.
6. Explain the role of exercise in blood pressure regulation and weight control.
7. Explain the relationship between stress and hypertension, factors that produce stress, and methods to modify stress.
8. Explain antihypertensive therapy, including name, rationale, dosage, and side effects of all medications.

Endocarditis

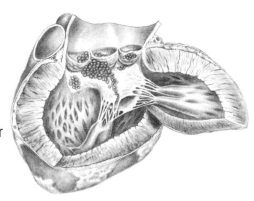

Endocarditis is an inflammatory process involving the endothelial layer of the heart, including the cardiac valves and septal defects if present.

Bacterial or fungal infection of the endocardium can compromise heart function if left untreated. Highly virulent pathogens produce acute endocarditis, which is characterized by sudden onset and rapid destruction of cardiac tissues. Subacute endocarditis typically starts insidiously. Because the infecting organisms are usually less virulent, the disease can be subclinical for as long as 8 weeks.

EPIDEMIOLOGY

The precise incidence of infective endocarditis (IE) is unknown. An estimated 5 of every 1000 patients admitted to the hospital have a diagnosis of endocarditis. Men are affected two to five times more often than women. The overall mortality rate is 20% to 30%, but among elderly patients mortality may be as high as 70%.[57]

Although the incidence of IE has not changed over the last two decades, epidemiologic patterns have shifted. In the preantibiotic era, it was considered a disease primarily of young adults, most of whom had damaged valves from rheumatic disease in childhood. The mean age of patients with endocarditis has risen to 55 years. Although the majority of infections still develop in people with preexisting heart disease, the number of cases of endocarditis in patients with functionally normal cardiac valves is increasing.[137] This can be attributed to the growing number of invasive diagnostic and therapeutic procedures, increased IV drug use, and an expanding elderly population. Immunosuppressed patients are susceptible to transient bacteremia.

PATHOPHYSIOLOGY

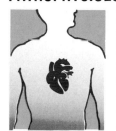

IE begins with the introduction of a pathogen into the circulation (see box on next page) causing bacteremia (or less commonly fungemia) (Table 4-3). Bacteremia is actually a common event that follows trauma to epithelial surfaces rich in indigenous bacteria. Normally it is subclinical, transient, and self-limited.

PORTS OF ENTRY FOR BACTEREMIA

Oral cavity—dental procedures, abscesses, oral irrigation, using unwaxed dental floss, bridgework

Upper respiratory tract—tonsilloadenoidectomy, orotracheal intubation, bronchoscopy, pneumonia

Gastrointestinal tract—barium enema, sigmoidoscopy, colonoscopy, percutaneous liver biopsy

Genitourinary system—catheterization, urethrotomy, prostatectomy, cystoscopy

Female reproductive tract—delivery, abortion, intrauterine devices, pelvic inflammatory disease

Skin—furuncles, infected or squeezed acne

Circulatory system—prolonged use of arterial polyethylene catheter, arteriovenous cannulas for hemodialysis, infection (e.g., hematogenous osteomyelitis, meningococcemia), IV drug use

For reasons not clearly understood, bacteria are attracted to damaged cardiac structures, particularly areas of turbulent blood flow. A sterile vegetation, or thrombus, composed of fibrin and platelets, forms on valves and adjacent areas when endocardial tissue is damaged. These vegetations are like magnets for circulating microorganisms, which attach to the thrombus and proliferate. The fibrin-platelet complexes surround the pathogen, forming a cyst-like structure to seal the colony from lymphocytes and other defensive cells that are ordinarily responsible for eradicating antigens.

Affected structures eventually become scarred, impeding function. Valve leaflets may retract and erode, which leads to valvular insufficiency. The infection may also burrow into the myocardium, causing conduction defects, fistulas, abscesses, and rupture of the chordae tendineae or ventricular septum.

The vegetations can break apart, since they are invariably located in areas of high velocity blood flow. Embolism produces infarctions and abscesses in other areas of the heart, brain, lung, kidneys, spleen, or extremities. Invasion of arterial walls may occur, causing mycotic aneurysms that can rupture at any time, even years after treatment.

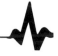

Table 4-3

INFECTING ORGANISMS

Organism	Comments
Staphylococci	
S. aureus	Highly virulent, associated with 45%-73% mortality; affects normal valves; responsible for 50% of acute cases; organism may enter from oral cavity, upper respiratory tract, or skin
S. faecalis	Causes both acute and subacute infection; *Enterococcus* is associated with advanced age, urologic procedures in men, and women of childbearing age
S. epidermidis	Implicated with valve replacement; associated with dental procedures; may also originate in upper respiratory tract and skin infections
Streptococcus	Low virulence, accounts for 40%-80% of subacute cases; *S. viridans* generally affects already damaged valves; organism is plentiful in the oral cavity and upper respiratory tract
Escherichia coli	May enter from gastrointestinal or genitourinary tract
Gram-negative organisms (*Klebsiella, Pseudomonas, Serratia marcescens*)	Occurs in elderly persons and IV drug users
Fungi (*Candida, Aspergillus*)	Incidence of fungal endocarditis has increased; IV drug users at high risk; inappropriate use of antimicrobials and corticosteroids may increase risk

This mechanism explains how endocarditis develops in patients who have damaged valves or a history of trauma to other areas of the endocardium. However, no underlying heart disease is found in between 20% and 40% of patients. It is not clear how microorganisms gain a foothold in apparently normal hearts. Indeed, it is possible that unrecognized endocardial trauma, however slight, is the underlying event in the majority of these cases.

SIGNS AND SYMPTOMS

Because the symptoms are highly variable, nonspecific, and often subtle, an initial presumptive diagnosis of IE is often made based on the patient's history of preexisting cardiac damage, recent medical or dental procedure, or known IV drug use.

General Signs and Symptoms

- In acute infection, high fever (102° to 104° F); in subacute infection, low-grade fever (102° F or less); occasionally normal temperatures are seen in the elderly and patients with renal failure, congestive heart failure, or severe disability
- Weakness, malaise, weight loss, anorexia, pallor, alternating chills and diaphoresis, arthralgia, and headache

Cardiac murmurs eventually develop but may be absent early in the infection. IV drug users often have vegetations on their tricuspid valves, which do not produce a murmur. In patients with valvular disease, a preexisting murmur can change sounds, or a new murmur can develop.

Although systemic emboli are often a complication of endocarditis, emboli are occasionally the first symptom. They can produce stroke, myocardial infarction, acute arterial insufficiency in an extremity, abdominal pain, or flank pain with hematuria.

COMPLICATIONS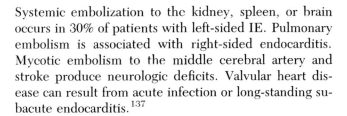

Systemic embolization to the kidney, spleen, or brain occurs in 30% of patients with left-sided IE. Pulmonary embolism is associated with right-sided endocarditis. Mycotic embolism to the middle cerebral artery and stroke produce neurologic deficits. Valvular heart disease can result from acute infection or long-standing subacute endocarditis.[137]

Systemic embolization
  Occurrence (30% of persons with left-sided IE)
  Infarction: kidney, spleen, brain
Pulmonary embolism, infarction (right-sided IE)
Mycotic embolism of middle cerebral artery
Stroke
Valvular heart disease

Signs of Embolization

- Petechiae of conjunctiva, buccal mucosa, and extremities—occur in 20% to 40% of patients
- Osler's nodes (small, tender nodules on the finger and toe pads)—occur in 10% to 20% of patients with subacute infection but are common in acute infection (also associated with typhoid fever and collagen vascular diseases)
- Splinter hemorrhages on nailbeds—also occur from local trauma
- Roth's spots (retinal hemorrhages with small white centers)—occur in fewer than 5% of patients (also associated with collagen vascular diseases and severe anemia)
- Janeway's lesions (nontender hemorrhagic macular lesions on the palms and soles)—more common in acute infection
- Splenomegaly—occurs in 23% of acute cases and 44% of subacute cases
- Clubbing of the fingers—most common in long-standing subacute infection

DIAGNOSIS

The only way to establish a definite diagnosis of IE is with blood cultures. Over several days, four to six cultures are made with samples obtained from different venipuncture sites. Diagnosis is based on at least two cultures positive for the same organism.

Bacteremia or fungemia is present in over 90% of cases. Sterile cultures do not necessarily rule out infective endocarditis, however. In long-standing subacute endocarditis, circulating levels of the microorganisms may be so low that culturing is nearly impossible. Prosthetic valves and right-sided endocarditis are frequently colonized by unusual bacteria that are difficult to culture.

Many fungi are also difficult to culture. Large emboli typically migrate to the lower extremities in fungal endocarditis. Because embolectomy is generally necessary in these cases, the pathogen may be identified by culturing the embolus.

Results of routine laboratory tests are nonspecific, showing a pattern of generalized immune response.

DIAGNOSTIC STUDIES AND FINDINGS

Diagnostic test	Findings
Laboratory tests	
Complete blood count	Normochromic, normocytic anemia
	Elevated ESR
	Leukocytosis in acute infection
Blood cultures	Identifies causative organism (negative cultures in 5%-15% of cases); 4-6 samples are drawn from different venipuncture sites over several days
Rheumatoid factor	Positive in 50% of patients with infection 6 wk or longer
Urine	Proteinuria
	Leukocyte casts
	Microhematuria
Blood chemistry	Elevated BUN and creatinine levels with renal complications
Echocardiogram	Vegetations or abscesses
	Valve involvement
	LV dysfunction
ECG	Early infection: normal
	Late infection: conduction defects, atrial fibrillation; or atrial flutter
Radionuclide studies	Gallium 67 citrate may accumulate in areas of inflammation

MEDICAL MANAGEMENT

GENERAL MANAGEMENT:

Rest: Hospitalization 2-6 wk during acute phase.

Vital Signs: Check q 4 h until clinically stable.

Diet: Regular diet if tolerated; force fluids while temperature elevated (unless ventricular failure develops); high-calorie supplemental feedings if unable to eat well.

IV therapy: Monitor for rate and amount as ordered; check frequently for localized inflammation and phlebitis.

DRUG THERAPY

Antibiotics: 4-6 wk, usually given IV, blood cultures; subacute cases—wait for cultures to identify pathogen before starting antibiotics; acute cases—start therapy immediately, negative cultures (10-20% of cases mostly subacute)—assume enterococcal infection, treat with combination penicillin and streptomycin, repeat blood cultures to monitor adequacy of coverage.

Antipyretics: For fever.

Anticoagulants: If large thrombus or atrial fibrillation develops.

Other agents: Dictated by complications (antiarrhythmics, diuretics, vasodilators).

Surgery: Excision of vegetations and thrombi indicated only if uncontrollable sepsis develops; valve replacement may be indicated in severe congestive heart failure.[134]

RECOMMENDED ANTIBIOTIC COVERAGE FOR ENDOCARDITIS PROPHYLAXIS

Drug	Dosage	Comments
Penicillin V (oral)		
Initial dose	2 g 1 h before procedure	Appropriate for most patients
Follow-up dose	1 g 6 h after initial dose	
Erythromycin (oral)		
Initial dose	1 g 1 h before procedure	For patients allergic to penicillin; may also be used for patients receiving oral penicillin as continuous rheumatic fever prophylaxis
Follow-up dose	500 mg 6 h after initial dose	
Ampicillin plus gentamicin (IM or IV)		
Initial dose	Ampicillin 1-2 g plus gentamicin 1.5 mg/kg 30 min before procedure	For patients at higher risk (especially those with prosthetic heart valves) who are not allergic to penicillin
Follow-up dose	Penicillin V 1 g orally 6 h after initial dose	
Vancomycin (IV)		
Initial dose	1 g over 1 h started 1 h before procedure	For higher risk patients (especially those with prosthetic valves) who are allergic to penicillin
Follow-up dose	Not necessary	

Modified from the American Heart Association, Circulation 56:139A, 1978.

1 ASSESS

ASSESSMENT	OBSERVATIONS

General complaints	Recurrent temperature elevation
	  Acute endocarditis: high fever 39-40° C (102 − 104° F)
	  Subacute endocarditis: low-grade fever >39.4° C (102° F)
	Alternating chills and diaphoresis
	Malaise, weakness, arthralgia, anorexia, weight loss, headache

Signs of embolization of vegetation (peripheral, cerebral, systemic)	Petechiae in conjunctiva, palate, buccal mucosa, and extremities Splinter hemorrhages on nail beds Osler's nodes Janeway lesions Roth's spots Neurologic changes
Heart sounds	Early infection: Usually normal Late infection: Murmurs apparent if valve damage occurs; ventricular gallop (S_3) indicates ventricular failure
Abdomen	Splenomegaly (occurs in 23% of patients with acute endocarditis; occurs in 44% of patients with subacute endocarditis)

→ 〉 〉 〉

2   DIAGNOSE

NURSING DIAGNOSIS	SUBJECTIVE FINDINGS	OBJECTIVE FINDINGS
Altered body temperature related to infectious process	Complains of flu-like symptoms, chills, weakness, irritability, myalgias, arthralgias	Elevated temperature, diaphoresis, tachycardia, leukocytosis, elevated ESR, positive blood cultures, anemia
Altered nutrition: less than body requirements related to biologic factors (fever, infection)	Reports appetite loss, nausea, decreased food intake	Weight loss, anorexia, vomiting, pallor of conjunctiva and oral mucosa
Diversional activity deficit related to prolonged hospitalization	Complains of boredom or restlessness	Confined to hospital (4-6 wk), disinterested, excessive sleeping, restlessness, irritability, anger
Potential altered cerebral tissue perfusion related to embolism	Complains of persistent headache	Altered mental status, aphasia, focal or general neurologic deficits, limb weakness, numbness, hemiplegia
Potential altered splenic tissue perfusion related to embolism	Complains of abdominal pain	Left upper quadrant abdominal tenderness
Potential altered renal tissue perfusion related to embolism	No specific complaints	Decreased urine output, hematuria
Potential altered pulmonary tissue perfusion related to embolism	Reports SOB, sudden chest pain	Tachypnea, dyspnea, orthopnea, hemoptysis, nonproductive dry cough, cyanosis, diminished breath sounds

3   PLAN

Patient goals

1. Patient will demonstrate normal body temperature.
2. Patient will obtain adequate nutrition to maintain body function.
3. Patient will engage in identified inpatient diversional activities.
4. Patient will demonstrate no signs of altered tissue perfusion.
5. Patient will increase knowledge regarding risk of reinfection and methods of prevention.

4 IMPLEMENT

NURSING DIAGNOSIS	NURSING INTERVENTIONS	RATIONALE
Altered body temperature related to infectious process	Assess for dehydration: diaphoresis, poor skin turgor, dry mucous membranes.	Perspiration reflects body's attempt to reduce temperature; as fever rises, water loss via skin increases.
	Obtain temperature q 4-8 h as indicated; monitor patients with chronic low-grade fever for elevated temperature.	Elevated temperature represents infectious process.
	Monitor fluid intake and output q 8 h noting water loss due to perspiration.	To avoid negative fluid balance from dehydration; however, loss of 2.2 lbs (1 kg) in 24 h may indicate need for fluid replacement, since 1 L of fluid equals about 1 kg.
	Encourage fluid intake as tolerated.	To maintain fluid balance.
	Administer antibiotics as ordered, ensuring they are given on time.	Interruption in dosage can prolong length of time patient must receive medication.
	Administer antipyretics as ordered.	To reduce temperature.
	Monitor laboratory reports on CBC with differential and blood cultures.	Persistent leukocytosis and positive blood cultures may indicate inadequate antibiotic coverage or formation of myocardial abscess.
	Monitor IV sites for redness and swelling; change site q 48 h.	To avoid parenteral line sepsis.
Altered nutrition: less than body requirements related to biologic factors (fever, infection)	Assess for progressive weight loss and signs of malnutrition: weight below normal for age and height, fatigue, decreased biceps skinfold thickness; weigh patient daily; decrease frequency as weight stabilizes.	Infectious process increases metabolic needs, but chronic illness leads to anorexia; malnourishment decreases body's resistance to infection.
	Weigh patient daily; decrease frequency as weight stabilizes.	To determine amount of weight loss and need to add supplemental feeding.
	Monitor daily caloric intake as indicated by patient's appetite and food intake.	To obtain a 1 lb weight gain, 3500 calories above metabolic needs must be taken.
	Offer supplemental feedings high in calories and protein; consult with dietitian to direct nutritional requirements.	To ensure adequate intake of nutrients during anorexic periods.
	Offer small, frequent feedings.	Large meals may contribute to nausea.
	Ensure patient comfort during meal times; encourage patient to select foods.	To stimulate appetite.

→ 〉 〉 〉

NURSING DIAGNOSIS	NURSING INTERVENTIONS	RATIONALE
Diversional activity deficit related to prolonged hospitalization	Assess for diversional deficit and differentiate from progression of disease process.	Reactive signs of boredom are similar to early signs of low cardiac output.
	Assess level and type of diversional interest to explore appropriate inpatient activities.	As condition improves, patient begins to exhibit signs of boredom, resulting in depression or feelings of being trapped.
	Provide diversional activities such as occupational therapy, reading, television, radio, passes to leave hospital, and daily structured exercise program (unless contraindicated by clinical status).	Varying daily routines will increase stimulation and interest to participate in self-care and activities.
	Ensure a daily structured exercise program unless contraindicated by clinical status.	To maintain muscle tone and to promote sense of well-being.
Potential altered tissue perfusion related to embolism	Assess for signs of embolization each shift and as often as indicated; report any changes to physician.	To facilitate recognition of complications associated with endocarditis.
Potential altered cerebral tissue perfusion related to embolism	Perform neurologic checks every shift or as indicated by patient condition.	CNS emboli have been reported in 6%-31% of patients with IE.
Potential altered splenic tissue perfusion related to embolism	Assess for splenomegaly; report signs and symptoms as indicated by tender or painful abdomen.	Splenic emboli have been discovered in 44% of cases but frequently go undetected.
Potential altered renal tissue perfusion related to embolism	Monitor intake and output q 8 h or as indicated by patient condition.	A decrease in urine output may reflect renal emboli or infarction.
	Monitor laboratory data: urinalysis.	Hematuria is associated with embolization.
Potential altered pulmonary tissue perfusion related to embolism	Auscultate lung sounds q 4-8 h or as indicated by patient condition.	Right heart endocarditis is associated with pulmonary embolism or infarction.
Knowledge deficit	See Patient Teaching.	

5 EVALUATE

PATIENT OUTCOME	DATA INDICATING THAT OUTCOME IS ACHIEVED
Inflammation has cleared.	Temperature, blood cultures, white cell count, and other laboratory values are normal. Patient's sense of well-being is improved. Patient reports feeling less fatigued, improved appetite, and absence of sweats and headache.

PATIENT OUTCOME	DATA INDICATING THAT OUTCOME IS ACHIEVED
Nutritional status is improved and maintained.	Baseline or normal weight is regained. Patient demonstrates improved appetite.
Boredom is reduced.	Patient actively engages in diversional activities, verbalizes decreased feelings of boredom, and appears alert and animated.
Tissue perfusion is maintained.	Patient is alert and oriented. No signs of embolism are present, lung sounds are clear, and urine output is normal.
Knowledge level is increased.	Patient verbalizes understanding of factors that contribute to endocarditis, need for antibiotic prophylaxis, nature of disease, and signs and symptoms of recurrence.

PATIENT TEACHING

1. Provide instruction about the disease process and the purpose of treatment procedures.
2. Explain precipitating factors that can lead to bacteremia and reinfection: poor oral hygiene, dental work (cleaning, gum treatment, extractions), gastrointestinal or genitourinary procedures, vaginal deliveries, furuncles, staphylococcal infections, and surgical procedures.
3. Explain importance of notifying all physicians and dentists of endocarditis risk before having any procedures performed.
4. Encourage regular follow-up care with a medical physician.
5. Explain the need for good oral hygiene and regular dental care, and stress the importance of notifying dentist at first signs of oral infection or gum disease.
6. Explain and reinforce the importance of antibiotic prophylaxis before procedures that may cause bacteremia.

Myocarditis

Myocarditis is an inflammatory response of the myocardium that can be diffuse or focal.

Giant-cell myocarditis

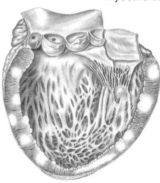

Histologically, the term **myocarditis** describes infiltration of myocardial cells by various forms of bacteria or viruses, which damage the myocardium by inciting an inflammatory response. Myocarditis generally occurs as the result of an infectious agent, but it also can be caused by radiation or other toxic physical agents such as lead. A variety of drugs—including phenothiazides, lithium, and chronic use of cocaine—may also lead to myocarditis.

In the United States the most common cause of myocarditis is viruses, (e.g., coxsackie Group B, ECHO), but a variety of bacterial, protozoal, and rickettsial diseases can produce inflammation of the heart. Myocarditis may also occur as a secondary complication to other diseases, including rheumatic fever, infectious mononucleosis, polio, mumps, or typhoid.

PATHOPHYSIOLOGY

The basic mechanism involved in myocardial damage begins with the acute phase, which involves the invasion of the myocardium by the offending agent or toxin. It is believed that antibodies against the toxin persist for several months, during which the inflammatory process is evident. In the late, or chronic, phase, myocardial damage occurs, probably the result of an immunologic response. Studies have implicated T-lymphocytes as the primary cause of cell-mediated toxic response that leads to myocardial destruction.[120]

COMPLICATIONS

Congestive heart failure
Dilated cardiomyopathy

DIAGNOSTIC STUDIES AND FINDINGS

Diagnostic test	Findings
Laboratory data	Leukocytosis with atypical lymphocytes; elevated ESR, viral titers; elevated CPK, LDH, SGOT
ECG	Conduction defects: LBBB
	Non-specific ST-T wave changes; Q-wave prolonged QT interval
	Tachyarrhythmias: atrial, ventricular ectopy
Chest x-ray	Normal C-T ratio; mild to moderate cardiomegaly, globular silhouette; pulmonary vascular congestion
Radionuclide studies	Detect inflammatory, necrotic changes in myocardium
Gallium 67; Technetium-99m-pyrophosphate	
Echocardiography	Regional wall abnormalities; dilated ventricles; hypokinesis of LV
Endomyocardial biopsy	Acute: appreciable lymphocyte, inflammatory cell infiltrates; myocyte necrosis (fraying of adjacent myocardial cells; myocardial fibrosis)
	Healing myocarditis: absence of myocyte necrosis; some persistent inflammatory cell infiltrate
	Healed myocarditis: absence of myocyte necrosis and active inflammatory cell infiltrate

MEDICAL MANAGEMENT

GENERAL MANAGEMENT

Physical activity: For acute myocarditis, bed rest with bathroom privileges during periods of fever, fatigue, and pain.

Cardiac monitoring: Used to evaluate and treat dysrhythmias.

DRUG THERAPY: Directed by clinical picture.

Antibiotics: If infecting agent can be isolated.

Immunosuppression therapy: Indicated for viral immune-mediated myocardial damage. Precise drug protocols are controversial but may include corticosteroids, azathioprine, or cyclosporine.

Antiarrhythmic agents

1 ASSESS

ASSESSMENT	OBSERVATIONS
General complaints	History of viral syndrome Fever, malaise, myalgias, fatigue, pericardial chest pain

Physical examination	Tachycardia
	Neck: lymphadenopathy; increased JVP
	Palpation: LV heave
	Pericardial friction rub
	Signs and symptoms of heart failure:
	    Breath sounds: crackles
	    Heart sounds:S_3
	Peripheral or dependent edema

2 DIAGNOSE

NURSING DIAGNOSIS	SUBJECTIVE FINDINGS	OBJECTIVE FINDING
Potential decreased cardiac output related to mechanical factors (preload, afterload, contractility) and electrical factors (dysrhythmias)	Increasing complaints of fatigue, exertional dyspnea, weakness	Tachycardia, tachypnea, orthopnea, pallor, diaphoresis, decreased urine output, increased JVD Breath sounds: crackles (rales); heart sound: S_3 chest x-ray: redistribution of blood to upper lobes; increased C-T ratio
Pain (chest) related to pericardial friction	Complains of chest pain with movement	Inability to rest quietly, need to sit up; Precordial chest pain, worsens with inspiration or movement Heart sounds: pericardial friction rub Chest x-ray: cardiac silhouette increased if pericardial effusion present

Other related nursing diagnoses

Fluid volume excess related to increased levels of aldosterone, sodium retention, and antidiuretic hormone

3 PLAN

Patient goals

1. Patient will demonstrate a stable and/or improved cardiac output.
2. Patient will verbalize absence of chest discomfort.

3. Patient will demonstrate increased level of knowledge.

→ > >

4 IMPLEMENT

NURSING DIAGNOSIS	NURSING INTERVENTION	RATIONALE
Potential decreased cardiac output related to mechanical factors (preload, afterload, contractility) and electrical factors (dysrhythmias)	Assess for signs and symptoms of decreased CO.	Clinical picture of each patient with myocarditis varies from no cardiac signs to congestive heart failure.
	Monitor vital signs q 4-8 h as indicated. Auscultate breath sounds and heart sounds q 8 h.	To detect increasing signs of pulmonary congestion and ventricular failure.
	Bed rest with head of bed elevated; encourage periods of rest throughout day.	To decrease cardiac workload.
	Administer medications as ordered.	Cardiac drugs are administered to increase contractility and decrease preload and afterload.
Pain (chest) related to pericardial friction	Assess quality of chest pain.	To distinguish pericardial pain from myocardial ischemia.
	Encourage bed rest; elevate head of bed; have patient lean forward on over-bed table.	Pericardial pain may be aggravated by turning or twisting; pain may be relieved by leaning forward.
	Administer analgesics as ordered.	To provide symptomatic relief.

5 EVALUATE

PATIENT OUTCOME	DATA INDICATING THAT OUTCOME IS REACHED
CO is maintained or improved.	Vital signs within normal limits. Patient reports absence of symptoms. Patient appears comfortable; activities are well tolerated.
Patient is free of pain.	Patient verbalizes absence of chest pain; appears relaxed, engages in hospital routines and activities without pain. There is no pericardial friction rub.
Patient's knowledge level is increased.	Patient demonstrates understanding of disease process and signs and symptoms to report to physician.

PATIENT TEACHING

1. Review nature of disease process and signs and symptoms to report to physician.
2. Review need to check with physician before resuming physical activities. **Caution** patient to avoid active physical exercise during and following viral or bacterial infection.
3. If the patient is on immunosuppression therapy, review drugs, dosages, and side effects.

Pericarditis

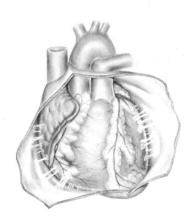

Pericarditis is an inflammatory process involving the parietal and visceral layers of the pericardium and outer myocardium.

Pericarditis may occur as an isolated process or as a complication of a systemic disease. Its designation as acute or chronic is based primarily on onset, frequency of occurrence, and symptoms. Acute pericarditis, which can occur within 2 weeks of the offending condition, lasts up to 6 weeks. It may be accompanied by effusion or tamponade. Chronic pericarditis may follow acute pericarditis and may last up to 6 months.

PATHOPHYSIOLOGY

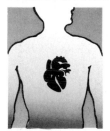

Because of the close proximity of the pericardium to structures such as the pleura, lungs, sternum, diaphragm, and myocardium, pericarditis may be the consequence of a number of inflammatory or infectious processes. The most common cause is idiopathic, probably viral; this generally has a favorable prognosis (Table 4-4).

Agents or processes causing pericardial inflammation do so by direct extension or by irritation. Under normal conditions the pericardial sac contains up to 50 ml of clear, serouslike fluid. When an acute injury occurs, an exudate of fibrin, white blood cells, and endothelial cells is released, covering the parietal and visceral layers of pericardium. Resultant friction between the pericardial layers causes irritation and inflammation of the surrounding pleura and tissues. This fibrinous exudate may localize to one region of the heart or be generalized. Acute pericarditis may be "dry" and fibrinous or obstruct the heart's venous and lymphatic drainage, causing seepage of fibrin exudate and serous fluid into the pericardial sac, which creates pericardial effusion.[165]

Serofibrinous exudates occur in varying amounts from 100 ml to 3L and may appear straw colored or turbid with fibrin strands. The exudate of pyrogenic pericarditis is purulent. The characteristics of pericardial exudate fluid are summarized in Table 4-5.

Table 4-4

COMMON ETIOLOGIES OF ACUTE AND CONSTRICTIVE PERICARDITIS

Etiologic agent	Comments
Virus (idiopathic)	Organism may never be isolated; most common offenders are coxsackie B, influenza A or B, infectious mononucleosis
Infection	Bacterial tuberculous; fungal, such as *Histoplasma nocardia*; parasitic
Neoplastic diseases	Primary: mesothelioma; secondary: either by direct extension or metastases from lung, breast, lymphoma
Radiotherapy	Radiation to chest
Drug therapy	Hydralazine, Procainamide, Minoxidil, Isoniazid
Autoimmune disorders	Systemic lupus erythamatosus, rheumatic fever (seen commonly in children), vasculitis, rheumatoid arthritis, dermatomyositis, scleroderma
Metabolic disorders	Uremia, spontaneous or in association with hemodialysis, myxedema; gout
Trauma	Chest trauma: blunt or penetrating, following CPR
	Myocardial infarction (Dressler's syndrome, postmyocardial infarction syndrome); cardiac surgery (postpericardiotomy syndrome)

Table 4-5

CHARACTERISTICS OF PERICARDIAL FLUID

Characteristic	Normal fluid	Exudate effusion
Appearance	Clear	Clear or turbid with fibrin sheds; straw or amber color; may appear hemorrhagic because of RBCs; may be purulent
Volume	50 ml	>100 ml (up to 3 L)
Specific gravity	<1.015	>1.015 (usually >1.017)
Total protein	<2 g/dl	>3 g/dl
Seromucin clot	Negative	Positive
Coagulation	Uncommon	Usual
Cells	Few	Few
Glucose	Nearly equal to plasma glucose	Nearly equal to plasma glucose
Culture	Negative	Negative

A slowly developing effusion of moderate amount (350 to 500 ml) may not alter cardiovascular dynamics. However, a rapidly accumulating effusion, regardless of amount, can interfere with diastolic filling and lead to cardiac tamponade.

The clinical syndrome of chronic pericarditis can occur in a variety of forms, including chronic pericardial effusion and constrictive or adhesive pericarditis. Chronic effusion may lead eventually to constrictive effusion, as described in the following paragraphs.

Constrictive pericarditis is characterized by pericardial thickening and scarring of the parietal or visceral pericardium. The layers become densely adherent to each other, obliterating the pericardial space. This adherence eventually involves the epicardial surface of the myocardium, causing the pericardium to become a totally noncompliant structure. In some cases the pericardium becomes calcified. Occasionally, the visceral layer attaches to the epicardium. A tense pericardial effusion develops. This form of constrictive pericardium is referred to as pericardium effusive "constricture pericarditis" (Goldberger).

As the pericardium becomes scarred and rigid, normal diastolic filling of the heart is impeded. In severe cases, left ventricular end-diastolic volume may be less than stroke volume, causing the stroke volume to be reduced with a subsequent drop in cardiac output. The normal compensatory tachycardia is unable to improve the cardiac output because of the constriction of the myocardium.

Constrictive pericarditis is usually generalized to all four chambers but may be localized to areas such as the right ventricle, pulmonary artery, or aortic root. When the chambers are uniformly involved, left and right ventricular diastolic pressure and atrial pressures equalize. As stroke volume diminishes, left and right filling pressures rise. When this is combined with reduced cardiac output, systemic and pulmonary congestion results.

COMPLICATIONS

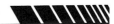

Pericardial effusion
Cardiac tamponade
Congestive heart failure

DIAGNOSTIC STUDIES AND FINDINGS

Diagnostic test	Findings
Laboratory studies	
Blood studies	Elevated WBC; elevated ESR; elevated viral titers
Urine cultures	Identification of organism in infectious process
Electrocardiogram (ECG)	**Acute pericarditis:**
	Stage I (Figure 4-26)—S-T segment elevation in LV leads V_5, V_6, I, II, aV_L, and aV_F during first few days; PR interval depression

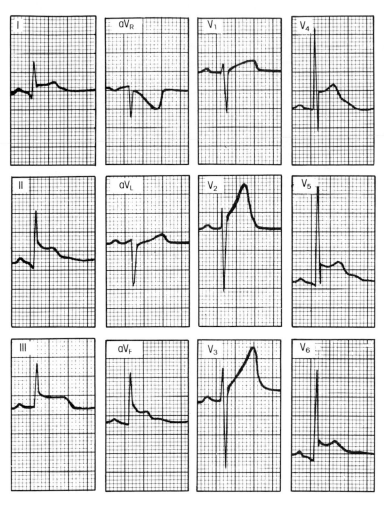

FIGURE 4-26
In acute pericarditis, ST segment elevation is typically upward and concave in leads I, II, aVF, and V₄ to V₆. (From Guzzetta.)[62]

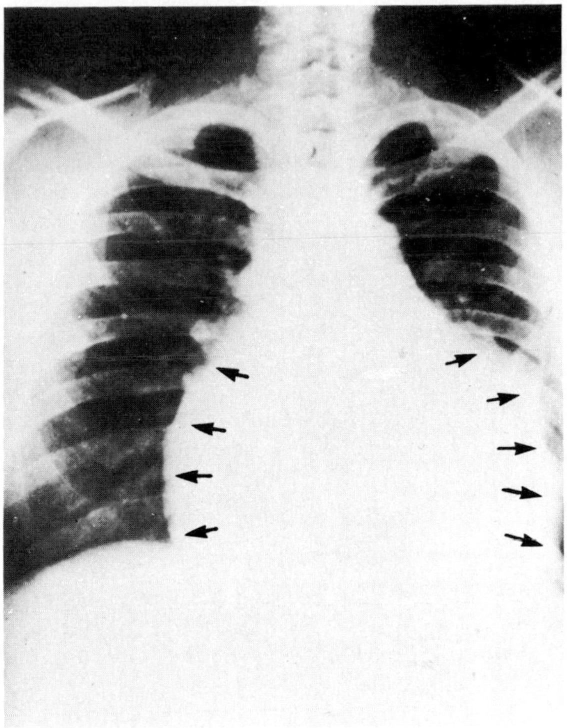

FIGURE 4-27
Chest x-ray showing pericardial effusion. Cardiac silhouette is enlarged and has globular shape *(arrows)*. (From Guzzetta.)[62]

Diagnostic test	Findings
	Stage II—return of ST segment to baseline; PR interval depression may persist
	Stage III—T wave inversions
	Stage IV—normalization of T waves
	Low-voltage QRS complexes in presence of pericardial effusion
	Atrial dysrhythmias
	Constrictive pericarditis:
	Wide P wave in leads I, II, and V; Q waves deep and wide; T waves flattened or inverted; low QRS voltage
Chest roentgenogram	Cardiac silhouette—normal or enlarged (enlarged with 250 ml or more of pericardial fluid) (Figure 4-27)
	Lung fields—clear
	Acute pericarditis:
	Normal if pericardial fluid < 250 ml

Continued.

Diagnostic test	Findings
Echocardiogram	**Constrictive pericarditis:** Normal or enlarged due to pericardial thickening or effusion; pericardial calcification Confirms presence of pericardial fluid (minimum of 20 ml can be detected) Abnormal echo—free space posterior to LV during systole (small effusion)
Radionuclide blood pool scanning (technetium-labeled macroaggregated albumin and thallium) **Magnetic resonance imaging (MRI)**	**Constrictive pericarditis:** Reduced LV posterior wall motion; abnormal movement of the septum characterized by flattening in systole and movement in diastole Demonstrates pericardial effusion outside of cardiac chambers; seen as abnormal space between heart and liver or heart and lungs Visualizes pericardium; can define thickened pericardium, thus differentiating acute vs chronic pericarditis
Cardiac catheterization	**Constrictive pericarditis:** Increased LA and RA pressures; loss of respiratory variation of the RA pressure curve; elevated pulmonary artery systolic pressure (35 - 40 mm Hg); elevated diastolic pressures equal in all four chambers, rarely differing by >5 mm Hg at rest or during exercise; CO normal in early stages, later decreased (<2.3 L/min/m^2); ejection fraction normal or decreased

MEDICAL MANAGEMENT

GENERAL MANAGEMENT

Physical activity:
Acute pericarditis—Bed rest with bathroom privileges during period of fever and pain; activity limited during acute period, with modification of all activities for 2 wk to allow inflammatory reaction of the pericardium to resolve.
Constrictive pericarditis—Bed rest with activity limitations before pericardiectomy; extent of limitation dictated by degree of hemodynamic compromise and symptoms

Diet: Acute pericarditis—Regular diet; encourage fluids during febrile period

Electrocardiography: Performed to rule out MI, when cardiac tamponade is suspected, and if patient demonstrates signs of cardiac decompensation.

Hemodynamic monitoring: Indicated if cardiac tamponade is evident for patients with constrictive pericarditis, closer monitoring of RAP, PAP, and CO; after pericardiectomy, elevated pressures may continue for several weeks or months.

MEDICAL MANAGEMENT—cont'd

DRUG THERAPY

Acute pericarditis:
Anti-inflammatory agents for symptomatic relief of chest pain, fever, and malaise in absence of clinical signs of cardiac tamponade.

Analgesic-antipyretics: Aspirin.

Nonsteroidal anti-inflammatory agents: Indomethacin (Indocin).

Corticosteroids: Less effective; given only in persistent recurring pericarditis and effusion.

Constrictive pericarditis: Chemotherapeutic agents aimed at specific cause—e.g., patients with known or suspected tuberculosis should receive antituberculous therapy before and after pericardiectomy.

SURGERY

Pericardiocentesis: Removal of pericardial fluid or blood by aspiration through needle or catheter inserted into parietal pericardium; indicated when persistent or large effusions are compromising LV function.

Pericardial window: Open pericardial drainage implemented for acute suppurative and chronic effusions; has certain advantages over pericardiocentesis: multiple aspirations can be avoided, pericardial tissue can be obtained for culture, pericardium can be visualized, and clots and fibrin deposits can be removed.

Pericardiectomy: Surgical removal of visceral and parietal pericardium; has excellent long-term benefits; operative mortality of about 10%; best results when myocardial fibrosis and ventricular atrophy are not far advanced and when total or near-total pericardiectomy is performed; if hemodynamic improvement not seen immediately, elevated pressures and abnormal waveforms continue for several weeks owing to atrophy of ventricles that have been immobilized for long periods—thus early pericardiectomy is encouraged before dense fibrosis and myocardial atrophy occur; postoperative care similar to that for any cardiac surgical patient.

1 ASSESS

ASSESSMENT	OBSERVATIONS	
	ACUTE PERICARDITIS	CONSTRICTIVE PERICARDITIS
General complaints	Chest pain: location—retrosternal or precordial radiating to neck and back, sudden pleuritic-like pain that worsens with deep inspiration, movement, or lying down and is relieved by sitting up or leaning forward; sharp, deep, persistent ache; tachypnea; shallow breathing; dyspnea in presence of pleural effusion or owing to impaired cardiac filling from compression of heart; restlessness; anxiety; malaise; dysphagia	Exertional dyspnea; fatigue; orthopnea; palpitations; PND; cough; peripheral edema

→ > >

ASSESSMENT	OBSERVATIONS	
	ACUTE PERICARDITIS	CONSTRICTIVE PERICARDITIS
Physical examination	Low-grade temperature (39° C [102° F]); may be associated with diaphoresis and chills; auscultation: pericardial friction rub—best heard with patient leaning forward, heard in second, third, or fourth intercostal space to left of sternal border or at apex, loudest during inspiration, varies in intensity (grade 4 to 5), may be transient, triphasic consisting of presystolic, systolic, and diastolic components, scratchy, grating	Afebrile; elevated JVP with presence of Kussmaul sign (increased distention during inspiration); arterial pressure normal or slightly reduced; diffuse precordial movement; decreased amplitude; absence of localized apical impulse; paradoxic pulse (rarely > 15 mm Hg); auscultation: quiet, distant heart sounds, pericardial knock—early diastolic sound, accentuated with inspiration and heard best along lower LSB; clinical signs of elevated venous pressure: peripheral edema, hepatomegaly, ascites

2 DIAGNOSE

NURSING DIAGNOSIS	SUBJECTIVE FINDINGS	OBJECTIVE FINDINGS
Anxiety related to actual or perceived threat to biologic integrity	Verbalizes apprehension; expresses concern and is fearful	Restlessness, diaphoresis
Pain (chest) related to pericardial inflammation	Reports chest discomfort and fatigue	Inability to rest quietly; orthopnea, dyspnea, elevated temperature
Potential decreased cardiac output related to reduced ventricular filling	Complains of restlessness agitation, SOB, weakness	Dyspnea; jugular venous distention Skin: pallor, cool, diaphoretic; tachycardia, tachypnea, dysphagia Pericardial effusion: muffled heart sounds Breath sounds: Ewart's sign—patch of dullness beneath tip of left scapula; crackles

Other related nursing diagnoses

Fluid volume excess related to increased levels of aldosterone, sodium retention, and ADH

3 PLAN

Patient goals

1. Patient will demonstrate reduced anxiety level.
2. Patient will verbalize absence of chest discomfort.
3. Patient will demonstrate stable CO.
4. Patient will demonstrate increased understanding of disease process.

4 IMPLEMENT

NURSING DIAGNOSIS	NURSING INTERVENTIONS	RATIONALE
Anxiety related to actual or perceived threat to biologic integrity	Assess level of anxiety and degree of understanding noting verbal and and nonverbal expressions regarding diagnoses and procedures.	To determine source of anxiety and to identify any misconceptions regarding disease process and treatment.
	Provide supportive care.	To ensure sense of trust and comfort as well as reassurance that feelings are appropriate to express.
Pain (chest) related to pericardial inflammation	Ensure quiet environment.	To reduce external stimuli.
	Assess quality of chest pain.	To distinguish pericardial pain from myocardial ischemia.
	Administer medications as ordered: nonsteroid anti-inflammatory drugs. Evaluate pain response.	To provide relief of pain and to suppress inflammatory symptoms of pericarditis.
	Encourage bed rest; elevate head of bed; position for comfort; have patient lean forward on over-bed table.	Pericardial pain is aggravated by movements such as turning in bed or twisting the body.
Potential decreased cardiac output related to reduced ventricular filling	Assess for signs and symptoms of decreased cardiac compression.	Cardiac compression is a complication of pericarditis, which can be caused by (1) pericardial effusions leading to tamponade or (2) development of fibrosis and/or calcification of pericardium, resulting in constrictive pericarditis.
	Check for pulsus paradoxus, narrowing pulse pressure, and respiratory filling of neck veins.	To detect early signs of increasing intrapericardial pressure and development of tamponade. Rate of fluid accumulation varies and may be of sudden onset in acute pericarditis.
	Monitor vital signs q 4-8 h as indicated.	To detect pericardial restriction, decreased BP, and tachycardia.
	Place on cardiac monitor checking rhythm q 1-2 h.	Pericarditis produces nonspecific changes due to superficial injury to epicardial surface of heart.
	Obtain 12-lead ECG as ordered.	To differentiate and monitor pericarditis vs ischemia. To detect reduced QRS voltage due to fluid accumulation that may interfere with electrical currents of heart.
	Auscultate heart sounds for presence of pericardial friction rub (may be distant).	Friction rub reflects friction between roughened pericardial and epicardial surfaces; it may also reflect presence of small or large effusion. Muffled heart sounds may be due to fluid accumulated between chest wall and heart chambers.

→ › ›

NURSING DIAGNOSIS	NURSING INTERVENTIONS	RATIONALE
Knowledge deficit	See Patient Teaching.	

5 EVALUATE

PATIENT OUTCOME	DATA INDICATING THAT OUTCOME IS REACHED
Patient demonstrates decreased anxiety.	Patient verbalizes relief of pain. Patient demonstrates ability to rest and sleep without complaint. Patient appears relaxed. Patient tolerates routine activities and procedures without complaining of pain or SOB.
Patient is free of chest discomfort.	Patient verbalizes absence of pericardial irritation. ECG is normal. There is no friction rub or chest pain. WBC count and ESR are normal. Temperature is normal.
CO is maintained.	Patient demonstrates hemodynamic stability. BP and pulse are maintained at baseline. Heart and breath sounds are normal. Absence of pulsus paradoxus. Chest x-ray is normal.
Patient shows an increased level of understanding.	Patient identifies signs and symptoms to report to physician. Patient verbalizes knowledge regarding disease, activity allowances and limitations, and medications.

PATIENT TEACHING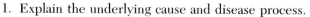

1. Explain the underlying cause and disease process.
2. Instruct the patient in signs and symptoms of recurring inflammation. Explain that signs and symptoms may continue up to 2 weeks and that during that time to avoid overexertion and heavy lifting. Instruct the patient to notify the physician if symptoms do not diminish and/or increase.
3. Explain the purpose, method of administration, and side effects of medication.

Cardiac Tamponade

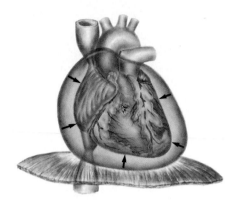

Hemopericardium and tamponade

Cardiac tamponade is acute cardiac compression caused when fluid accumulation within the pericardial sac exerts increased pressure around the heart. The result is restriction of flow in and out of the ventricles.

PATHOPHYSIOLOGY

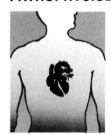

Tamponade is most commonly caused by acute pericarditis but is quite common in patients with malignant and uremic pericardial effusions. A hemopericardium, bleeding into the pericardial spaces, may occur as a result of chest trauma, cardiac surgery, myocardial rupture, aortic dissection, or anticoagulant therapy.

The pericardial sac normally holds 30 to 50 ml of fluid, creating subatmospheric intrapericardial pressures of approximately -1 to -3 mm Hg during expira-

tion and -5 mm Hg with inspiration. An increase in pericardial fluid can cause a rise in intrapericardial pressure, first to 0 mm Hg and eventually to a positive value. However, it is the rate of accumulation, not the volume, that determines the degree to which ventricular filling becomes restricted and whether cardiac tamponade will ensue.

When pericardial fluid accumulates slowly, large volumes (1 to 2 L) can be readily accommodated because of the stretching of pericardial fibers. During rapid filling, however, the pericardium fails to stretch, causing intrapericardial pressure to rise to a level ex-

---

PULSUS PARADOXUS

Pulsus paradoxus is a phenomenon in which there is an abnormally large drop in arterial pulse during inspiration; normal pulse reappears during expiration. In normal persons, the arterial pulse falls 4-5 mm Hg during inspiration. An inspiratory decrease in systolic arterial pulsations exceeding 10 mm Hg is considered abnormal.

Causes of pulsus paradoxus

1. Cardiac tamponade
2. Constrictive pericarditis
3. Acute or chronic respiratory distress
4. Hypovolemic shock
5. Restrictive cardiomyopathy
6. Massive pulmonary emboli
7. Intubated patients undergoing positive pressure ventilation

Technique for determining pulsus paradoxus

1. Inflate BP cuff 20 mm Hg above systolic pressure instructing patient to breathe normally.
2. Begin to deflate cuff slowly and evenly until the first BP sounds (Korotkoff) are heard. During deflation, it becomes evident that some sounds are audible during expiration but not during inspiration.
3. Continue deflating the cuff until the BP sounds are heard throughout the respiratory cycle.
4. Pulsus paradoxus is measured as the difference between the first intermittently heard BP sounds (heard only during expiration) and the appearance of all the sounds (heard throughout the entire respiratory cycle).

ceeding normal filling pressure of the ventricles. When this occurs, filling of the ventricles is restricted, stroke volume decreases, and cardiac output falls. These hemodynamic alterations are followed by hypotension and shock. Pulsus paradoxus, an important hemodynamic feature of tamponade, is an abnormally large inspiratory fall in arterial pressure. When left ventricular filling and stroke volume are decreased with inspiration, blood pools in the lung and right side of the heart, increasing intrapericardial pressure. Therefore, during inspiration a greater negative intrathoracic pressure occurs, resulting in a dramatic fall in systolic blood pressure and pulse volume. The arterial blood pressure may normally fall 4 to 5 mm Hg during inspiration, but a decrease of 10 mm Hg or more is considered abnormal.

COMPLICATIONS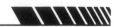

Heart failure
Cardiogenic shock
Cardiac arrest

DIAGNOSTIC STUDIES AND FINDINGS

Diagnostic test	Findings
Chest roentgenogram	Enlarged cardiac silhouette (globular configuration depending on degree of effusion); lung fields clear
ECG	Nonspecific ST and T wave changes; diminished voltage with altering voltage of both P wave and PRS; (electrical alternans) alternating voltage of QRS complex only is also seen; peaked T waves in precordial leads associated with hemopericardium
Echocardiogram	Increased pericardial fluid; paradoxic septal motion (septum moves toward LV during inspiration as RV fills); may be possible to estimate fluid volume
Radionuclide scan	May be possible to identify presence of pericardial fluid by demonstrating increased space between inferior border of the heart and liver
Magnetic resonance imaging (MRI)	May be used to show loculated effusions
Right heart catheterization	Documents hemodynamic parameters associated with tamponade: decreased ventricular filling pressures, elevated RAP, alteration (equalization) of pressures during inspiration

MEDICAL MANAGEMENT

GENERAL MANAGEMENT

Physical activity: Bed rest with head of bed elevated to position of comfort.

Nutrition: Nothing by mouth (NPO) in anticipation of pericardiocentesis; parenteral therapy as ordered to maintain adequate BP.

ECG and hemodynamic monitoring: Continuous monitoring of clinical signs and symptoms, as well as changes in hemodynamic parameters, to support patient until definitive treatment is initiated; arterial pressure monitored for pulsus paradoxus and hypotension.

Pericardiocentesis or pericardial window (subxiphoid incision and placement of tube for continuous drainage): To remove pericardial fluid and relieve cardiac compression.

MEDICAL MANAGEMENT—cont'd

DRUG THERAPY

Supportive therapy: Volume expansion with normal saline and infusion of inotropic agents to increase myocardial contractility and improve CO and BP.

SURGERY

Pericardiectomy: Removal of both parietal and visceral layers of pericardium—procedure is indicated as treatment for chronic, constrictive pericarditis.

1 ASSESS

ASSESSMENT	OBSERVATION
General complaints	Clinical presentation may vary from asymptomatic to dramatic and severe and is often non-specific; anxiety; tachypnea; mild dyspnea to marked respiratory distress; lightheadedness; fatigue; chest discomfort (fullness, heaviness); peripheral pallor and/or cyanosis; tachycardia; weak, absent peripheral pulses
Arterial pressures	Decreased systolic blood pressure; pulsus paradoxus greater than 10 mm Hg; soft or absent pulse during inspiration
Venous pressure	Elevated venous pressure; distended neck veins on inspiration (positive Kussmaul's sign)
Heart sounds	Auscultate for distant, often inaudible heart sounds, due to accumulation of pericardial fluid; diminished heart sounds
Cardiac pressures	Lowered left atrial pressure
Cardiac output	Decreased

2 DIAGNOSE

NURSING DIAGNOSIS	SUBJECTIVE FINDINGS	OBJECTIVE FINDINGS
Decreased cardiac output related to restricted ventricular filling	Feeling of heaviness, SOB Normal HR; normal BP Light-headedness, fatigue	Mild tamponade Moderate to severe tamponade Pallor, hypotension, tachycardia, oliguria, stupor
Anxiety (moderate to severe) related to perceived and/or actual threat to biologic integrity	Apprehension, anxiety, fear progressing to panic	Restlessness, tachycardia, tachypnea, diaphoretic

→ › › ›

3   PLAN

Patient goals

1. Patient will demonstrate hemodynamic stability.
2. Patient will demonstrate reduced anxiety.
3. Patient will demonstrate increased level of knowledge.

4   IMPLEMENT

NURSING DIAGNOSIS	NURSING INTERVENTIONS	RATIONALE
Decreased cardiac output related to restricted ventricular filling pressure	Assess for and estimate degree of pulsus paradoxus and increased JVP.	Reflects presence of tamponade and increasing intrapericardial pressure.
	Monitor arterial pressure, pulse pressure, pulse volume, ECG, and level of consciousness q 5-15 minutes.	To evaluate signs of progressive impairment of ventricular filling, decreased stroke volume.
	Assist with pericardiocentesis.	Removal of pericardial effusion causes drop in intrapericardial pressure.
	Administer inotropic and chronotropic medications as ordered.	To increase myocardial contractility and HR and reduce PVR.
	Administer colloid or crystalloid infusions as ordered.	To increase stroke volume and improve CO by increasing ventricular pressure.
Anxiety (moderate to severe) related to perceived and/or actual threat to biologic integrity	Assess level of anxiety, noting both verbal and nonverbal expressions.	Extreme anxiety leads to further release of catecholamines, which increase HR.
	During this period, remain with patient offering realistic assurances; use simple explanations.	Perception may become reduced, patient becomes highly distractible. Remaining with patient increases sense of trust and comfort in knowing staff is available.
Knowledge deficit	See Patient Teaching.	

5   EVALUATE

PATIENT OUTCOME	DATA INDICATING THAT OUTCOME IS REACHED
Improved ventricular compliance is shown by absence of tamponade.	Pulsus paradoxus decreases. Jugular venous distention decreases. Ventilation is improved. Pulse pressure and arterial pressure are normal. Kussmaul's sign is absent.
Anxiety level is reduced.	Patient appears relaxed; is able to tolerate routine activities and procedures without complaining of SOB.

PATIENT OUTCOME	DATA INDICATING THAT OUTCOME IS REACHED
Patient's level of knowledge is increased.	Patient verbalizes understanding of condition and need for medical intervention.

PATIENT TEACHING

1. Provide an explanation of the condition.
2. Explain the need for and procedures regarding pericardiocentesis or pericardiectomy as ordered.

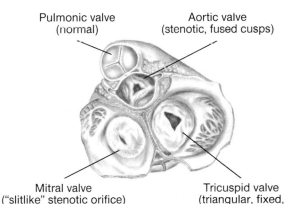

Pulmonic valve (normal)

Aortic valve (stenotic, fused cusps)

Mitral valve ("slitlike" stenotic orifice)

Tricuspid valve (triangular, fixed, stenotic orifice)

Valvular Heart Disease

Valvular heart disease is an acquired or congenital disorder of a cardiac valve, characterized by stenosis and obstructed blood flow or by valvular degeneration and regurgitation of blood.

With the introduction of antibiotic therapy and with improved diagnostic procedures, the incidence of valvular heart disease (VHD) has declined over the past three decades. It is most commonly a chronic illness, and symptoms requiring therapy may take years to develop. VHD may also occur as an acute illness following trauma or myocardial infarction.

PATHOPHYSIOLOGY

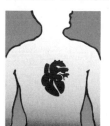

The etiology of VHD can be classified into congenital and acquired disorders.

Congenital disorders include bicuspid aortic valve and pulmonary stenosis. Although not usually classified as VHD, tricuspid and mitral pulmonary atresia and Ebstein's anomaly are all defects involving valvular function. Mitral valve prolapse (MVP) may also fall into this category.

Rheumatic fever and endocarditis account for the greatest number of cases of acquired VHD, but other disorders—such as Marfan's syndrome, cardiomyopathy, myocardial infarction, and myxomatous degeneration of the mitral valve, as well as trauma—can also lead to valvular dysfunction.

Two basic valve abnormalities exist: stenosis and regurgitation. In stenosis, narrowing of the valve orifice occurs as a result of thickening and rigidity of the valve leaflets. Stenosis produces an obstruction to flow across the valve, increasing the pressure gradient. In regurgitation (insufficiency, incompetency), calcification, scarring, and retraction of the leaflets or adjacent structures lead to an incomplete valve closure that results in retrograde blood flow. This can occur as a result of perforation of the leaflets, rupture of the chordae tendineae or papillary muscle, or dilatation of the left ventricle. Mixed lesions, in which both problems exist, can also occur. In addition, more than one valve may be affected.

The burden placed on the ventricles by valvular lesions can be classified in terms of pressure and volume overload. Pressure overload leads over a period of years to an increase in intramyocardial wall tension, which enables the heart to pump more blood through the highly resistant valve opening. This results in an increase in left ventricular wall thickness, and ventricular hypertrophy. Volume overload, on the other hand, leads to dilatation of the affected chamber and hypertrophy as the work of the ventricle increases proportionally to the volume of regurgitated blood. In the early stages, the stroke volume will compensate by increasing in order to maintain an effective stroke volume that is within normal limits. But, over time, a gradual decline in the contractile state of the ventricular myocardium begins to occur, and heart failure develops.

In the following sections, five valvular disorders are presented.

Mitral Stenosis

The most common cause of mitral stenosis is rheumatic valvulitis that leads to fibrotic thickening and fusion of the valve commissures. In addition, scarring of the free margins of the anterior and posterior leaflets occurs with shortening and thickening of the chordae tendineae, which may contribute to the mitral regurgitation often seen with mitral stenosis.

The normal mitral valve orifice is 4 to 6 cm^2. When this opening is reduced, flow across the valve is obstructed, increasing the pressure gradient necessary to eject blood from the left atrium to the left ventricle. The pressure gradient rises to ensure maintenance of cardiac output. When the mitral orifice is decreased to 1.5 cm^2, cardiac output drops and symptoms appear with exertion. As the disease progresses, the mean left atrial pressure rises, causing left atrial chamber enlargement. The increased left atrial pressure is reflected in the pulmonary capillaries and pulmonary artery. As pulmonary capillary pressure rises, fluid flows back across the alveolar membrane, eventually exceeding oncotic pressure of the plasma proteins in the blood and forcing fluid out of the capillaries into the lung. Pulmonary edema develops if this fluid cannot be removed by lymphatic drainage.

Mitral Regurgitation

Rheumatic fever, the usual cause of mitral regurgitation, produces thickening, scarring, rigidity, and calcification of the valve leaflets. The commissures become fused with the chordae tendineae, causing shortening and retraction of the leaflets, which prevents them from complete closure during systole. A nonrheumatic cause of mitral regurgitation is myocardial infarction, which causes dilation of the left ventricle and displacement of the papillary muscles. Papillary muscle dysfunction may also occur as a result of rupture or fibrosis caused by ischemia, infarction, and ventricular aneurysm at the base of a papillary muscle. In addition, annular dilation may lead to an incompetent mitral apparatus. The most common cause is left ventricular dilation resulting from coronary artery disease or congestive cardiomyopathy.

As mitral valve incompetence progresses, the retrograde flow to the left atrium causes left atrial pressure to rise. This pressure is reflected in the pulmonary veins, leading to transudation of fluid into the lungs.

The progressive increase in backward flow causes atrial dilation and enlargement. The left ventricle becomes hypertrophied, since it must deal with the larger volume of blood that is lost to the left atrium during systole.

Aortic Stenosis

Aortic stenosis can be classified as occurring at the supravalvular, valvular, and subvalvular levels. Of the three, valvular aortic stenosis is the most commonly seen, occurring most frequently as result of a congenital bicuspid or unicuspid valve and degenerative changes associated with aging. Congenital bicuspid valve occurs in 1% to 2% of the population, with a preponderance in males (3:1).[128] A less common cause of aortic stenosis is rheumatic heart disease. In rheumatic aortic stenosis, the cusps become thickened and develop commissural fusion. Degenerative stenosis, which is found in persons over age 65, is caused by thickening and calcifications of aortic cusps.

The normal aortic valve orifice measures 2.6 to 3.5 cm^2. Valve narrowing results from calcification of the leaflets. Calcification may extend into the aortic wall or onto the anterior leaflet of the mitral valve, which accounts for the mitral disease commonly occurring with aortic stenosis. Calcification may also extend into the conduction system, leading to conduction defects. As the disease progresses, calcification makes the valve inflexible, reducing the opening to a small slit.

As the aortic valve orifice decreases, left ventricular pressure rises to generate pressures sufficient to eject a normal stroke volume and propel flow across the valve into the aorta. This obstruction to left ventricular outflow leads to a pressure gradient between the aorta and left ventricle during systole. To maintain flow across the narrowed valve orifice, wall thickness gradually increases in the pressure-overloaded left ventricle, leading eventually to hypertrophy. In time the flow across the valve becomes fixed, and cardiac output does not increase in response to demand. During exercise the increased flow to extremities in the setting of fixed cardiac output causes a decreased cerebral blood flow, resulting in dizziness or syncope.

Left atrial hypertrophy occurs in a compensatory attempt to increase cardiac output. To produce a forceful atrial contraction, left ventricular end-diastolic pressure (LVEDP) rises, which in turn increases the myocardial fiber stretch and leads to increased contraction and improvement in stroke volume.

The clinical course of aortic stenosis depends on the size of the valve orifice and the compensated left ventricle. When myocardial contractility falls, the left ventricle dilates, causing diastolic and left atrial pressures to increase further.

The onset of symptoms of heart failure indicates moderate to severe disease, and death often occurs less than 5 years after symptoms appear. Sudden death is associated with severe aortic stenosis (0.5 to 0.7 cm^2).

Aortic Regurgitation

Incompetency of the aortic valve is attributed to numerous causes. Rheumatic fever, syphilis, and infective endocarditis are common causes. Connective tissue disorders such as Marfan's syndrome are also implicated in this disease.

The basic hemodynamic problem in aortic regurgitation is a volume-overloaded left ventricle. Blood ejected during normal systole reenters the left ventricle in diastole. To compensate for this regurgitant volume, the left ventricle must produce a higher stroke volume by increasing the systolic pressure, resulting in eventual hypertrophy of the left ventricle.

With time, LVEDP and left atrial pressure increase. As myocardial contractility diminishes and failure occurs, mitral regurgitation may result from malposition of papillary muscles.

Mitral Valve Prolapse

Mitral valve prolapse (MVP) is a term that describes superior systolic displacement of the mitral leaflets. First described by Barlow in 1963, various terms* have been used to describe what has come to be one of the most commonly found disorders involving the mitral

*Billowing mitral valve syndrome, Barlow's syndrome, systolic click-late systolic murmur syndrome, and floppy mitral valve syndrome

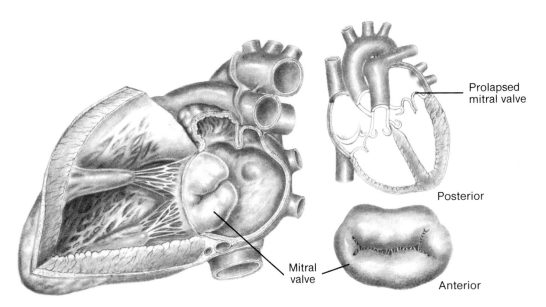

Prolapsed mitral valve

Posterior

Anterior

Mitral valve

FIGURE 4-28
Mitral valve prolapse.

valve. Reports have indicated that as many as 15% of otherwise normal healthy young persons will demonstrate some bowing or arching upward of the mitral leaflets during systole.[130,146,187] It is becoming increasingly clear that a large number of these cases reflect what is considered to be normal superior systolic displacement of the mitral leaflets. However, when there is excessive valvuloventricular disproportion, it is believed that the findings reflect the primary connective tissue abnormality of the mitral leaflets, the anulus, and chordae tendineae referred to as MVP (Figure 4-28).

MVP can occur as an isolated abnormality or in individuals with other connective tissue abnormalities such as Marfan's syndrome and Ehler-Danlos syndrome. It can also occur in association with patent ductus arteriosus, atrial septal defects, Ebstein's anomaly, or in persons with skeletal abnormalities such as pectus excavatum and pectus carinatum. While it is found in people of all ages and both sexes, it is detected more frequently in females under 40 years.

In MVP, either the posterior leaflet alone or the posterior and anterior leaflets bulge or billow up into the left atrium during ventricular systole. This billowing is due to the redundancy of the valve tissue resulting from myxomatous degeneration of the middle layer (spongiosa) of the mitral valve's three layers. This redundancy, which makes the mitral valve too large for the ventricle, intrudes on the fibrosa layer, weakening the valve's ventricular surface, and allows the bulging of the weakened valve toward the atrium. In addition, elongation and thinning of chordae tendineae and an enlarged valve orifice may occur.

The clinical findings are dependent on the degree to which the leaflets prolapse in the atrium. If the mitral leaflets prolapse to such an extent that the contact between the two leaflets is impaired, then mitral regurgitation will result.[182]

COMPLICATIONS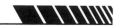

Infective endocarditis
Embolism
LV failure
RV failure
Ruptured papillary muscles of chordae tendineae
Pulmonary edema

DIAGNOSTIC STUDIES AND FINDINGS

Diagnostic test	Findings				
	Mitral stenosis	Mitral regurgitation	Aortic stenosis	Aortic regurgitation	Mitral valve prolapse
ECG	LA enlargement; notched P wave (P mitrale); RV hypertrophy	LA enlargement; LV hypertrophy; atrial fibrillation	LV hypertrophy; conduction defects: first-degree A-V block, LBBB	LV hypertrophy	Normal; may show ST segment and T-wave abnormalities, especially in inferior leads or prominent U waves; dysrhythmias, supraventricular tachyarrhythmias, premature atrial or ventricular beats
Chest roentgenogram	LA and RV enlargement; pulmonary venous congestion; interstitial pulmonary edema	LA and LV enlargement; pulmonary vascular congestion	Poststenotic aortic dilation; aortic valve calcification	Aortic valve calcification; LV enlargement; dilation of ascending aorta	Identifies or confirms presence of skeletal abnormalities
Echocardiogram	Decreased excursion of leaflets; diminished E to F slope	LA enlargement; hyperdynamic LV	Nonrestricted movement of aortic valve; thickening of LV wall	LV dilation; diastolic fluttering of anterior leaflet	2-D records mild to moderate degree superior systolic displacement of posterior and/or both mitral leaf-

Diagnostic test	Findings				
	Mitral stenosis	Mitral regurgitation	Aortic stenosis	Aortic regurgitation	Mitral valve prolapse
					lets, and the coaptation of point of the cusps; records atrial size, chordal rupture; Doppler records degree of mitral regurgitation
Radionuclide studies	To determine resting and exercise ejection fraction	To determine resting and exercise ejection fraction	To determine resting and exercise ejection fraction	To determine resting and exercise ejection fraction	To determine resting and exercise ejection fraction
Cardiac catheterization	Pressure across mitral valve increased; LA pressure increased; PCWP increased; low CO	LVEDP increased; LAP increased; angiography with contrast media performed to quantify regurgitation	Pressure gradient in systole across aortic valve; LVEDP increased	Pulse pressure increased; LVEDP increased; LAP increased; angiography with contrast media performed to quantify regurgitation	Normal unless mitral regurgitation present; LV angiogram shows the prolapsed mitral valve

MEDICAL MANAGEMENT

GENERAL MANAGEMENT: Dictated by severity of valvular disorder

Diet therapy: Sodium restriction for patients with mild to moderate signs of pulmonary congestion.

Percutaneous balloon catheter dilation: A palliative procedure that is still under investigation; used in treatment of calcific valvular stenosis. The procedure involves passing a catheter under fluoroscopy across the stenosed valve. Once in place the balloon is inflated repeatedly until valve gradient is relieved. At present, procedure is limited to patients who may be at some risk for valve surgery, including children, the elderly, and women of childbearing age.

Cardioversion: Indicated for patients with mitral stenosis in atrial fibrillation.

DRUG THERAPY: Guided by patient's clinical signs and symptoms.

Digitalis and diuretics: For heart failure

Quinidine, procainamide, propranolol: For dysrhythmias.

Anticoagulants: For patients in atrial fibrillation who are at risk for systemic or pulmonary embolization; warfarin sodium (Coumadin) in doses titrated to maintain prothrombin time at two times control.

Antibiotic prophylaxis: Before any procedure that increases risk of endocarditis. (see page 140)

SURGERY: Indicated when medical therapy no longer alleviates clinical symptoms or when there is diagnostic evidence of progressive myocardial failure (e.g. progressive enlargement of heart).

MEDICAL MANAGEMENT—cont'd

Open mitral commissurotomy (valvulotomy): Surgical splitting of stenotic and fused valve leaflet by inserting expandable dilator into the mitral orifice and separating fused commissures; palliative procedure performed only for pure mitral stenosis that involves leaflets and not chordae; contraindicated in patients with history of emboli.

Valvular annuloplasty: Reparative procedure of valve ring, chordae, or papillary muscle performed primarily for mitral and tricuspid regurgitation.

Valve replacement: Replacement on stenotic or incompetent valve with bioprosthetic or mechanical valve; commonly used valves include pynolite tilting disks, porcine heterografts, pericardial valves, and ball-in-cage valves.

Assessment of the patient with VHD varies depending on the presenting symptoms. In the early stages, VHD may be identified only by the presence of a specific murmur, but over the course of time, the patient may become progressively more symptomatic. Therefore it becomes necessary to establish a baseline assessment to determine both the progression of the disease process and the effectiveness of the medical plan.

1 ASSESS

	OBSERVATIONS				
ASSESSMENT	MITRAL STENOSIS	MITRAL REGURGITATION	AORTIC STENOSIS	AORTIC REGURGITATION	MITRAL VALVE PROLAPSE
General complaints	Fatigue; DOE; palpitations; hemoptysis; hoarseness; orthopnea; PND	Dyspnea; fatigue; exercise intolerance; orthopnea; palpitations	Fatigue; dyspnea; orthopnea; angina pectoris; dizziness; syncope	DOE; palpitations; orthopnea; exertional chest pain	Atypical chest pain, fatigue, palpitations, dizziness, dyspnea that may be accompanied by light headedness and giddiness, syncopo
Physical examination	Resting tachycardia; irregular pulse; jugular venous distention increased in presence of RV failure; prominent "a" wave with pulmonary hypertension (absent in atrial fibrillation)	Irregular pulse; sharp upstroke of arterial pulse; jugular venous distention increased in presence of RV failure; prominent "a" wave with increased RV pressure	Early: normal BP blood pressure; late: systolic pressure decreased; narrow pulse pressure; carotid pulse slow with small pulse volume	Arterial pulsations: bounding pulse with rapid rise and fall (water-hammer pulse); widened pulse pressure; head bobbing (de Musset's sign); skin warm, damp, and flushed	Skeletal abnormalities—pectus excavatum, pectus carinatum, scoliosis, or kyphosis

	OBSERVATIONS				
ASSESSMENT	**MITRAL STENOSIS**	**MITRAL REGURGITATION**	**AORTIC STENOSIS**	**AORTIC REGURGITATION**	**MITRAL VALVE PROLAPSE**
Cardiac palpation	Diastolic thrill at apex	Apical impulse forceful and displaced downward and to left	Systolic thrill palpable at base of heart; apical pulse strong and sustained throughout systole	Diastolic thrill along LSB; laterally displaced apical impulse; systolic thrill in jugular notch and along carotid arteries	Normal unless there is evidence of mitral regurgitation
Heart sounds	Loud S_1; opening snap; low snap; low-pitched, rumbling diastolic murmur	Diminished or absent S_1; wide splitting of S_2; S_3, S_4 heard in severe regurgitation; holosystolic murmur heard best at apex	Diminished or absent A_2; crescendo-decrescendo harsh systolic murmur heard best at base (2nd ICS to right of sternum); aortic ejection sound	Decrescendo diastolic murmur (blowing), high pitched and heard best at base (2nd ICS to right of sternum); systolic ejection murmur heard best at base	Mid to late systolic click and apical systolic murmur heard best alone or in combination at apex or along LSB; auscultory findings can be accentuated or decreased by postural changes, including squatting; holosystolic murmur at apex relects presence of mitral regurgitation

2 DIAGNOSE

Decreased cardiac output related to mechanical factors (preload, afterload) secondary to valvular dysfunction	*Preload:* Early: none Late: fatigue, DOE, palpitation
	Afterload: Early: none Late: exertional chest pain; dizziness, syncope
		Orthopnea; PND
		  Heart rate: rapid, irregular pulse
		  Heart sounds: murmurs; ejection sounds
		  Breath sounds: crackles (rales)

Potential altered cerebral tissue perfusion related to interruption of arterial blood flow secondary to embolization	Complains of disturbances, syncope	Restlessness; Increased BP with widened pulse pressure; altered breathing pattern; altered mental status; unequal or dilated pupils; paresthesia; aphasia; hemiparesis, hemiplegia

→ > >

NURSING DIAGNOSIS	SUBJECTIVE FINDINGS	OBJECTIVE FINDINGS

Other related nursing diagnoses

Fluid volume excess related to cardiac decompensation
Activity intolerance related to diminished cardiac reserve
Anxiety related to altered heart action
Decreased cardiac output related to electrical factors (alteration in rate, rhythm conduction)

3 | PLAN

Patient goals

1. CO is restored and/or maintained.
2. Patient demonstrates adequate cerebral blood flow.
3. Patient demonstrates increased level of knowledge.

4 | IMPLEMENT

NURSING DIAGNOSIS	NURSING INTERVENTIONS	RATIONALE
Decreased cardiac output related to mechanical factors (preload, afterload)	**For preload and afterload:** Establish baseline assessment of cardiovascular status.	To evaluate disease process and development of RV or LV failure. To evaluate response to medical therapy.
	Monitor vital signs q 4 1-8 h or as indicated: BP, heart rate and rhythm.	Tachycardia is a compensatory mechanism reflecting decreased LV contraction. Changes in rhythm may reflect development of dysrhythmia, which can interfere with ventricular filling.
	Auscultate heart sounds q 4-8 h as indicated. Record quality and severity of murmurs.	Any increase or changes in baseline characteristics reflect progressive valvular dysfunction.
	Record pressure or absence of gallop sounds.	Gallop rhythms reflect noncompliance or distention of heart chambers.
	During acute phase, monitor and record ECG rate and rhythms.	Development of atrial dysrhythmias reflects an increase in atrial pressure and leads to further decrease in CO.
	Observe and record dysrhythmia.	Presence of uncontrollable dysrhythmias can lead to further reduction in CO.
	Prepare for cardioversion for atrial fibrillation.	To restore sinus rhythm. Loss of atrial systole can decrease the CO 25% to 33%.
	Limit and/or modify activities during acute phase.	To conserve energy and decrease myocardial oxygen demand.

NURSING DIAGNOSIS	NURSING INTERVENTIONS	RATIONALE
	Administer medications as ordered—antiarrhythmics and vasodilators.	Antidysrhythmics restore sinus rhythm to decrease ventricular rate in presence of atrial fibrillation with ventricular rates > 100-150 bpm. Vasodilators increase CO by decreasing PVR and/or decrease LVEDP.
	Restrict and monitor dietary intake of sodium.	To excrete excess fluid from body, need to excrete sodium; therefore, must minimize sodium retention.
	For afterload only: Assess for signs of decreased CO secondary to increased afterload (e.g., exertional angina).	Progressive valvular stenosis leads to higher afterload, increased wall tension, and compensatory LV hypertrophy.
	Limit and/or modify activities; instruct patient to avoid strenuous physical activities.	Hypotension and diminished cerebral perfusion can occur with reduced CO.
	Administer diuretics as indicated.	Must be given cautiously; excessive use may deplete volume necessary to maintain left atrial pressure and an adequate CO.
	Administer nitroglycerin for chest pain.	Must be given cautiously for first dose because it decreases circulating blood volume, which can result in decreased CO.
Potential altered cerebral tissue perfusion related to interruption of arterial blood flow	Assess and record baseline data observing for signs of embolization.	Thrombi can form a left atrial appendage; risk of systemic embolization increases in presence of atrial fibrillation. Symptoms may be transient or persistent.
	In the presence of atrial fibrillation check neuro signs q 8 h or as indicated.	Patients with mitral valve disease, enlarged left atrium, and atrial fibrillation are considered at high risk for emboli.
	Monitor BP, HR, and respiratory rate.	Indicators of intracranial collapse.
	Administer anticoagulants as ordered.	May be indicated for patients with atrial fibrillation in mitral regurgitation or history of systemic emboli.
Knowledge deficit	See Patient Teaching.	

→ > >

5 EVALUATE

PATIENT OUTCOME	DATA INDICATING THAT OUTCOME IS REACHED
CO is adequate.	Lungs are clear. Patient reports improvement of symptoms. HR is within acceptable limits.
Cerebral tissue perfusion is maintained.	Patient is alert and oriented. Pupils equal and normally reactive to light. Intact motor and sensory function. BP, HR, and respiratory rates within normal limits.
Patient's level of knowledge is increased.	Patient verbalizes understanding of disease and need to make appropriate changes in lifestyle. Patient is compliant with medical therapy. Patient is free of complications.

PATIENT TEACHING

1. Teach patient about disease, including etiology, possible complications, and associated symptoms to report to physician.
2. Assist patient during diagnostic workup and assist with decision for medical or surgical treatment.
3. Include patient's family in teaching and decision-making process.
4. Instruct the patient in the name, dose, and purpose of medications.
5. Explain activity allowances and limitations.
6. Explain diet and fluid restrictions.
7. Instruct the patient about antibiotic prophylaxis to prevent infective endocarditis.
8. Explain importance of notifying dentist, urologist, and gynecologist of valvular heart disease.
9. Provide instruction to women regarding appropriate choice of contraception and risk associated with pregnancy.
10. Instruct the patient about maintaining good oral hygiene, daily care, and regular visits to dentist.

Congenital Heart Disease

A congenital cardiac anomaly is any structural or functional abnormality or defect of the heart or great vessels existing from birth.

Congenital heart disease is considered a specialty of pediatrics. With advances in surgical techniques, however, persons with congenital defects are living to adulthood. Seven defects in which survival to adulthood is possible are presented.

Although the incidence of congenital cardiac malformations has decreased over the decades, they continue to occur at a rate of 5 to 8 per 1000 live births.[2]

The etiology of congenital heart disease remains unclear. However, it is now thought that rather than a singular cause, congenital heart defects occur as a result of several factors:

Genetics. While studies have demonstrated genetic transmission of cardiac defects among siblings and blood relatives, chromosomal or genetic abnormalities only account for 10% of all cardiac abnormalities.[55,118] Examples of chromosomal abnormalities associated with cardiac defects include Down Syndrome (trisomy 21) and Turner Syndrome (XO).

Environmental factors. Environmental factors known to contribute to the development of congenital heart disease include exposure by the mother to rubella during the first 8 weeks of pregnancy. Altitude at birth has been implicated in failure of the ductus arteriosus to close after birth.

Teratogens. Use of certain drugs (e.g., warfarin, trimethadone, hydantoin, and alcohol) by the mother during gestation has been shown to cause not only cardiac malformations but also widespread injury to the embryo.

Patent Ductus Arteriosus (PDA)

The ductus arteriosus is a vascular connection that during fetal life directs blood flow from the pulmonary artery to the aorta, bypassing the lungs. Functional closure of the ductus occurs after birth. In some cases it takes 6 months to several years before complete closure occurs. If the ductus remains patent, the direction of blood flow is reversed to left to right because of high systemic pressure in the aorta (Figure 4-29). Blood is shunted through the ductus to the pulmonary artery during both systole and diastole, raising pressure in the pulmonary circulation and increasing the pressure against which the right ventricle must work.

Survival into adulthood is common. Patent ductus arteriosus (Figure 4-29) occurs more frequently in girls and can be associated with other anomalies such as ventricular septal defect and coarctation of the aorta.

Pathophysiology. A patent ductus functions as an arteriovenous fistula, increasing the work of the left ventricle. Patients with large shunts and relatively low pulmonary vascular resistance (PVR) are at risk for developing left ventricular failure and increased pulmonary pressure. With progressive pulmonary hypertension, reversed shunting with cyanosis and clubbing may develop. Once pulmonary pressure exceeds systemic pressure, the patient becomes inoperable.

Atrial Septal Defect (ASD)

Defects in the atrial septum allow blood flow between the right and left atria (Figure 4-30). ASDs account for 10% of all congenital heart defects. Defects that occur in the higher portion of the septum wall near the fossa ovalis are the most common and are referred to as secundum defects. Less common are ostium primum defects, which are found in the lower portion of the atrial septum. They result from failure of the septum primum to fuse with the endocardial cushions during septation of the atrium. Ostium primums are frequently associated with a deformed mitral valve that includes a cleft defect in the anterior leaflet, which can lead to mitral regurgitation.

ASDs often go undetected until the third, fourth, or fifth decade.

Pathophysiology. The hemodynamic effects of an unrepaired ASD depend on the size and direction of the shunt, the compliance of the ventricles, and the

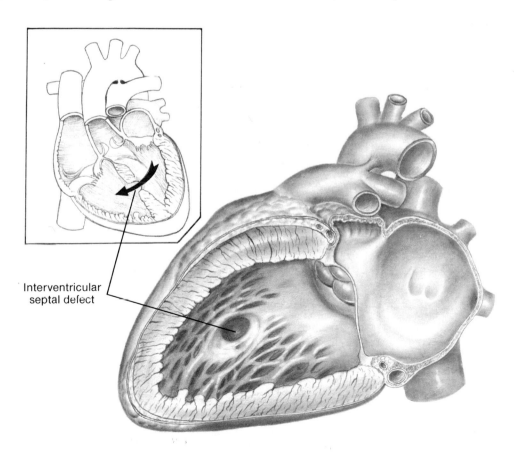

Interventricular
septal defect

EISENMENGER REACTION

Eisenmenger Reaction is a complication that results from the development of high pulmonary vascular resistance (PVR) that is greater than 800 dynes-sec/cm−5. As a result, reversed or bidirectional shunts occur at the aorticopulmonary, ventricular, or atrial levels. It is associated with decrease oxygen saturation, cyanosis, and polycythemia.

The term *Eisenmenger reaction* applies to a number of shunting defects, such as VSD and ASD, which are similar because of the presence of pulmonary hypertension and an associated right to left shunt. It usually occurs as a result of delayed operation and may go undiagnosed until adolescence or adulthood, when surgical correction is no longer possible.

Clinically, the most common complaint is effort intolerance, probably due to decreased arterial oxygen saturation. In later stages, symptoms are more commonly due to ventricular failure. Other common features include cyanosis, with clubbing, and polycythemia.

Most patients survive and live reasonably active lives throughout the fourth and fifth decades. Sudden death, presumably from dysrhythmias, is the most common cause of death. Other causes of death include heart failure and pulmonary infarction from arterial thrombosis.

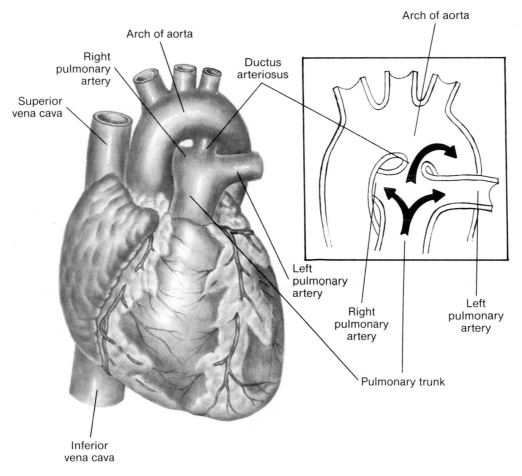

FIGURE 4-29
Patent ductus arteriosus

adaptive response of the pulmonary vascular bed to the increased flow of blood. After birth, because PVR is high and the right and left ventricles are equally compliant, there is little shunting at the atrial level. However, with increasing age, the PVR falls, the RV becomes less resistant, and systemic resistance rises, leading to the development of a left-to-right shunt.

This increased volume load to the RV and increased pulmonary blood flow are generally well tolerated. However, the persistent elevation in PVR can lead eventually to reversal of the shunt, cyanosis (Eisenmenger syndrome), and heart failure.

Ventricular Septal Defect (VSD)

A ventricular septal defect is an abnormal communication or opening between the right and left ventricles (Figure 4-31). VSDs vary in size (7 mm to 3 cm in diameter) and can occur either in the membranous (upper) or in the muscular (lower) portion of the ventricular septum. Three fourths of all defects are membranous. VSDs are found to occur in 2 of every 1000 live births.[69]

Pathophysiology. The size of the defect determines the clinical findings and the extent of the shunt from left to right ventricle. The larger the shunt, the greater the volume of blood ejected into the right ventricle and lungs. Therefore large defects cause a volume overload for both ventricles. Large defects can also lead to an increase in PVR, producing pulmonary hypertension. If this occurs, the shunt may be reversed to right to left, causing systemic cyanosis and producing the Eisenmenger syndrome, which renders the patient inoperable.

Pulmonic Valvular Stenosis

Congenital pulmonic valvular stenosis may occur as an isolated anomaly, in conjunction with other defects such as atrial or ventricular septal defect, or as part of tetralogy of Fallot (Figure 4-32). If it is an isolated anomaly, the chance of survival to adulthood is good. Pulmonic stenosis may occur as one of three types: valvular, subvalvular (infundibular), or supravalvular. Survival to adulthood with mild unrepaired pulmonic stenosis is common.

Pathophysiology. The severity of right ventricular obstruction dictates the clinical presentation. Most patients with mild to moderate pulmonic stenosis remain asymptomatic. However, over time, changes in the right ventricle, such as myocardial fibrosis or subvalvular muscular hypertrophy, can occur, leading to an alteration in RV function. This alteration contributes to the obstruction to RV outflow. Furthermore, over time, the congenitally deformed pulmonic valve can become thickened, fibrotic, and calcified, thus reducing valve mobility and increasing valve obstruction.

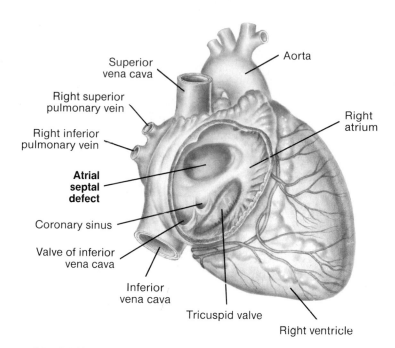

FIGURE 4-30
Atrial septal defect.

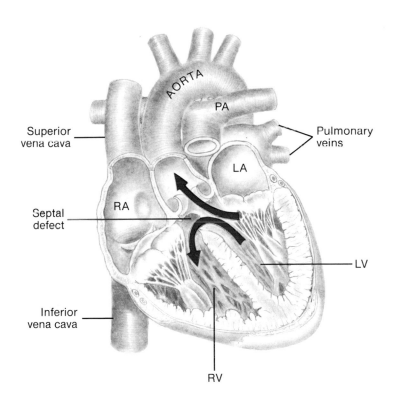

FIGURE 4-31
Ventricular septal defect.

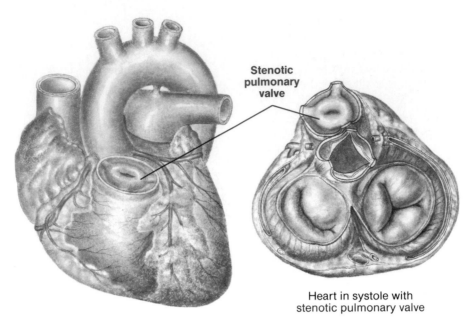

Stenotic
pulmonary
valve

Heart in systole with
stenotic pulmonary valve

FIGURE 4-32
Pulmonic valvular stenosis.

Coarctation of the Aorta

Coarctation of the aorta is defined as a narrowing or partial obstruction of a section of the aorta (Figure 4-33). Although a coarctation can occur at any point along the aortic wall, the majority occur near or distal to the left subclavian artery near the ligamentum arteriosum. Coarctations account for 10% of congenital heart malformations and are associated with other congenital cardiac anomalies, including bicuspid aortic valve and VSD.

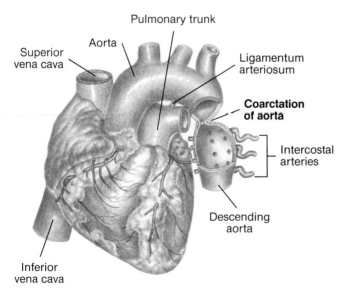

Pulmonary trunk

Aorta

Superior
vena cava

Ligamentum
arteriosum

**Coarctation
of aorta**

Intercostal
arteries

Descending
aorta

Inferior
vena cava

FIGURE 4-33
Coarctation of the aorta.

Pathophysiology. Aortic narrowing produces increased systemic resistance. This increase results in increased pressure in the aorta proximal to the zone of obstruction and decreased pressure distal to the narrowing. Because arterial renal blood flow is diminished, plasma renin is stimulated, contributing to the development of arterial hypertension and pressure overload on the left ventricle. However, aortic pressure distal to the coarctation is not increased. As a means of supplying blood to the lower extremities, collateral vessels develop from the arteries above the obstruction, usually the anterior or posterior branches of the subclavian artery.

Ebstein's Anomaly

Ebstein's anomaly involves the tricuspid valve and is characterized by a downward displacement of the tricuspid valve leaflets into the RV (Figure 4-34). A portion of the RV becomes mechanically part of the right atrium and is referred to as an atrialized RV. As a result the right atrium is exceptionally large, the right ventricle is small, and the tricuspid valve is incompetent. Typically, the right atrium is dilated and either a patent foramen ovale or secundum ASD is present.

Ebstein's anomaly occurs in less than 1% of all congenital heart malformations, with survival into adulthood being expected.[128]

Pathophysiology. Abnormal functioning of the right heart occurs as a result of an incompetent tricuspid valve, a poorly contracting and dilated right atrial chamber, and a small RV with reduced pumping capac-

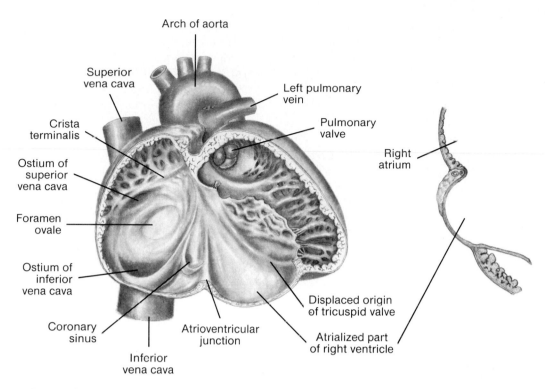

FIGURE 4-34
Ebstein's anomaly.

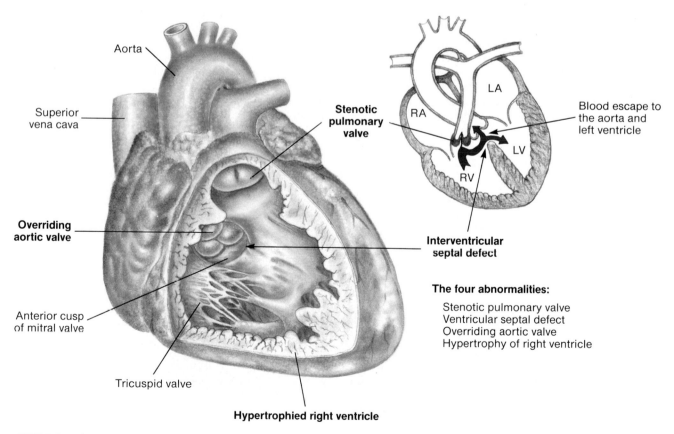

The four abnormalities:

Stenotic pulmonary valve
Ventricular septal defect
Overriding aortic valve
Hypertrophy of right ventricle

FIGURE 4-35
Tetralogy of Fallot.

ity because of its decreased muscle mass. Right-to-left shunting through a foramen ovale or ASD may occur as a result of ineffective emptying of the right atrium.

Tetralogy of Fallot

Tetralogy of Fallot is an anomaly characterized by four defects: ventricular septal defect, right ventricular outflow obstruction (pulmonic stenosis), deviation (dextroposition) of the aorta so it overrides the ventricular septum, and right ventricular hypertrophy (Figure 4-35). Tetralogy of Fallot, the most common cyanotic lesion in which survival to adulthood is expected, accounts for 10% of all congenital heart defects.

Pathophysiology. The severity of symptoms depends on the size of the ventricular septal defect, degree of pulmonic stenosis, and position of the aorta. Right ventricular outflow is obstructed, resulting in hypertrophy of the right ventricle and a right-to-left shunt. This produces a decrease in systemic arterial oxygen saturation, cyanosis, reduced pulmonary blood flow, and in some cases a hypoplastic pulmonary artery.

COMPLICATIONS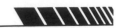

Endocarditis
Cardiac dysrhythmias
Congestive heart failure
Eisenmenger reaction (for cyanotic patients)

DIAGNOSTIC STUDIES AND FINDINGS

Diagnostic test	Patent ductus arteriosus	Atrial septal defect	Ventricular septal defect	Pulmonic stenosis	Coarctation of aorta	Ebstein's anomaly	Tetralogy of Fallot
Electrocardiogram (ECG)	Normal (small ductus); LVH; PR interval may be prolonged; atrial fibrillation	Normal; RVH; RBBB; PR interval may be prolonged; left axis deviation (ostium primum); normal or right axis (ostium secundum)	Normal if defect is small; if moderate to large, LVH; LVH/RVH in presence of pulmonary hypertension	Normal if stenosis is mild; if moderate to severe, RVH and right axis deviation; if severe, right atrial hypertrophy (RAH)	Normal; LVH (in older patients); T-wave inversion, S-T depression (V_5V_6)	Normal; atrial flutter with one-to-one response or atrial fibrillation with rapid ventricular response via a right bypass tract; pre-excitation (WPW) occurs in 20%-25% of patients	RVH
Chest x-ray	Normal; with moderate to large shunt, enlarged cardiac silhouette with enlarged LA, LV, and pulmonary artery (PA); enlarged aorta; enlarged pulmonary trunk and increased pulmonary flow	Enlarged RA, RV, PA; increased pulmonary vascular markings; LA, LV, and aortic knob may be small	Mild LVH with small shunt; with large shunt, increased LV, dilation of PA, increased pulmonary vascular markings, enlarged LA	Enlarged RV and PA; if severe, decreased peripheral pulmonary vascular markings	Normal; rib-notching due to dilated intercostal collaterals; prominent ascending aorta; indentation below aortic knob at site of coarctation (3-sign); LV enlargement	Normal or cardiomegaly with enlarged RA; normal or decreased pulmonary vascularity	Small cardiac silhouette; small PA; prominent aorta (may arch to right in 25% of cases)

Diagnostic test	Patent ductus arteriosus	Atrial septal defect	Ventricular septal defect	Pulmonic stenosis	Coarctation of aorta	Ebstein's anomaly	Tetralogy of Fallot
Echocardiogram	Ductus not visualized; enlarged LA and LV owing to left-to-right shunt	With ostium secundum, enlarged RV, paradoxic movement of septum during systole; with ostium primum, mitral valve displaced inferiorly and anteriorly	Defect not visualized; large shunt; enlarged LA	Normal if stenosis is mild; if moderate to severe, enlarged RA and RV	Normal; confirms presence of bicuspid aortic valve; increased LV thickness associated with bicuspid aortic valve	12-dimensional: delayed closure as well as increased amplitude of anterior tricuspid leaflet and displaced septal leaflet; atrialized RV	Overriding aorta visualized; pulmonary stenosis visualized with degree of obstruction; enlarged ventricular septum (septal motion remains normal)
Laboratory tests	No specific findings	No specific findings	No specific findings unless patient is cyanotic, then increased Hct value, decreased HgB level and arterial oxygen saturation	No specific findings	No specific findings	No specific finding unless patient is cyanotic, then increased Hct	Increased Hct value; degree depends on amount of deoxygenated systemic blood
Cardiac catheterization	Increased pulmonary blood flow; increased oxygen saturation in PA; intracardiac pressures normal; RV and PA pressures may be slightly elevated	Left-to-right shunt; increased oxygen saturation in RA; RA pressure usually normal; mitral regurgitation	Left-to-right shunt; study determines degree of shunt; increased pulmonary blood flow, oxygen saturation in RV, and systolic pressure in RV and PA	Increased RA pressure, which determines systolic pressure gradient between RV and PA	Aortography confirms obstruction and determines pressure gradient	Done to evaluate degree of tricuspid regurgitation	RV outflow obstruction; increased RV pressure; RV to LV shunt; decreased PA pressure as catheter crosses obstruction

MEDICAL MANAGEMENT

GENERAL MANAGEMENT

Indicated by complications such as heart failure, dysrhythmias, or effects of polycythemia in cyanotic patient.

DRUG THERAPY

Dictated by patient's clinical picture and presence of ventricular failure and dysrhythmias.

SURGERY

Patent ductus arteriosus: Ligation of ductus.

MEDICAL MANAGEMENT—cont'd

Atrial septal defect: Direct closure by suturing or placement of Dacron patch across defect. In ostium primum ASD, correction of mitral regurgitation by valvuloplasty or replacement (depends on degree of regurgitation).

Ventricular septal defect: Direct closure by suturing or with placement of Dacron patch across defect.

Pulmonic stenosis: Valvotomy—Resection of excess infundibular muscle; valve replacement.

Coarctation of aorta: Excision of coarctation area followed by end-to-end anastomosis; patch angioplasty—incision is made longitudinal across area of narrowing, and then a Dacron or polytetrafluroethylene patch is sewn into place.

Ebstein's anomaly: Reconstruction or replacement of tricuspid valve (depends on severity of symptoms related to regurgitation). Closure of any ASD if present.

Tetralogy of Fallot: Palliative procedures performed on infants to enhance blood flow to lungs, thereby reducing hypoxia.
  Blalock-Taussig procedure—anastomosis between subclavian artery and pulmonary artery.
  Potts' anastomosis—side-to-side anastomosis of left pulmonary artery to descending aorta.
  Waterston-Cooley procedure—anastomosis of right pulmonary artery to descending aorta.
  Corrective surgery—intracardiac repair of VSD and pulmonic stenosis; contraindicated if pulmonary artery is hypoplastic.

1 ASSESS

ASSESSMENT	PATENT DUCTUS ARTERIOSUS	ATRIAL SEPTAL DEFECT	VENTRICULAR SEPTAL DEFECT	PULMONIC STENOSIS	COARCTATION OF AORTA	EBSTEIN'S ANOMALY	TETRALOGY OF FALLOT
History	Small shunt: asymptomatic; large shunt: exertional dyspnea, decreased exercise tolerance	Small shunt: asymptomatic; moderate to large shunt: exertional dyspnea, decreased exercise tolerance, palpitations	Small to moderate shunt: asymptomatic, exertional dyspnea; large shunt	Asymptomatic; If develops symptoms: exertional dyspnea; decreased exercise tolerance	Asymptomatic; symptoms may be related to high BP or increased failure	Clinical symptoms vary from asymptomatic to mild to moderate exertional dyspnea and fatigue; complaints of palpitations and light-headedness	In adulthood (following palliation): exertional dyspnea, cyanosis with clubbing
Physical examination						Cyanosis: absent to moderate; mean JVP	

ASSESSMENT	PATENT DUCTUS ARTERIOSUS	ATRIAL SEPTAL DEFECT	VENTRICULAR SEPTAL DEFECT	PULMONIC STENOSIS	COARCTATION OF AORTA	EBSTEIN'S ANOMALY	TETRALOGY OFFALLOT
Palpation	Neck vessels dilated and pulsating	Left parasternal lift	Large shunt: left parasternal lift	Left parasternal heave; subxiphoid pulsation	Delayed; diminished femoral pulsations; lag in timing of arterial pulses in lower extremities compared to upper extremities; presence of forceful carotid and suprasternal pulsations; visible collateral arterial pulses over scapula Precordium; suprasternal thrill, normal to sustained LV impulse	Normal; RV impulse absent	Precordial prominence; parasternal heave
Auscultation	Systolic pressure normal; diastolic pressure low; wide pulse pressure; harsh, loud, continuous murmur in 1st, 2nd, 3rd ICS at lower LSB; machinery-like murmur best heard	Soft blowing systolic murmur at 2nd ICS at LSB	Small shunt: holosystolic at 3rd, 4th, and 5th ICS, systolic thrill; large shunt: holosystolic murmur at 3rd, 4th, and 5th ICS, splitting of S_2 during expiration, widening during inspiration, systolic ejection sound at 2nd ICS at LSB	S_1 normal; early systolic ejection click heard at base; midsystolic murmur at 2nd and 3rd ICS at LSB, radiates to suprasternal notch and to left side of neck; S_2 widely split	Systolic pressure > diastolic, wide pulse pressure, differences in arterial pressure between right and left arms; continuous murmur in interscapular area and/or over upper thorax anteriorly and posteriorly; S_2— normal with	S_1 is widely split with a loud delayed S_2: S_3 may be present due to abnormal filling of RV; early systolic or holosystolic murmur; short mid-diastolic murmur occurs, especially in prolonged P-R interval	Single S_2; systolic ejection murmur at 3rd ICS; may radiate upward to left side of neck

ASSESSMENT	PATENT DUCTUS ARTERIOSUS	ATRIAL SEPTAL DEFECT	VENTRICULAR SEPTAL DEFECT	PULMONIC STENOSIS	COARCTATION OF AORTA	EBSTEIN'S ANOMALY	TETRALOGY OFFALLOT
	when patient is lying, becoming fainter when patient is standing				loud aortic component; with bicuspid aortic valve—a systolic ejection murmur		

2 DIAGNOSE

NURSING DIAGNOSIS	SUBJECTIVE FINDINGS	OBJECTIVE FINDINGS
Anxiety related to threat to biologic integrity	Verbalizes fear, anxiousness; repetitive questioning; reports feelings of isolation; verbalizes uncertainty about future	Restlessness; facial tension; somatic complaints; tachycardia; sleeplessness
Potential activity intolerance related to immobility, lack of knowledge; or progressive decreased cardiac reserve	Complains of fatigue and weakness; verbal report of avoiding activities, or inability to perform ADLs	Abnormal response to exercise: HR, BP, dysrhythmias, decreased exertional tolerance, dyspnea, increased cyanosis during activity, dizziness
Ineffective individual and family coping related to (1) inadequate or incorrect information regarding clinical diagnosis, (2) progressive life-style and role changes imposed by disease process	Patient/family members verbalize inability to deal with life-style changes imposed by clinical diagnosis: verbalize fear, anxiety, or anger; verbalize incorrect information regarding clinical diagnosis and imposed limitation; make direct or subtle appeal for assistance with various aspects of care	Patient argumentative over various aspects of prescribed care; displays sudden outbursts of emotion Family members display destructive bickering; overprotectiveness

Other related nursing diagnoses

Decreased cardiac output related to mechanical factors (preload, afterload, and contractility) and electrical instability (dysrhythmias)

3 PLAN

Patient goals

1. Patient will exhibit decrease in anxiety level.
2. Patient will be able to identify factors that contribute to activity intolerance; to identify activities that are age appropriate and within physical limitations; and to support increased tolerance of activity.
3. Patient (or family) will demonstrate ability to cope with changes imposed upon life-style and/or family structure and dynamics.
4. Patient will verbalize understanding regarding clinical status, any imposed limitations, and prescribed treatment regime.

4 IMPLEMENT

NURSING DIAGNOSIS	NURSING INTERVENTIONS	RATIONALE
Anxiety related to threat to biologic integrity	Assess level of anxiety and determine primary cause. Assess patient's information level to identify any misconceptions related to condition. Elicit questions and concerns.	These data provide information about the patient's appraisal and perception of his/her clinical condition. An inadequate or incorrect knowledge base contributes to anxiety and increased stress levels.
	Assess usual coping mechanisms for dealing with stress.	Established methods of dealing with stress may be inappropriate or insufficient to control anxiety and fear.
	Provide, clarify, and validate information relative to condition, any restrictions, or prognosis.	Anxiety can be the result of misinterpretation of what congenital heart disease means. Commonly diagnosed in childhood, these patients are often the product of overprotective parents, who may have imposed unnecessarily severe restrictions on physical and social activities.
	Assist patient to deal realistically with anxiety, providing alternative methods for dealing with stress, (e.g., guided imagery, progressive muscle relaxation).	Explain effects of anxiety and stress on cardiovascular system (e.g., increased HR and BP) and importance of identifying a means of anxiety reduction that is appropriate for patient.
	Provide positive reinforcement about prognosis. Assist patient in attaining realistic goals and life-style.	Setting achievable goals promotes a sense of wellness and optimism about future.
Potential Activity intolerance related to immobility, lack of knowledge, or progressive decreased cardiac reserve	Assess activity level. Determine if activity is appropriate for medical condition.	Frequently patients with congenital heart disease are misinformed about appropriate activity allowances and limitations. They may be either severely limited or have failed to be told to avoid strenuous work in presence of postoperative residual gradient as in aortic stenosis or coarctation of aorta.
	Assess and monitor response to activity noting type of activity, intensity, frequency, and type of symptoms that develop.	To determine reasons for signs of activity intolerance.
	For patients with reduced cardiac reserve implement measures that will improve activity tolerance by minimizing fatigue.	To limit myocardial oxygen demand that is in excess of the amount of oxygen available.

NURSING DIAGNOSIS	NURSING INTERVENTIONS	RATIONALE
Ineffective individual and family coping related to (1) inadequate or incorrect information regarding clinical diagnosis or (2) progressive lifestyle and role changes imposed by disease process	Assess patient's/family's perceptions of condition. Identify any misconceptions, associated guilt, fears or tendency for inappropriate overprotectiveness.	Poor emotional adjustment often seen in adults with congenital heart disease has been related to parental anxiety rather than to degree of severity of disease.
	Determine the degree of emotional and financial stress placed on family by patient's condition. Refer to appropriate support services: social service, vocational counseling.	Issues of occupation and insurability are often faced by these patients and present a constant source of strain on family.
	Include family/spouse in teaching plan. Acknowledge and encourage verbalization of feelings individually, and together as a family.	It is important that each family member (including children and siblings) has an opportunity to express concerns without fear of recrimination.
	Provide opportunity for family group sessions.	Discussions in a setting in which all members are present encourage open discussion of common fears and help to clarify any misconceptions.
Knowledge deficit	See Patient Teaching.	

_5_   EVALUATE

PATIENT OUTCOME	DATA INDICATING THAT OUTCOME IS REACHED
Anxiety is decreased.	Patient and/or parent verbalize reduction in anxiety level. Patient demonstrates appropriate behavior in self-care management. Patient able to verbalize source of anxiety and identify anxiety-reducing measures.
Optimum level of activity is maintained.	Patient adopts activities appropriate to clinical status. Patient verbalizes absence of fatigue, weakness. Patient reports ability to perform ADLs, work, and leisure activities.
Copes with changes in life-style and/or family structure and dynamics.	Patient and/or family verbalizes understanding and expresses concerns regarding changes in life-style or family structure and dynamics imposed by disease. Patient and/or family recognize role changes needed to maintain family integrity. Patient and/or family seeks help to adjust to imposed changes in family dynamics.
Level of knowledge is increased.	Patient and/or parent verbalize knowledge regarding defect, prescribed care, medication, need for return visits, and endocarditis prophylaxis.

PATIENT TEACHING

1. Provide patient and family with a description of primary defect (explaining expected signs and symptoms) and a description of any palliative or corrective surgical interventions.
2. Review activity allowances and limitations as indicated by clinical status.
3. Provide counseling with respect to schooling, sports, and employment.
4. Explain dietary restrictions as indicated.
5. Explain need to prevent endocarditis (see page 140).
6. Explain importance of regular or periodic clinical follow-up.
7. For adolescents and adults, provide counseling concerning genetics, marriage, and childbearing.
8. For women, provide information regarding risks of pregnancy and delivery according to type of defect, surgical interventions and clinical status. Discuss importance of obtaining prepregnancy counseling and need for appropriate type of contraceptive use.

CHAPTER 5

Vascular Diseases and Disorders

The prevalence of peripheral vascular disease is not precisely known. With few exceptions, the incidence of disorders of peripheral vessels increases with age, occurring most often in people over age 65 who have some form of cardiovascular disease. Patients usually seek treatment because of pain. Frequently, the diagnosis is made on the basis of characteristics of the pain. Vascular disorders may involve the arteries and veins.

Atherosclerosis, certain cardiac disorders, and hypertension are major contributing factors to the development of peripheral vascular disease. For example, chronic arterial insufficiency is a progressively debilitating disorder usually caused by atherosclerotic plaques. In contrast, thrombi resulting from cardiac disorders account for most cases of acute arterial insufficiency.

Vessels also may suffer trauma that results in chronic disease. Venous thrombosis partly arises from injury to the vessel epithelium, although other factors, such as hypercoagulability and prolonged immobility, are also involved.

Thromboangiitis obliterans is seen mainly in men between the ages of 20 and 40. This is a form of chronic arterial insufficiency caused by an inflammatory reaction to cigarette smoking.

Occasionally, peripheral vascular disorders are congenital, as may occur in arteriovenous fistula or varicose veins, in which venous valves are absent.

Acute Arterial Insufficiency

Acute arterial insufficiency is a sudden decrease in the arterial blood supply to an extremity. Obstruction of any major artery can precipitate symptoms.

The most common causes of acute arterial insufficiency are thrombosis, embolism, and trauma. Cardiac disorders, such as mitral valve disease, rheumatic heart disease, atrial fibrillation, left atrial myxoma, and prosthetic valves are the primary sources of thrombi on the left side of the heart.

The lower extremities are most commonly involved in arterial occlusions. The femoral artery is most frequently affected (46%), followed by the popliteal tibial tree (11%) and the iliac arteries (18%). The terminal segment of the aorta is affected 14%. Only 5% of arterial occlusions involve the upper limbs.[195]

Acute arterial obstruction may also occur as a result of traumatic injury produced by compression, shearing, or laceration of a vessel. Severe hypothermia also may produce sudden severe vasoconstriction.

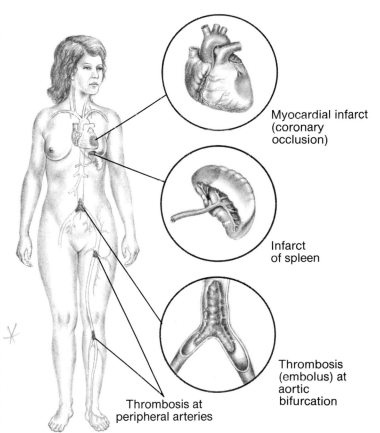

Myocardial infarct (coronary occlusion)

Infarct of spleen

Thrombosis (embolus) at aortic bifurcation

Thrombosis at peripheral arteries

PATHOPHYSIOLOGY

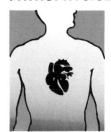

Once dislodged, an embolus may travel throughout the systemic circulation, lodging in an arterial branch and stagnating flow in the distal circulation. This leads to the formation of a soft coagulum proximal and distal to the area of stagnant blood flow.[111] The result is the formation of a secondary thrombus, which extends along the arterial wall and progressively compromises collateral circulation. Without adequate collateral circulation, the distal tissues are deprived of oxygenation, a situation which leads to ischemia, pain, and paresthesia in the affected area. With prolonged ischemia, cellular damage occurs, leading to muscle necrosis.

COMPLICATIONS

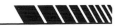

Gangrene
Muscle necrosis
Limb amputation

DIAGNOSTIC STUDIES AND FINDINGS

Diagnostic test	Findings
Doppler ultrasonography	Abnormal blood flow pattern proximal to occlusion; "pistol shot" sound characterizes absence of diastolic flow component; ankle/brachial index <0.25 reflects severe ischemia and impending gangrene
Echocardiography	Done to determine if heart is source of emboli
Arteriography	Determines location of obstruction and character of arterial circulation proximal and distal to obstruction

MEDICAL MANAGEMENT

GENERAL MANAGEMENT

Percutaneous transluminal angioplasty: Nonsurgical procedure involving mechanical dilation of occluded artery performed under local anesthesia with fluoroscopy; lesions considered suitable are stenotic vessels with intraluminal diameter of 2.5 mm and length of not >10 cm.

Laser thermal angioplasty: Nonsurgical procedure that is still under development; obliterates atheromatous lesions by applying "heat" energy from a laser source.

DRUG THERAPY

Anticoagulants

   Heparin sodium (Lipo-Hepin and others). Indications: used once diagnosis of embolization is made and before surgical treatment is performed. Dosage is given to keep PTT to 2× normal.

Fibrinolytic agents

   Streptokinase (Streptase), urokinase (Abbokinase). Indications: Thrombolytic agents instilled by intra-arterial infusion into site of occlusion; method of action is fibrinolysis causing fibrin dissolution.

SURGERY

Embolectomy: Embolus can be removed directly via femoral arteriotomy using soft balloon-tipped catheter known as Fogarty catheter. Catheter is passed distal to occlusion, carefully inflated, and withdrawn. Successful restoration of arterial blood flow and limb salvage is best achieved if embolectomy is done early, before advanced ischemia occurs.

Amputation of limb: For severe advanced ischemia.

1 ASSESS

ASSESSMENT	OBSERVATIONS
Peripheral extremity	**Moderate obstruction** Pain, sudden in onset; numbness; "embolic syndrome" characterized by five Ps (pain, pallor, paresthesia, pulselessness, and paralysis) Temperature: decreased Skin: pale yellow color Pulses: absence of distal arterial pulsations of affected extremity; Poor capillary filling **Severe obstruction** Leg muscle (gastrocnemius) becomes firm; dorsiflexion of foot produces pain

2 DIAGNOSE

NURSING DIAGNOSIS	SUBJECTIVE FINDINGS	OBJECTIVE FINDINGS
Altered peripheral tissue perfusion related to interruption of arterial blood flow	Complains of pain and numbness in lower extremities	Pallor, swelling, cool to touch, and paresis in lower extremities
Pain related to peripheral ischemia	Complains of pain in affected area; reports inability to concentrate	Guarded position of affected area. Fear, restlessness. Facial expression of discomfort with movement

Other related nursing diagnoses

Anxiety related to perceived/actual biologic threat (loss of limb)
Decreased cardiac output related to mechanical factors secondary to embolization

3 PLAN

Patient goals

1. Patient will demonstrate increased arterial blood flow.
2. Patient will be free of pain.
3. Patient will demonstrate increased level of knowledge.

4 IMPLEMENT

NURSING DIAGNOSIS	NURSING INTERVENTIONS	RATIONALE
Altered peripheral tissue perfusion related to interruption of arterial blood flow	Assess arterial pulses distal to occlusion q 1-2 h.	To assess arterial blood flow to extremity.
	Auscultate pulses using Doppler ultrasound.	To evaluate presence of soft or hard to palpate pulses.
	Evaluate signs of advanced ischemia by checking the color and temperature of extremity, or absence of sensation and levels of motor deficit.	An increase in clinical signs may indicate the onset of advanced ischemia: rigor, gangrene.

→ > >

NURSING DIAGNOSIS	NURSING INTERVENTIONS	RATIONALE
	Monitor and record HR, BP q 4-8 h or as indicated. Monitor ECG recording for cardiac dysrhythmias.	Arterial embolus is frequently associated with myocardial disease; therefore need to detect signs and symptoms that may contribute to increased morbidity and mortality.
	Maintain patient on bed rest during acute phase.	To reduce oxygen demand of extremity.
	Do not raise extremities above level of heart.	To maintain optimal gravitational flow.
	Administer anticoagulation as ordered.	To prevent distal propagation of thrombus and further embolization.
	Monitor PTT, HgB, and Hct daily or as indicated.	To maintain therapeutic range (twice normal) and avoid hemorrhagic complications.
Pain related to peripheral ischemia	Assess quality and degree of pain to determine if acute vs chronic. Determine if onset is sudden or associated with other symptoms and if increased by dorsiflexion of foot.	It is believed that pain is a sign of embolic occlusion, whereas numbness is an initial sign of acute in situ thrombosis.
	Maintain on bed rest during acute phase. Provide for position of most comfort. *Do not* raise knee gatch, elevate extremity, or allow hips to be maintained in prolonged flexion.	Flexion and elevation of affected extremity can interfere with arterial circulation and increase pain.
	Administer analgesics as ordered.	To provide some measure of pain relief. NOTE: Pain relief usually occurs once obstruction and ischemia are relieved.
	Protect affected extremity by using a bed cradle, cotton blankets, or sheepskin.	To protect extremity from injury.
Knowledge deficit	See Patient Teaching.	

5 EVALUATE

PATIENT OUTCOME	DATA INDICATING THAT OUTCOME IS REACHED
Peripheral perfusion is improved.	Pain is relieved; distal and proximal pulses are present; extremity has normal color; normal motor function returns in affected extremity.
Comfort level is achieved.	Pain is relieved or improved. Patient states he is more comfortable. Patient requires less analgesic.
Level of knowledge is increased.	Patient demonstrates understanding of disease process and need to avoid situations that cause blood pooling or interruption of blood flow.

PATIENT TEACHING

1. Instruct patient and family about the disease process, possible causes, and therapeutic modalities.
2. At discharge, explain anticoagulant therapy and the need for follow-up monitoring with clotting studies as indicated.
3. Instruct patient to avoid situations that cause blood pooling or interruption of blood flow, e.g., crossing legs or sitting or standing for extended periods of time.

Chronic Arterial Insufficiency

Chronic arterial insufficiency   is inadequate blood flow in arteries, caused by occlusive atherosclerotic plaques or emboli, damaged or diseased vessels, aneurysms, hypercoagulability states, or heavy use of tobacco.

Arteriosclerosis obliterans is the primary cause of chronic arterial insufficiency. Other causes, although rare, may lead to arterial insufficiency of the lower extremities. These include thromboangiitis obliterans (Buerger's disease), cystic degeneration of the popliteal artery, popliteal entrapment, and some connective tissue disorders.

Arteriosclerosis obliterans is a progressive ischemic syndrome. It is more prevalent in men, and the incidence rises with age. It is a diffuse process but is generally confined to short segments of arteries near bifurcations and origins. The aortoiliac and femoropopliteal areas are common sites.

PATHOPHYSIOLOGY

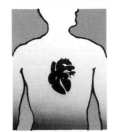

Progressive narrowing of the arterial tree by atherosclerotic plaques gives rise to collateral vessels that tend to ensure adequate blood supply and prevent peripheral ischemia. However, the effectiveness of these collateral pathways is limited by their small size and high resistance and by the extent of occlusive disease. Clinically, progressive occlusion leads to hypoperfusion and ischemia, which are related directly to the number of occlusions and the adequacy of collateral vessels to counteract the reduced blood flow. The distal extremities are the most vulnerable to ischemia. The course of the disease may be a gradual progression or may be complicated by development of thrombosis or a minor traumatic event.

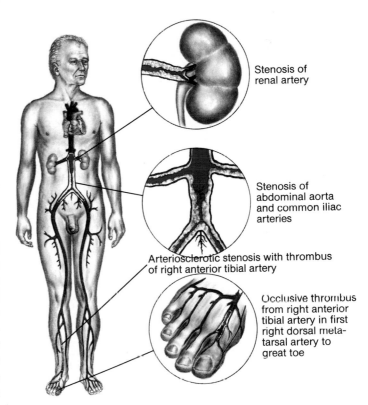

Stenosis of renal artery

Stenosis of abdominal aorta and common iliac arteries

Arteriosclerotic stenosis with thrombus of right anterior tibial artery

Occlusive thrombus from right anterior tibial artery in first right dorsal metatarsal artery to great toe

COMPLICATIONS

Peripheral ischemia
Gangrene
Limb amputation

DIAGNOSTIC STUDIES AND FINDINGS

Diagnostic test	Finding
Doppler ultrasonography	Quantitates degree of ischemia; ankle/brachial index: arterial pressure < pressure in brachial artery
Plethysmography	Decreased peripheral circulation
Angiography	Shows exact localization of arterial obstruction

MEDICAL MANAGEMENT

GENERAL MANAGEMENT

Risk reduction program: Weight reduction for the obese patient; smoking cessation; a low-cholesterol, low saturated fat diet.

Evaluation and control of diabetes and hyperlipidemia should be carried out to slow the progression of the atherosclerotic process.

Daily foot care: Inspection, cleaning, use of cotton socks; attention to nails, corns, calluses.

Regular walking program: To point of claudication—done several times a day may improve patient's walking distance. It is thought that this improvement may be due to development of increased collateral arterial flow, progressive adaptation to discomfort and/or gait modification, metabolic changes in the muscles, or redistribution of blood flow to the muscles.[40,186]

Peripheral angioplasty (percutaneous transluminal angioplasty, or PTA):   Using an inflatable balloon-tipped catheter, the atheromatous plaque is mechanically compressed, allowing for increased lumen patency. Vessels of the iliac or femoral arteries are reported to respond best to PTA, but success has been reported for vessels of the aorta, popliteal, superior mesenteric, subclavian, and brachial systems as well as stenoses in peripheral arterial grafts.[139]

Laser thermal angioplasty (LTA):   A new, experimental method of obliterating the atheromatous plaque by heat vaporization. Using a fiberoptic catheter, energy from a laser source is applied to the occlusive lesion. Often performed in conjunction with PTA.

DRUG THERAPY

Several drugs, such as anticoagulants, vasodilators, and antiplatelets, have been used but are of questionable help; they may be used as a palliative measure.

Peritoxifylline (Trental)   Indications: To increase claudication distance.

SURGERY

Arterial revascularization and/or reconstruction: Performed to restore unimpeded pulsatile blood flow, usually beginning with proximal segments (aortoiliac-femoral).

Endarterectomy: Removal of atheromatous intima from artery.

Bypass graft surgery: Use of Dacron conduit to deliver blood from aorta to femoral vessels, bypassing diseased segments.

Femoropopliteal reconstruction

Profundoplasty: Local endarterectomy of proximal profunda femoris artery.

Lumbar sympathectomy: Removal of second and third lumbar ganglia; performed to improve blood flow to skin.

Amputation of limb: For severe, irreversible ischemia (gangrene).

1 ASSESS

ASSESSMENT	OBSERVATIONS

General complaints	*Mild to moderate obstruction*
	
	Intermittent claudication (inability of arterial circulation to meet oxygen demand during exercise)
	    Discomfort varies from mild to severe
	    Can occur in calves, thighs, buttocks depending on occlusive lesions (foot rarely involved)
	    Described as cramping, ache, squeezing, burning sensation; relieved with rest
	Location of claudication may be diagnostic of artery involved:
	    Hip claudication—bilateral iliac artery
	    Thigh claudication—common femoral artery
	    Calf claudication—superficial femoral artery
	
	Severe obstruction
	
	Ischemic "rest" pain (due to low-grade tissue necrosis): continuous burning pain confined to toes or to area of ulceration; may appear first at night, waking patient; occurs at rest and improves with walking, or by maintaining leg in dependent position; due to loss of gravitational blood flow, elevation increases pain
	Edema (secondary) of affected extremity—occurs with prolonged leg dependence
	    Sensory changes:
	        Numbness—toes, foot, or lower portion of leg
	        Paresthesias—tingling, burning
	Palpation: measure on a 0-4 scale (see Chapter 2, p. 25), pulse volume and quality may range from slightly reduced to absent
	Auscultation: the presence of bruits, commonly at abdominal aorta and iliac and femoral arteries

Skin	Mild: dry, shiny, loss of hair
	Moderate to severe:
	    Color: pallor at rest—elevation of limb causes an abnormal pallor to appear, which will take from 5-60 sec to return to normal color once limb is lowered; rubor (abnormal redness) with leg in dependent position reflects maximal arterial dilation
	    Temperature: varies; a decrease in one limb must be compared with other before attributing to occlusive disease and not environment
	    Fissures on toes, heels, soles
	    Ulceration: usually begins over the toes and the heels above the lateral malleolus, which are the most distal parts of the arterial tree
	    Gangrene

Trophic changes	Nails: opacificaton, thick, brittle Hair loss: toes, leg
Sexual function	Impotence in men (reflects decrease in arterial blood flow to branch of the internal iliac [hypogastric] artery, which may interfere with penile erections)

→ › ›

2 DIAGNOSE

NURSING DIAGNOSIS	SUBJECTIVE FINDINGS	OBJECTIVE FINDINGS
Altered peripheral tissue perfusion (chronic) related to interruption of blood flow	Reports pain in calf, thigh, and/or buttock at rest or with exercise; fatigue; numbness; impotence	Diminished or absent peripheral arterial pulses. Poor capillary filling. Changes in skin color and temperature. Muscle wasting.
Pain related to peripheral ischemia	Reports intermittent or continuous pain in extremities	Guarded position of affected limb. Facial expression of discomfort at rest or with activity. Reflex abnormalities.
Impaired skin integrity related to impaired circulation	Reports discomfort from injury	Changes in skin's tissue integrity, e.g., blisters, excoriation, redness and inflammation, fissures, ulcers, necrosis

Other related nursing diagnoses

Noncompliance related to inadequate knowledge vs inadequate motivation
Sexual dysfunction related to reduced blood flow to iliac artery
Activity intolerance related to pain and discomfort

3 PLAN

Patient goals

1. Patient will demonstrate improved arterial blood flow to lower extremities.
2. Patient will demonstrate pain relief.
3. Patient will demonstrate progressive healing of skin breakdown.
4. Patient will demonstrate increased level of knowledge.

4 IMPLEMENT

NURSING DIAGNOSIS	NURSING INTERVENTIONS	RATIONALE
Altered peripheral tissue perfusion (chronic) related to interruption of arterial flow.	Assess extremities for adequacy of peripheral arterial blood flow.	Severity of symptoms reflects the extent of arterial obstruction and amount of collateral blood flow.
	Assess and record degree and quality of pain.	Often the only measure of disease progression is appearance of claudication with progressively decreased amounts of exercise.
	Assess arterial pulses noting location, quality, and volume. Auscultate for bruits before and after exercise.	Presence or absence of peripheral pulse reflects adequacy of peripheral circulation; systolic bruits confirm presence of regional atherosclerotic lesion.
	Inspect skin color, changes with elevation and dependency procedures, and tropic changes.	Presence of these changes in association with claudication indicates advanced state of arterial insufficiency and estimates degree of ischemia.

NURSING DIAGNOSIS	NURSING INTERVENTIONS	RATIONALE
	Maintain affected extremity in a dependent position; avoid procedures or bed positions that interfere with gravitational blood flow (arterial flow is downward), such as elevating affected extremity, use of knee gatch.	Proper positioning of extremities helps to maintain optimal and/or improve arterial blood flow and reduces the pain.
	Place bed cradle over affected areas. Avoid use of heating devices on lower extremities.	To protect extremity from injury. Heat increases tissue metabolism, which can increase oxygen demand in excess of supply.
	Instruct patient to avoid smoking or use of other nicotine products (chewing tobacco, pipe).	Nicotine causes vasoconstriction and damages intimal cells of both large and small blood vessels.
	Initiate a progressive walking program: 20 min twice a day, increasing to first sign of pain; do not force beyond pain level.	To promote development of collateral circulation.
	Administer medications as ordered (analgesics, vasodilators).	Reduction of pain will allow patient to continue walking program, thereby promoting development of collateral circulation.
	For involvement of iliac artery, monitor urine output q 8 h or as indicated.	To detect signs of decreased perfusion to kidneys.
Pain related to peripheral ischemia	Assess quality and degree of pain. Assist patient to identify activities that precipitate or aggravate pain.	To determine degree of claudication and exercise tolerance. To identify factors that aggravate or interfere with arterial blood flow.
	Provide position of most comfort; elevate head of bed on block.	Frequent position changes may be helpful during periods of restlessness brought on by pain.
	Administer pentoxifylline as ordered.	Pentoxifylline facilitates blood flow in microcirculation by increasing red cell flexibility and preventing platelet aggregation, which decreases viscosity of blood and improves flow properties.
	Instruct patient on methods of relieving pain: stand or dangle at side of bed to obtain relief from ischemic pain; use bed cradle if weight of bed covers increases pain.	To promote circulation and reduce factors that contribute to or aggravate pain.
	Encourage patient to participate in a variety of activities to distract patient from persistent discomfort.	Chronic and persistent pain generates a depressive state, and patient begins to internally focus increasingly on chronic illness.

→ › ›

NURSING DIAGNOSIS	NURSING INTERVENTIONS	RATIONALE
Impaired skin integrity related to impaired circulation	Inspect skin daily noting tissue integrity; observe for signs of necrosis.	To detect signs of skin breakdown and/or signs of tissue necrosis.
	Provide daily skin care: wash with mild soap, rinse, and pat dry; ensure that skin is thoroughly dried; lubricate skin with lanolin lotions.	To maintain skin integrity and avoid development of fissures.
	Treat ulcerations as they occur: bed rest, administer saline soaks; topical and/or systemic antibiotics and dressings as ordered.	To limit development or extension of ulceration.
	Avoid using adhesive tapes directly on skin.	To avoid stripping of epidermis when removing tape.
	Avoid use of tight constricting socks or hose; avoid use of knee gatch; reposition extremities frequently.	To avoid pressure, which will interfere further with an already compromised circulation.
	Use natural sheepskin padding.	To reduce friction and irritation; provides resistance to shear and even pressure distribution.
	Use cotton or woolen socks that are proper length and size.	Cotton and wool absorb moisture, thereby preventing skin breakdown caused by moisture.
	Instruct patient to wear properly fitting shoes when out of bed; avoid going barefoot.	To avoid injury.
Knowledge deficit	See Patient Teaching.	

5 EVALUATE

PATIENT OUTCOME	DATA INDICATING THAT OUTCOME IS REACHED
Peripheral perfusion is improved.	Patient reports relief of pain (no claudication). Pulses are present, equal, and bilateral. Skin color is normal; Skin is warm to touch
Comfort level is achieved.	Patient verbalizes absence or control of pain and verbalizes and demonstrates appropriate use of pain relief measures to control pain.
Skin integrity is maintained.	Skin shows no signs of ulcerations. Patient verbalizes and demonstrates appropriate care of skin and feet.
Level of knowledge is increased.	Patient verbalizes understanding of disease and reports appropriate changes in life-style.

PATIENT TEACHING

1. Provide information regarding disease and associated risk factors.
2. Explain the need to stop or avoid smoking or use of nicotine products.
3. Instruct the patient in a daily progressive walking program.
4. Discuss positioning of extremity to promote maximum circulation.
5. Explain skin care. Discuss the need to avoid heat, such as very warm showers or baths.
6. Provide weight counseling for obese patients.
7. Explain dietary limitations of a low-cholesterol, low-fat diet.

Aortic Aneurysm

An **aneurysm** is a circumscribed dilation of an artery or a blood-containing tumor connecting directly with the lumen of an artery.

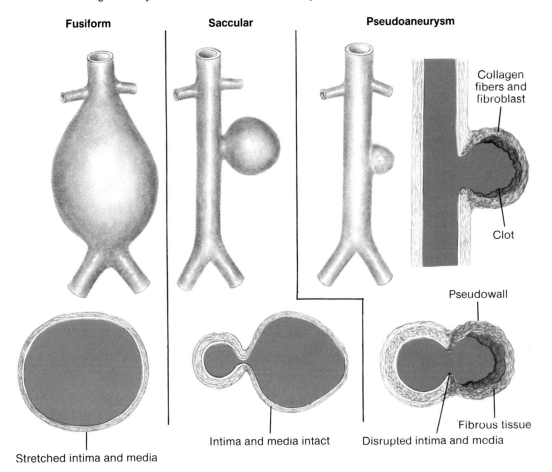

Fusiform — Stretched intima and media

Saccular — Intima and media intact

Pseudoaneurysm — Collagen fibers and fibroblast; Clot; Pseudowall; Fibrous tissue; Disrupted intima and media

INCIDENCE

Although an aneurysm can be located anywhere along the aorta and the iliac vessels, the infrarenal, abdominal aortic aneurysm is the most common. It occurs four times more frequently than the thoracic aneurysm. White men in the fifth and sixth decades of life are most likely to develop aneurysms; however, women are also at risk for developing aneurysmal disease.

Approximately 30% of abdominal aortic aneurysms (AAA) are diagnosed during routine physical examinations; 70% of the AAAs are discovered during clinical workup for other problems.[53] Generally a palpable mass is felt at the level of the umbilicus, extending toward the epigastrium. At this point the aneurysms are small, less than 5 cm, and difficult to palpate. If symptoms are present, abdominal and intermittent back pain are usually noted. If the aneurysm ruptures, the pain becomes intense.

Thoracic aneurysm, on the other hand, presents with more acute symptoms, causing the patient to seek medical evaluation. Chest pain is most commonly experienced with thoracic aneurysms. It is generally substernal but may radiate to the neck, lower back, shoulders, or abdomen. Increasing intensity of pain suggests dissection or rupture. However, as the aneurysm enlarges, adjacent thoracic structures may be compressed, causing a variety of symptoms. For example, difficulty in breathing can occur if the trachea or bronchus is compressed. If there is pressure on the recurrent laryngeal nerve, the patient may experience hoarseness and cough. Difficulty in swallowing results from compression of the esophagus. Edema of the upper extremities and head and a cyanotic appearance may be evident if there is superior vena cava obstruction. Aortic valvular insufficiency is seen as the aneurysm encroaches on the heart.

ETIOLOGY

The most common cause of aneurysms is atherosclerosis. Less common causes include cystic medial necrosis, infections leading to abscesses or mycotic aneurysms, and syphilitic aortitis, which is not frequently seen since the development of modern antibiotics. Chronic aortitis and trauma can also lead to aneurysms.

PATHOPHYSIOLOGY

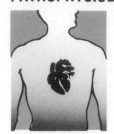

The primary structural defect that results in development of an aneurysm is a weakened aortic wall secondary to destruction of the media. As the aneurysm increases, so does the wall tension, which contributes further to enlargement until eventual rupture. The majority of aneurysms (80% to 90%) rupture into the retroperitoneal space, while others will rupture into the peritoneal cavity.

There are three main categories of aneurysms. The saccular aneurysm is described as a localized outpouching of the vessel wall. While the saccular aneurysm affects only one side of the artery, the fusiform aneurysm is a diffuse circumferential dilation of the artery. The false, or pseudoaneurysm, results from a complete tear of all three arterial coats. Blood fills the surrounding tissues, producing a pulsatile hematoma.[36,53]

COMPLICATIONS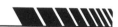

Aortic dissection
Aortic rupture—with a potential fatal hemorrhage

DIAGNOSTIC STUDIES AND FINDINGS

Diagnostic test	Findings
Plain chest and abdominal x-rays	Calcium within the aneurysm wall (diagnostic 55-85% of the time)
Chest x-ray	Widened mediastinum suggests enlargement of thoracic aneurysm
Ultrasound	Determines presence and size; used to follow patients over time to track growth of the aneurysm; not useful for thoracic aneurysms
CT scan	Accurate for size determination; better able to distinguish periaortic hematomas than ultrasound; diagnostic for thoracic aneurysms
Aortography	Useful to define anatomy and perfusion of the renal arteries, patency of the inferior mesenteric artery, iliac artery involvement and distal perfusion

MEDICAL MANAGEMENT

GENERAL MANAGEMENT

Dictated by clinical presentation. Patients with aortic aneurysms <4.5 cm in diameter may be treated medically.

Symptomatic aneurysm: Cardiac monitor.
Diet—sodium restriction.
Hemodynamic monitoring—arterial line, PAP, PCWP, urine output.

DRUG THERAPY

Antihypertensives: Nipride diuretics.

Pain management: Morphine sulfate.

Sedation

SURGERY

Elective: Indicated for aneurysms >4.5 cm. Repair of an aortic aneurysmal involves cross clamping above and below the aneurysm, incising the aneurysmal wall, and laying a synthetic graft inside the aneurysmal wall and attaching it to the native aorta. If necessary, the inferior mesenteric artery is reimplanted into the graft to protect perfusion to the bowel. The aneurysmal wall is then sewn over the graft. This protects the new graft from coming into contact with the bowel.

1 ASSESS

ASSESSMENT*	OBSERVATIONS
Abdomen	Palpable mass at level of umbilicus that may be pulsatile and expansile
Abdominal or back pain	May be vague, intermittent; increasing pain may be due to sudden aneurysm enlargement, dissection, or rupture
Aortic rupture	Sudden, severe pain to anterior chest, back, or epigastric area; hypertension; decreased or absent peripheral pulses
Aortic dissection	Hypovolemic shock; peritoneal irritation

NOTE: Patient may be completely asymptomatic.

2 DIAGNOSE

NURSING DIAGNOSIS	SUBJECTIVE FINDINGS	OBJECTIVE FINDINGS
Anxiety related to perceived/actual threat to biologic integrity secondary to upcoming surgery	Verbalizes fears, being scared	Restlessness Sympathetic response: hypertension, hyperventilation, tachycardia, diaphoresis

→ 〉 〉

NURSING DIAGNOSIS	SUBJECTIVE FINDINGS	OBJECTIVE FINDINGS
Potential decreased cardiac output related to possible dissection/rupture	Complains of increased pain, restlessness, SOB, fatigue	Hypertension, followed by falling BP and narrowed pulse pressure Changes in mentation: lethargy, semiconsciousness Tachycardia; pulse weak, thready Skin: pallor, diaphoresis, cool Increasing size of abdomen (if aneurysm ruptures anteriorly into the peritoneal space)
Potential fluid volume deficit related to possible rupture of aneurysm	Complains of increased thirst, restlessness	Hypotension, tachycardia, pulse weak and thready Flat neck veins; hemodynamic findings: decreased PAP, PCWP, CO Decreased urine output Tachypnea—shallow respiration Poor skin turgor

3 PLAN

Patient goals

1. Patient will demonstrate reduced anxiety.
2. Patient will have adequate or improved cardiac output.
3. Patient will demonstrate stable fluid balance.
4. Patient will demonstrate knowledge and understanding of condition and contributing factors, and proposed medical and surgical plan.

4 IMPLEMENT

NURSING DIAGNOSIS	NURSING INTERVENTIONS	RATIONALE
Anxiety related to perceived/actual threat to biologic integrity secondary to upcoming surgery	Assess level of anxiety. Provide brief explanations about routines, procedures. Administer sedative medications as ordered.	Sympathetic response to anxiety can have detrimental effects on the hemodynamics in the perioperative period.
	Remain with patient offering realistic assurance.	Perceptions may become reduced; remaining with patient increases sense of trust and comfort.
Potential decreased cardiac output related to possible dissection/rupture	Assess and monitor for signs and symptoms of decreased CO q 1h; report subtle and sudden changes to physician.	Survival depends on careful and early recognition of deteriorating cardiac hemodynamics.
	Maintain bed rest with patient in supine position.	To prevent further drop in BP.
	Initiate and monitor hemodynamic parameters as ordered: arterial pressure, PAP, PCWP.	To detect signs of circulatory collapse; drop in aortic pressure and increased LVEDP can lead to hypoperfusion of coronary and renal arteries.

NURSING DIAGNOSIS	NURSING INTERVENTIONS	RATIONALE
	Measure and calculate CI/CO and SVR.	To evaluate cardiac function, preload, and afterload.
	Initiate and maintain patent IV line.	To facilitate vein access to deliver emergent drugs.
Potential fluid volume deficit related to hemorrhage if the aneurysm ruptures	Assess components of CO q 1 h. Assess for signs and symptoms of fluid volume deficit.	If the aneurysm ruptures, the patient will exhibit signs of hypovolemia as the vascular space becomes depleted.
	Monitor BP, pulse, and respirations q 1 h during acute phase.	To determine stabilization vs progressive deterioration.
	Administer fluids as ordered—blood plasma, volume expanders, saline solutions, and dextran.	To restore blood volume.
	Monitor hemodynamic parameters—RAP, PAP, PCWP.	To accurately monitor response to fluid replacement.
	Maintain intake and output q 1 h or as indicated.	To assess kidney function as well as circulating fluid volume.
	Maintain on bed rest, supine; in absence of head injury elevate legs.	To increase venous return.

5 EVALUATE

PATIENT OUTCOME	DATA INDICATING THAT OUTCOME IS REACHED
Exhibits signs of decreased anxiety.	Patient appears calm, resting quietly; HR, respirations are within normal limits. Patient is able to verbalize fears and asks appropriate questions.
Cardiac output is maintained or improved.	Vital signs are at baseline or normal; mentation: alert and oriented; skin: color good, warm, and dry. CO, PA, PCWP at baseline or normal.
Remains normovolemic.	Patient is normotensive. PCWP is 10-15 mm Hg. Urine output is increased.
Knowledge level is increased.	Patient is able to describe disease process, associated risk factors, and signs and symptoms to report to physician.

PATIENT TEACHING

1. Provide information regarding disease, and contributing risk factors.
2. Discuss importance of maintaining blood pressure under control and restricting salt in diet as ordered.
3. Review signs and symptoms to report, including chest or back pain.

Aortic Dissection

Aortic dissection is a precipitous disruption of the medial layers of the vessel wall that travels along a course parallel to blood flow resulting in medial hemorrhage and the formation of a false channel between the intima and the adventitia.

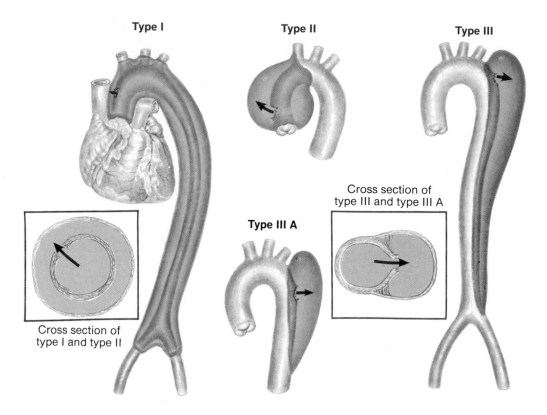

Type I

Type II

Type III

Cross section of type III and type III A

Type III A

Cross section of type I and type II

Acute dissection is the most lethal problem involving the aorta. In describing dissections, various classification systems have been used. The most widely used is the DeBakey I-II-III system, which includes the following classifications:

Type I—The intimal tear starts just above the aortic valve and often involves the valve leaflets and extends beyond the arch of the aorta as far as the abdominal aorta. Type I dissections are seen in 60% of all reported cases.

Type II—Begins the same as type I, but dissection is limited to the ascending aorta and does not extend into the arch. Most often seen with Marfan's syndrome and pregnancy, type II dissections account for 10% of all dissections.

Type III—Begins beyond the aortic arch distal to the left subclavian artery and extends down to the aortic bifurcation and beyond. Type III is often seen in older hypertensive persons. It accounts for 20% to 30% of the dissections.

INCIDENCE

It is estimated that there are 5 to 10 dissections per million population per year. Many go unrecognized or diagnosed as aneurysms, MIs, or CVAs. Dissections tend to occur 2 to 3 times more frequently in men between the ages of 50 and 70 than in women of that age range. Below the age of 40 the incidence is about the same in men and women. Half the dissections in women occur during pregnancy.[36]

ETIOLOGY

The exact cause of aortic dissection is yet to be known. However, intrinsic weakness and damage of the media, atherosclerosis, and hydraulic shear stresses all may play a role.

1. **Medical degeneration**—associated with Marfan's syndrome, the normal aging process and hypertension
2. **Intimal damage**—resulting from arteriosclerosis, trauma, and infection
3. **Result of shearing stress**—related to the heart beating; the ascending aorta being affected most often resulting from the hemodynamic forces of the pulse wave.[40,183]

Though the exact cause of aortic dissection is unknown and the triggering event for medial degeneration is unclear, exposure to certain disorders does place the aorta at risk for dissection.[40]

Hypertension—More than 90% of the patients with aortic dissections have a history of systemic hypertension. Hypertension stresses the vasa vasorum and the media, causing degeneration and necrosis. However, medial abnormalities must first be present for the degeneration to occur.

Marfan's syndrome—Marfan's syndrome is an inherited connective tissue disorder. The hallmark of this problem is an increased elasticity of the aortic wall because of the deficiency of connective tissue and an ineffective cross-linking of collagen.[40]

Cystic medial necrosis—This involves the proximal aorta and is characterized by the disruption of the media, with the accumulation of cyst-like spaces filled with mucoid material, that leads to degeneration of the elastic tissue and structural abnormalities. It is commonly found in Marfan's syndrome, but may be found in any patient with connective tissue disease.

Pregnancy—Hormonal changes, together with increased blood volume and hypertension, may disrupt the integrity of the media, which then leads to degeneration. Risk of dissection is usually in the last trimester.[53]

Traumatic dissection—Deceleration injuries are frequently responsible for disruption of the aortic wall distal to the left subclavian artery. Tears occur at the aortic isthmus where the aortic arch joins the thoracic aorta. Other traumatic causes of aortic dissection include those caused by direct injury during special procedures such as arteriography, cardiopulmonary bypass, and intra-aortic balloon pump procedures.

PATHOPHYSIOLOGY

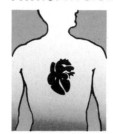

A primary tear in the intima or rupture of the vasa vasorum permits blood to enter the medial layer and results in hemorrhage and hematoma formation. The intimal tear may be the result of shearing stresses and hemodynamic forces, which allow blood to enter the media from the aortic lumen. The hematoma develops and the degenerated medial layer separates, producing an acute dissection. This longitudinal separation of the media is the pathophysiologic hallmark of aortic dissection. The dissection will then propagate for varying distances. The progressing dissection may undermine the aortic valve leaflets, occlude branch vessels, then reenter the circulation producing a double lumen to rupture through the adventitia, resulting in fatal hemorrhage. Autopsy studies have shown that one third of patients will die 24 hours after acute dissection and rupture.

COMPLICATIONS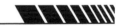

Fatal hemorrhage

DIAGNOSTIC STUDIES AND FINDINGS

Diagnostic test	Findings
Complete blood count	Decreased Hct
	Increased WBC
Chest x-ray	Superior mediastinal widening
	Widening of the distal aortic knob
	Increased aortic diameter
	Right deviation of the trachea
	Pleural effusions
	NOTE: Aortic dissection may be present even when there is a normal CXR
CT scan and angiography	Demonstrates the site of intimal tear and the extent of the false lumen

MEDICAL MANAGEMENT

The overall goal is to halt the progression of the dissection through pain and BP control and surgical intervention.

GENERAL MANAGEMENT

ECG: Nonspecific ST-T changes, not usually diagnostic.

DRUG THERAPY

Pain management: Morphine sulfate.

Nitroprusside with a beta-blocker (e.g., propranolol):   To decrease afterload and contractility.

Trimethaphan camsylate (Arfonad):   A ganglionic blocking agent; lowers BP and contractility.

Loop diuretics (e.g., furosemide):   Aid in limiting contractility (secondary to decreasing preload), which results in slowing of the dissection process.

NOTE: Hydralazine (Apresoline) is contraindicated in aortic dissection because it increases the shearing force on the heart.

SURGERY

Surgery is indicated immediately if any of the following conditions are present:

Inability of drug therapy to control/prevent further dissection.
Aortic valve regurgitation
Tamponade
Decreased perfusion to a major aortic branch
Threatened aortic rupture

Types I and II dissection repair: Resection of the aorta with graft placement; aortic valve repair if indicated and necessary revascularization to restore perfusion to affected aortic branches.

Type III dissection management: Many of these can be effectively managed medically. If distal dissections ultimately require surgery, the dissection is resected and a graft is placed after the false lumen is obliterated.

1   ASSESS

ASSESSMENT	OBSERVATIONS
Pain	Sudden onset begins in the anterior chest, back or epigastric area (the identification of the point of dissection may be estimated based on the location of the pain) Radiation of chest pain to the back may indicate distal progression; Described as sharp or tearing sensation
BP	Generally hypertensive (>200 systolic) Hypotension may mean that the aorta has already ruptured and is most commonly seen with dissections of the ascending aorta May be a difference in auscultated BP bilaterally
Heart sounds	Murmur related to aortic insufficiency if valve leaflets are disrupted

ASSESSMENT	OBSERVATIONS
Pulses	Decreased, unequal or absent pulses (potential) arterial bruits (potential)
Jugular veins	If distended may be suggestive of CHF, tamponade, or mediastinal hemorrhage
Level of consciousness	May be decreased if there is occlusion of the carotid arteries; also possible—syncope, CVA
Motor movement	Paresthesias and paralysis
Abdomen	Abdominal pain, distended abdomen, and hypoactive or absent bowel sounds
Urine output	Oliguria or hematuria (the symptoms of renal failure may also be present after prolonged hypotension)

2 DIAGNOSE

NURSING DIAGNOSIS	SUBJECTIVE FINDINGS	OBJECTIVE FINDINGS
Potential altered tissue perfusion related to aortic dissection	Complains of restlessness; verbalizes discomfort	Variability of pulses, decreased loss of pulse; peripheral bruits. Changes in level of consciousness. Abdominal pain. Decreased urine output. Heart sounds: aortic regurgitation murmur. Shock state.
Pain related to aortic dissection	Describes sharp pain	Hypertension. Tachycardia, decreased pulses. Hyperventilation. Guarding of chest.
Anxiety related to pain, pending emergent surgery, and threat of loss of life	Verbalizes fears, concerns	Tachycardia, tachypnea, hypertension, agitation, inability to rest

Other related nursing diagnoses

Decreased cardiac output related to mechanical factors secondary to aortic valve disruption
Potential impaired skin integrity related to impaired perfusion
Potential impaired gas exchange related to hyperventilation and mechanical factors secondary to the dissection

3 PLAN

Patient goals

1. Patient will exhibit evidence of perfusion adequate to meet bodily needs.
2. Patient will be pain-free.
3. Patient will demonstrate behavior indicative of lessened anxiety.
4. Patient will demonstrate understanding of condition and associated risk factors and interventions.

→ > >

4 IMPLEMENT

NURSING DIAGNOSIS	NURSING INTERVENTIONS	RATIONALE
Pain related to aortic dissection	Assess and document the location, quality, and radiation of pain.	Pain that increases or subsides then returns indicates propagation of the dissection.
	Administer medications as ordered.	Narcotics are used to relieve pain; nitrates and beta blockers are given to decrease systemic BP and myocardial contractility, which will decrease shearing effect that produces dissection.
	Obtain a 12-lead ECG.	To rule out myocardial ischemia due to CAD.
	Obtain chest x-ray and compare with previous studies.	Serial chest x-rays may show changes in width or shape of aorta.
	Maintain patient on bed rest in a quiet environment.	To reduce excessive stimulation and sympathetic response, which helps reduce BP.
Altered tissue perfusion (acute) related to aortic dissection	Assess for signs of propagation of dissection. Monitor and record BP, HR, peripheral pulses and movement q 1h.	Evidence of deterioration in vascular status may reflect further dissection.
	Auscultate heart sounds and check neurologic status q 1 h.	Aortic insufficiency is a symptom of a valve disruption. Decreased LOC may be the result of decreased cerebral perfusion due to hypotension or dissection propagation.
	Assess motor function q 1 h.	Decreased motor function may suggest intercostal or lumbar artery involvement.
	Administer medications as ordered.	Antihypertensive agents are given to reduce BP, which must be lowered to prevent dissection propagation.
	Monitor and document hemodynamic pressures q 1 h (PAP, CO/CI).	Changes in hemodynamic pressures may be suggestive of progression of dissection of aortic rupture.
	Measure urine output q 1 h.	Oliguria may indicate renal artery dissection or be the result of prolonged hypotension.
	Auscultate bowel sounds and palpate abdomen q 2-4 h.	Signs of acute abdomen may indicate mesenteric artery involvement.

NURSING DIAGNOSIS	NURSING INTERVENTIONS	RATIONALE
Anxiety related to pain, pending emergent surgery, and threat of loss of life	Assess for signs and verbal expressions of anxiety and fear.	Heightened anxiety levels stimulate sympathetic release of catecholamines, which can increase BP.
	Allow for as much rest as possible, keeping the environment as quiet as possible.	Reduces anxiety level by decreasing unnecessary external stimuli.
	Provide patient with brief explanation about procedures to decrease fear of the unknown as much as possible.	Providing information increases sense of control and decreases uncertainty, thereby reducing level of anxiety.

5 EVALUATE

PATIENT OUTCOME	DATA INDICATING THAT OUTCOME IS REACHED
Tissue perfusion is improved.	Pulses are present bilaterally. Skin is warm and dry. Renal output is at least 30 ml per hour. Abdomen is soft and nontender with positive bowel sounds.
Pain is relieved.	Patient verbalizes pain relief. Physiologic signs of pain (e.g., tachycardia, tachypnea, hypertension) decrease.
Demonstrates decreased anxiety.	Patient appears calm and rests quietly—heart rate and respiration are normal.
Knowledge level is increased.	Patient verbalizes increased knowledge and understanding regarding condition and factors that increase risk of dissection and demonstrates understanding of self-care management.

PATIENT TEACHING

1. Provide information regarding condition and possible contributing factors.
2. Discuss signs and symptoms to report to physician: 5 Ps—pain, pallor, paresthesia, paralysis, and pulselessness.
3. Review medications, dosage, and side effects.
4. Review activity allowances and limitations. Instruct patient to avoid isometric activities such as heavy lifting.
5. Review importance of blood pressure control—low-sodium diet, weight control, taking prescribed medication; self-monitoring of BP.
6. Review importance of avoiding smoking and use of tobacco products.

Venous Thrombosis

Venous thrombosis is an abnormal vascular condition in which a thrombus develops within a blood vessel.

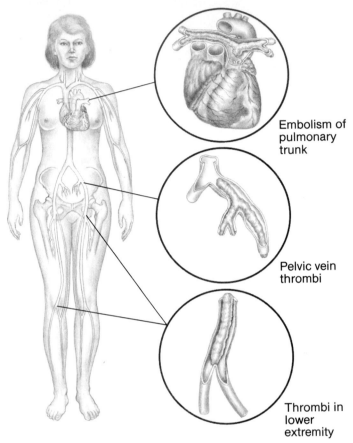

Embolism of pulmonary trunk

Pelvic vein thrombi

Thrombi in lower extremity

COMPLICATIONS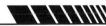

Venous ulcers
Pulmonary embolism
Chronic venous insufficiency

EPIDEMIOLOGY

Venous thrombosis is the most common venous disorder. The greatest morbidity and mortality occur among surgical patients (30% to 60%) and in patients receiving intravenous therapy, because of the associated embolization of a thrombus to the lungs. The incidence of pulmonary embolism in surgical patients has been estimated to be between 7.3% and 54%, with the estimated number of deaths 200,000 per year.[111]

PATHOPHYSIOLOGY

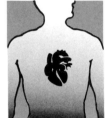 The triad of stasis, intimal damage, and hypercoagulability is responsible for most venous thrombosis.

Venous stasis occurs in persons who are inactive for a time because of bed rest or immobilization of the lower extremities. Thrombus formation results from a reduction of flow-induced dilution and a decrease in natural circulating anticoagulants (antithrombin III, platelet factor IV, and some prostaglandins). Stasis caused by reduced flow increases the contact between platelets and coagulation factors that enhance platelet aggregation.

Intimal damage may occur as a result of internal or external trauma. Venipuncture and traumatic or long-term intravenous therapy are common offenders. Endothelial damage leads to exposure of the subintimal collagen membrane, which promotes platelet adherence, and activation of intrinsic coagulation factors, which contribute to thrombus formation.

Hypercoagulability reflects an alteration in blood coagulability, which occurs in some patients with hematologic disorders (such as polycythemias and anemias), excessive estrogen or steroid use, or malignancies.

Once formed, the thrombus initiates an inflammatory process leading to fibrosis. The enlarging thrombus eventually occludes the lumen of the vein or detaches and embolizes to the systemic circulation.

Frequent sites for venous thrombus formation are the soleal and gastrocnemius venous sinus and the larger veins, such as the venae cavae and the femoral, iliac, and subclavian veins. Thrombosis of these veins is associated with increased risk of embolization. Thrombosis in superficial (subcutaneous) veins rarely leads to pulmonary embolism.

DIAGNOSTIC STUDIES AND FINDINGS

Diagnostic test	Findings
Plethysmography	Decreased circulation distal to affected area
Doppler ultrasonography	Reduced blood flow to specific area; shows obstruction to venous flow
Phlebography	Confirms diagnosis; shows filling defects
^{125}I fibrinogen scan	Defines location of clot and any emboli that may have dislodged

MEDICAL MANAGEMENT

GENERAL MANAGEMENT

Physical activity: Bed rest with elevation of affected extremity above level of RA.

Other: Warm, moist heat; custom-fitted elastic stockings when ambulatory; monitoring of PTT and/or PT while patient is receiving anticoagulant therapy.

DRUG THERAPY

Anticoagulants:

Heparin sodium. Indications: Initially administered IV to augment fibrinolytic activity and aid in thrombolysis.

Warfarin. Indications: Given later to maintain prothrombin time to twice control level; usually for 3 mo.

Fibrinolytic agents:

Streptokinase (Streptase).Indications: Produces total clot lysis and restores normal venous valve function.

Antiplatelet agents: Used in prevention of thrombus.

Antiplatelet agents (to prevent thrombus formation).
Dipyridamole (Persantine)

SURGERY

Rarely indicated.
Techniques used for deep vein thrombophlebitis necessitating venous interruption—ligation, vein plication, or clipping.
Iliofemoral thrombectomy—may be considered for patients with acute iliofemoral thrombosis and compromised arterial perfusion that fail to respond to conventional therapy.

Procedures to prevent distal embolization:

Extravascular vena caval interruption—application of a partitioning clip around the vein; used prophylactically for patients considered high risk for embolization who are undergoing abdominal surgery for another reason.

Intracaval filters (Mobin-Uidden umbrella, Kimray-Greenfield filter) are interruption devices inserted into the right internal jugular vein and advanced to the vena cava via a catheter; once in place, the devices permit continuous venous flow while filtering clots, thus preventing further embolization.

1 ASSESS

ASSESSMENT	OBSERVATIONS
Lower extremity (deep veins)	Calf pain and tenderness; Homan's sign (calf pain on dorsiflexion of foot); dilated superficial veins; edema of involved extremity (30%-50% of DVTs may be clinically silent); pain and tenderness over involved vein (e.g., groin); increased size compared with nonaffected side
Upper extremity (superficial veins)	Redness, warmth, and tenderness over affected vein; veins visible and palpable

2 DIAGNOSE

NURSING DIAGNOSIS	SUBJECTIVE FINDINGS	OBJECTIVE FINDINGS
Impaired skin integrity related to venous stasis and fragility of small blood vessels	Complains of discomfort in extremities	Erythema, swelling, edema, drainage, ulceration in extremities
Altered peripheral tissue perfusion related to interruption of venous flow	Complains of pain: ache, cramping, tenderness	Skin changes: 　Color—cyanosis 　Temperature—warm 　Swelling Positive Homan's sign; asymmetry between legs
Potential impaired gas exchange related to pulmonary embolism	Reports SOB; dyspnea; chest or shoulder pain	Changes in mental acuity (restlessness, confusion, somnolence, syncope); cough; hemoptysis; diaphoresis; tachypnea; tachycardia; arterial blood gas (decreased Pa_{O2}, decreased P_{CO2}) Chest x-ray: elevated diaphragm, pleural effusions

Other related nursing diagnoses

Pain related to affected extremity
Impaired physical mobility related to imposed activity restrictions

3 PLAN

Patient goals

1. Patient will demonstrate minimal tissue disruption; if present, will demonstrate progressive healing.
2. Patient will demonstrate improved venous blood flow in affected extremity.
3. Patient will demonstrate no signs of pulmonary embolism.
4. Patient will demonstrate understanding of disease process and methods of preventing recurrence.

4 IMPLEMENT

NURSING DIAGNOSIS	NURSING INTERVENTIONS	RATIONALE
Impaired skin integrity related to venous stasis and fragility of small blood vessels	Assess skin integrity of affected extremity daily, noting development of stasis ulcers.	Development of ulcerations is reflective of venous stasis and transudation of fluid into the interstitial space.
	Raise affected extremity above level of heart as ordered.	To avoid venous hypertension.
	Use elastic compression gradient stocking.	To minimize peripheral edema, which is necessary for wound healing.
	Administer daily skin care to affected area. Use mild soap; rinse well; dry gently, but thoroughly.	To prevent development of ulceration.
	Avoid vigorous massage or rubbing of reddened area.	Massaging may lead to dislodgment of clot and pulmonary embolism.
	If ulceration present, initiate treatment as indicated: administer warm saline soaks.	To limit extension of wound and prevent infection. Warm saline soaks relieve discomfort and decrease inflammation.
	Administer topical antibiotics and sterile dressing; use bed cradle as indicated.	Topical antibiotics and dressings prevent and/or control infection. Bed cradles relieve pressure from bed linens and protect affected extremities.
Altered peripheral tissue perfusion related to interruption of venous flow	Assess circulation of affected extremity, noting changes in leg circumference; measure and record size of affected extremity every day.	To identify presence of DVT.
	Maintain on bed rest during acute phase if thrombosis present.	To stop thrombotic process and prevent embolization.
	Elevate affected limb above level of heart unless contraindicated.	To lessen venous stasis and improve venous flow.
	Avoid use of knee gatch or pillows behind knees; instruct patient not to cross legs and to avoid elastic stockings above the knees.	These activities restrict venous blood flow by causing venous compression, which results in venous pooling and edema.
	Administer medications as ordered: anticoagulants and fibrinolytic agents.	Anticoagulants are given prophylactically to minimize risk of embolization. Fibrinolytic agents help dissolve the clot.
	Instruct patient to stop smoking.	Tobacco causes vasoconstriction, which interferes with peripheral circulation.
	Monitor laboratory values: Warfarin—prothrombin. Heparin—partial thromboplastin time.	To reduce risk of bleeding when taking anticoagulants.

→ > >

NURSING DIAGNOSIS	NURSING INTERVENTIONS	RATIONALE
	Initiate a progressive exercise program as ordered. Never dangle extremities; apply support stockings prior to ambulating; avoid standing for long periods; alternate position by standing on toes then on heels.	Normal muscle activity facilitates venous return. Prolonged standing or sitting decreases venous flow, causing increased venous pooling.
Potential impaired gas exchange related to pulmonary embolism	Assess daily for signs of impaired gas exchange.	Early signs of embolism may be very subtle going undetected unless carefully evaluated.
	Auscultate lung sounds q 8 h or as indicated.	Diminished breath sounds or crackles may be heard over affected lung.
	Administer anticoagulants as ordered.	To promote thrombolysis.
	Maintain on bed rest during acute phase.	To avoid dislodgment of clot from venous thrombosis.
	Use elastic support stockings when ambulatory or sitting for prolonged period.	To maintain venous circulation and avoid venous pooling.
Knowledge deficit	See Patient Teaching.	

5 EVALUATE

PATIENT OUTCOME	DATA INDICATING THAT OUTCOME IS REACHED
Skin integrity is maintained or improved.	Absence of skin ulcerations; patient demonstrates management of home skin care.
Inflammation is decreased and venous blood flow is improved.	Patient reports relief of pain, swelling, and redness.
Exhibits no sign of respiratory distress due to embolization.	ABGs are within normal limits; chest x-ray normal; respirations at baseline.
Level of knowledge is increased.	Patient is able to describe the disease process and demonstrates methods to improve venous blood flow.

PATIENT TEACHING

1. Instruct the patient and family about the nature of the disorder and methods of preventing recurrence.
2. Instruct the patient to avoid constrictive clothing and crossing legs when sitting.
3. Explain the value of rest periods with legs raised.
4. Explain the need to lose weight if the patient is obese.
5. Instruct the patient to avoid use of oral contraceptives.
6. Explain the need for a regular or moderate exercise program, the need to avoid prolonged standing or sitting, and the need to use elastic stockings when walking.
7. Explain the importance of avoiding tobacco products: smoking cigarettes, cigars, or chewing tobacco.
8. Explain anticoagulant therapy, stressing the following:

    Importance of returning for regularly scheduled laboratory tests: Heparin—prothromboplastin time (PTT). Warfarin—prothrombin time (PT). To report signs of overmedication: Bleeding gums. Easy bruising. Heavy menstrual period. Need to avoid use of aspirin, alcohol, which influence effects of medications.
9. Instruct patient about skin care.

CHAPTER 6

Surgical and therapeutic procedures

CARDIAC SURGERY

Surgical interventions for cardiac disorders may be employed as a corrective measure in congenital heart disease or as an alternative treatment modality when a patient's clinical course becomes refractory to medical management.

Cardiac surgery may be broadly classified as an open or a closed procedure. Open heart techniques were made possible with the development of the cardiopulmonary bypass machine (extracorporeal circulation) in the early 1950s. Since that time, advances in myocardial preservation, in preoperative and postoperative support devices, and in pharmacology have contributed to improved mortality and morbidity and to increases in the number of operative procedures for cardiac disorders.

Procedures for acquired disorders include:

Coronary artery bypass grafting (CABG) (Figures 6-1 and 6-2)—direct method of increasing myocardial coronary blood flow; provides symptomatic relief in 80% of patients with significant angina and has low operative mortality. Indications include disabling angina that is refractory to medical therapy, significantly abnormal electrocardiogram (ECG) response to exercise, 50% or greater obstruction of left main coronary artery, and significant obstructive lesions in all three coronary arteries.

Valve surgery—valvulotomy (commissurotomy), valvuloplasty (repair of valve), and replacement with prosthetic valve

Resection of ventricular aneurysm—resection of nonviable myocardium

Septal defects—closure of atrial or ventricular septal defect by direct suturing or placement of Dacron patch across defect

Antiarrhythmic surgery—mapped, directed endocardial resection; aneurysmectomy

Procedures for congenital defects include:

Closure of patent ductus arteriosus
Closure of atrial or ventricular septal defect
Repair of coarctation of aorta
Repair of tetralogy of Fallot
Fontan or modified Fontan procedure for tricuspid atresia and single ventricle
Mustard procedure for transposition of great vessels

Extracorporeal circulation (heart-lung machine) assumes the function of the heart and lungs, providing a bloodless operative field. The procedure involves cannulation of great vessels, allowing drainage of unoxygenated blood that is emptied into the venous reservoir. Blood is then passed to oxygenator, where it is fully saturated. To reduce tissue oxygen requirements, temperature of blood circulating in extracorporeal unit is lowered; cold blood is returned to patient, reducing total body temperature and slowing metabolic processes. Myocardial preservation is required while the heart is arrested and includes coronary perfusion, topical cooling (profound hypothermia), and cold cardioplegia arrest. To prevent coagulation in the extracorporeal circuit, anticoagulation with heparin is administered before cannulation. At the end of cardiopulmonary bypass, protamine sulfate is given to reverse the effect of heparin.

INDICATIONS

See page 214.

CONTRAINDICATIONS

Bleeding disorders
Acute (recent) cerebrovascular accident (CVA, stroke)

CAUTIONS

Cardiac surgery may be performed with added risk in patients with pulmonary hypertension, with an active infectious process, or in refractory ventricular failure.

COMPLICATIONS

Bleeding
Dysrhythmias
Myocardial failure
Respiratory failure

PREPROCEDURAL NURSING CARE

1. Determine the type of surgical procedure—palliative, corrective, repair, bypass, or transplant—and associated risks.
2. Initiate preoperative instruction for the patient and family, including information about the surgical procedure and associated risks. Review postoperative care: routine intensive care unit (ICU) procedures (suctioning, turning, monitoring of vital signs); various tubes (endotracheal, chest, gastrointestinal, urinary catheter, intravenous); equipment (respirators, monitors); pain management; level of consciousness and emotional response; and visitor policies.
3. Obtain written informed consent.
4. Obtain baseline data: chest x-ray; ECG; laboratory work—complete blood count (CBC), blood type and cross-match, electrolytes, serum chemistries, and urinalysis; weight; height; and vital signs.
5. Perform skin preparation: chest; legs for vein harvesting.
6. Hold or modify preoperative medications:
   Digoxin—discontinue 24 to 36 hours before surgery.
   Antiplatelets—instruct patient not to take these up to 1 week before surgery.
   Anticoagulants—discontinue warfarin; initiate heparin therapy.

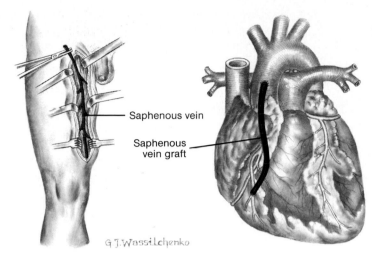

FIGURE 6-1
Coronary artery bypass graft using saphenous vein. (From Thelan.)[169]

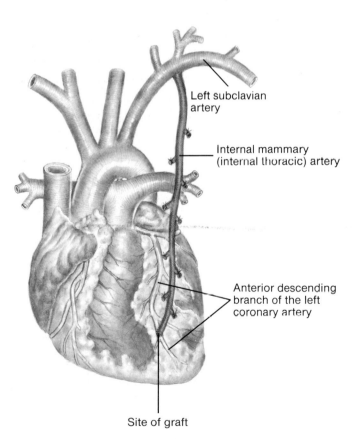

FIGURE 6-2
Coronary artery bypass graft using internal mammary artery. (From Thelan.)[169]

Antiarrhythmics, antihypertensives—in most patients continue until hours before surgery.
7. Initiate pulmonary preparation by instructing the patient to stop smoking, teaching the patient methods for coughing and deep breathing, and using an incentive spirometer. Encourage return demonstration.

8. Deal with preoperative anxiety, offering reassurance and support.
9. Assist with insertion of balloon flotation catheter, if ordered, before surgery.
10. Administer preoperative sedation.

MEDICAL MANAGEMENT

GENERAL MANAGEMENT

Immediate postoperative: Hemodynamic monitoring—arterial, LAP, PAP, and PCWP pressures; CO; CI; and SVR are usually required measurements
  ECG monitoring: continuous evaluation of HR and rhythm
  Pacemakers
  Intra-aortic balloon pump—used when severe ventricular dysfunction occurs as patient is removed from bypass; provides circulatory support to failing myocardium
  Ventricular assist devices
  Mechanical assisted ventilation
  Nasopharyngeal suctioning
  Endotracheal suctioning
  Chest tubes—one or two placed in mediastinum to maintain free flow of drainage and to monitor amount of bleeding from surgical site

Laboratory/diagnostic studies: HgB, Hct, electrolytes, ABG, PT, PTT, platelets

Ongoing postoperative: Diet therapy—sodium and fluid restrictions on basis of patient's clinical status
Pulmonary toilet—encourage coughing, deep breathing, and use of incentive spirometry

DRUG THERAPY

Preoperative management: Cardiac glycosides
  Digoxin (Lanoxin)—Indications: atrial fibrillation and flutter
Antiarrhythmics
  Lidocaine (Xylocaine)—Indications: ventricular ectopy, tachycardia
  Quinidine sulfate (Quinora, others)—Indications. ventricular ectopy, tachycardia
  Procainamide (Pronestyl)—Indications: ventricular ectopy, tachycardia
Potassium replacement
  Usual dosage: IV or PO to maintain serum levels at 4-5 mEq/L

Postoperative management (based on clinical symptoms, complications, and progress of patient): Parenteral fluids
  Usual dosage (calculated on basis of procedure performed and patient's body surface area): CABG, 50 ml/h; valve replacement, 1000-1500 ml/24 h; pediatric dosage, 60 ml/kg for first 10 kg body weight, 30 ml/kg for next 10 kg, 15 ml/kg for remainder of weight
  Blood/blood components: Packed cells, plasma, platelets
  Drugs to correct coagulopathy: protamine sulfate, 6-aminocaproic acid (Amicar), epsilon aminocaproic acid (EACA), vitamin K
  Pain medication: Morphine 0.1 ml/kg; Tylenol with codeine
  Antibiotics
  Anticoagulation therapy—for patients with prosthetic valves or valved conduits; Heparin; Coumadin

1 ASSESS

ASSESSMENT	OBSERVATIONS
Level of conscious-ness	Early: arousable Late: alert and oriented
Pupils	May be small but reactive to light
Sensory motor func-tion	As patient awakens, moves all extremities
Respiratory function	Early: atelectasis; diminished breath sounds at base Late: clear with full aeration; ABGs normal

Cardiovascular sys-tem	Complications:
	  Low CO
	    Narrow pulse pressure; thready, rapid pulse; decreased urine output; labored respira-tion; disorientation; increased PCWP and LAP
	  Dysrhythmias
	    Atrial fibrillation and flutter; junctional rhythms; heart block; ventricular rhythms—premature ventricular contractions (PVCs), tachycardia, fibrillation
	  Cardiac tamponade
	    Hypotension, narrowed pulse pressure (10 mm Hg), pulsus paradoxus, widened medi-astinal shadow on chest x-ray, increased venous pressure
	  Bleeding
	    Chest tube drainage at least 250 ml/h, hypotension, disorientation, prolonged PT and PTT, decreased platelet levels
	  Infection
	    Elevated temperature, purulent drainage from suture sites, chills, diaphoresis, malaise
	  Pericarditis, postpericardiotomy syndrome
	    Pericardial friction rub, low-grade fever, chills, diaphoresis, malaise, chest pain

2 DIAGNOSE

NURSING DIAGNOSIS	SUBJECTIVE FINDINGS	OBJECTIVE FINDINGS
Decreased cardiac output related to mechanical factors (changes in preload, afterload, contractil-ity) or electrical in-stability		Decreased mentation, dyspnea Skin—pallor, cool, diaphoresis Hypotension, tachycardia/bradycardia Decreased peripheral pulses Decreased urine output ECG—dysrhythmia: premature atrial con-traction (PAC), premature ventricular con-traction (PVC), supraventricular tachycardia (SVT), junctional atrioventricu-lar (AV) conduction Hemodynamic measurements—decreased CO, CI, SVR; increased LAP, PCWP Laboratory values—decreased/increased potassium level

NURSING DIAGNOSIS	SUBJECTIVE FINDINGS	OBJECTIVE FINDINGS
Impaired gas exchange related to hypoventilation and to ventilation/perfusion abnormalities	Reports inability to rest, SOB	Changes in mentation—anxious, restless, confused Respiratory distress—tachypnea, bradypnea, use of accessory muscles of respiration, labored breathing, diaphoresis Pallor, cyanosis Breath sounds—decreased, crackles
Ineffective breathing pattern related to decreased lung expansion and to incisional pain and anxiety	Complains of fatigue, SOB, chest pain; anxious	Tachypnea, SOB, tachycardia, absent or decreased breath sounds, pleural friction rub, elevated temperature
Fluid volume excess related to postoperative expanded extracellular fluid volume and to postoperative sodium and water retention	Complains of fatigue, SOB	Dyspnea, orthopnea, cough, tachypnea, tachycardia, weight gain, decreased urine output Heart sounds—S_3, S_4 Breath sounds—crackles Increased jugular venous distention (JVD) Elevated PAP, PCWP Laboratory values—increased sodium level
Potential for infection related to compromised host defense and increased exposure to invasive lines	Verbalizes discomfort	Elevated temperature, chills, diaphoresis Sternotomy—redness, swelling, drainage, tenderness, dehiscence Leg incisions (vein graft)—redness, swelling, drainage Invasive lines and suture sites—redness, swelling, tenderness Systemic—elevated WBC count, positive blood cultures
Potential for injury (hemorrhage) related to disruption in platelet function and clotting factor secondary to effects of heart-lung machine	Reports apprehension, restlessness	Altered mentation, tachycardia, tachypnea, hypotension Significant oozing around dressing sites Decreased HgB, Hct Increased chest drainage (>300 ml/h) Thrombocytopenia (platelets <50,000/mm^3) Activated clotting time—increased
Anxiety related to actual or potential threat to biological integrity, fear of dying, ICU environment	Verbalizes fears, concerns; increased questioning, anger	**Mild to moderate anxiety** Discomfort or tension; increased verbalization; increased muscle tension; facial tension Preoperatively—increased concentration on upcoming surgery Postoperatively—verbalizes fear of being discharged **Severe anxiety** Sense of impending doom, uncertainty, ineffective functioning, lack of clear comprehension of immediate situation

Other related nursing diagnoses: Activity intolerance related to generalized weakness; **Fluid volume deficit** related to postoperative fluid shifts or bleeding; **Pain** related to incisions (sternotomy, leg)

3   PLAN

Patient goals

1. Patient will improve and maintain adequate CO.
2. Patient will demonstrate improved gas exchange.
3. Patient will demonstrate an effective breathing pattern.
4. Patient will demonstrate normal fluid balance.
5. Patient will demonstrate no signs of infection and normal wound healing.

6. Patient will not demonstrate signs of bleeding.
7. Patient will demonstrate reduced anxiety.
8. Comfort level is achieved.
9. Patient demonstrates increased knowledge regarding procedure and associated risks and will demonstrate adequate skills necessary to support self-care activities during and following hospital stay.

4   IMPLEMENT

NURSING DIAGNOSIS	NURSING INTERVENTIONS	RATIONALE
Decreased cardiac output related to mechanical factors (changes in preload, afterload, contractility) or electrical instability	Assess and monitor for signs of decreased CO, documenting changes and response to therapy. Report any signs of increased afterload, decreased preload, or electrical instability.	To detect *early* trends and changes in CO. Prompt reporting enhances early interventions.
	Monitor PAP, PCWP, arterial pressures, and mixed venous oxygen saturation (SV_{O_2}) q 15 min during immediate postoperative period; decrease frequency as clinical status stabilizes. Then monitor vital signs q 2-4 h. Obtain CO measurements q 2 h; calculate CI and SVR as indicated.	Baseline hemodynamic measurements assist to determine patient's hemodynamic stability and appropriate response to therapy; also provide information regarding effectiveness of myocardial contractility and vascular response. These data guide the administration and initiation of medication to maximize CO.
	Monitor and record ECG rate and rhythm q 4-6 h; initiate pacing as ordered.	Dysrhythmias, which frequently occur in first 72 h postoperatively, may reflect hypoxia, electrolyte/acid-base abnormalities, or underlying myocardial dysfunction; therefore early detection enhances appropriate treatment and avoids hemodynamic compromise.
	Measure urine output q 1 h; note output of <30 ml/h.	Decreased urine output may reflect decreased circulating volume and hypoperfusion of kidneys.
	Check peripheral perfusion: pulses, skin temperature, and color.	Decreased pulses reflect decreased tissue perfusion related to low CO.
	Administer fluids and medications as ordered: inotropic agents, vasodilator therapy, and antiarrhythmics.	Inotropic agents increase myocardial contractility; vasodilators decrease SVR (afterload); antiarrhythmics control dysrhythmias.
	Initiate intra-aortic balloon pump as ordered.	To decrease afterload and to increase myocardial perfusion by decreasing cardiac workload.

→ › ›

NURSING DIAGNOSIS	NURSING INTERVENTIONS	RATIONALE
	Obtain laboratory values as ordered.	To monitor for changes.
	Check temperature on admission to unit and q 1 h until temperature within normal limits; continue rewarming methods until temperature within normal limits.	Persistent postoperative hypothermia increases vasoconstriction, which can lead to increased SVR.
Impaired gas exchange related to hypoventilation and to ventilation/perfusion abnormalities	Assess and monitor respiratory function while patient is on ventilator. Assess rate and quality of respirations as patient is being weaned.	To determine return of spontaneous respiration and/or to detect early signs of abnormal ventilation/perfusion that may result from effects of anesthesia, hypoxia, acid-base abnormalities, secretions, or lung abnormalities (atelectasis, pneumothorax).
	Obtain and monitor ABGs and SV_{O2} as ordered.	To assess signs of respiratory acidosis/alkalosis; low levels of SV_{O2} reflect decreased O_2 delivery and increased tissue O_2 extraction.
	Administer O_2 therapy with assisted ventilation as ordered.	Controlled ventilation and oxygenation produce gas exchange during initial postoperative period while patient remains under influence of anesthesia and drugs.
	Auscultate lung sounds q 1-2 h.	To detect atelectasis and pulmonary congestion.
	Suction q 1-2 h; hyperoxygenate before suctioning procedure per institutional policy; monitor and record any dysrhythmias during procedure.	Postoperative suctioning is necessary to remove secretions that can interfere with effective gas exchange. Hyperoxygenation before suctioning prevents hypoxia, which can result in dysrhythmias.
	Elevate head of bed 30°.	To promote oxygenation.
	Obtain serial chest x-rays as ordered.	To detect signs of pulmonary complication; to verify correct endotracheal placement.
	After extubation, administer O_2 via high-humidity face mask.	To avoid hypoxemia.
	Encourage coughing and deep breathing; encourage use of incentive spirometer.	To loosen secretions and maintain effective airway clearance.
	Encourage early ambulation and/or repositioning; perform chest percussion as ordered.	To promote removal of secretions, which improves gas exchange.
	Auscultate lung sounds q 4-8 h or as indicated.	To assess resolving atelectasis and pulmonary congestion.

NURSING DIAGNOSIS	NURSING INTERVENTIONS	RATIONALE
Ineffective breathing pattern related to decreased lung expansion and to incisional pain and anxiety	Assess rate and quality of respiration.	To detect signs of decreased lung expansion or splinting.
	Observe and maintain patency of chest tubes.	To ensure proper drainage.
	Auscultate chest for dimimished breath sounds, initially q 1-2 h and later q 4-6 h.	Initially to detect signs of atelectasis; later to determine resolution and improvement of breathing and gas exchange.
	Reposition patient from one side to other during immediate postoperative period.	To encourage lung expansion; to mobilize secretions.
	Assist and encourage patient to cough and deep breathe q 2-4 h; encourage use of incentive spirometer; use pillow to splint chest when coughing.	To mobilize secretions; to increase lung expansion; to prevent and correct atelectasis.
	Administer pain medications as required before pulmonary toilet.	To facilitate and ease breathing pattern.
Fluid volume excess related to postoperative expanded extracellular fluid volume and to postoperative sodium and water retention	Assess for signs of fluid volume excess; monitor filling pressures (RAP, pulmonary artery diastolic pressure, LAP). Inspect for increased JVD and dependent edema.	Fluid volume excess results from several factors, including an expanded extracellular fluid volume caused by hemodilution perfusion or by elevation of ADH and aldosterone levels, which favors sodium and water retention in early postoperative phase.
	Auscultate heart sounds (S_3) and breath sounds.	Sudden development of S_3 reflects an increase in central blood volume, which may result from cardiac dysfunction; presence of adventitious sounds indicates pulmonary congestion.
	Monitor intake and output q 24 h for first 3 days or as ordered; measure specific gravity.	Mobilization of extracellular fluid is demonstrated by spontaneous decreases on day 3 or 4 postoperatively.
	Weigh patient daily (same time of day, same amount of clothing).	To determine accurate fluid loss or retention.
	Follow fluid restrictions as ordered.	To prevent further fluid retention during period when total body sodium content is elevated.
	Administer diuretic therapy as ordered.	To reduce body fluid excess.
Potential for infection related to compromised host defense and increased exposure to invasive lines	Observe suture sites and invasive line sites for local redness, drainage, and swelling. Check temperature q 2 h for 48 h, then q 4 h for 48 h, then q 8 h.	To detect developing infectious process; incisional wound infections are associated with poor aseptic techniques.
	Observe for signs of elevated temperature, chills, and diaphoresis.	May indicate sepsis.

→ > >

NURSING DIAGNOSIS	NURSING INTERVENTIONS	RATIONALE
	Obtain CBC, with differential blood cultures as ordered.	To identify infecting organisms; to guide medical therapy.
	Change IV and pressure lines, solutions, and dressings according to protocol, maintaining sterile technique.	To prevent nosocomial infection and cross-contamination; to inhibit bacterial growth in tubings and solution.
	Remove indwelling urinary catheter as soon as patient is awake and stable (1-2 h).	To prevent urinary tract infection.
Potential for injury (hemorrhage) related to disruption in platelet function and clotting factor secondary to effects of heart-lung machine	Observe for signs of hemorrhage and co-agulopathy: blood oozing from incision, bloody secretions from endotracheal tube, and hematuria.	Effects of heparin given intraoperatively (heparin rebound) can appear postoperatively; platelet function is decreased.
	Observe color and measure chest tube drainage q ½-1 h. Report output in excess of 150 ml/h for an adult.	Chest drainage should begin to decrease and become more serous in color within 4-6 h after surgery; excessive drainage indicates possible coagulopathy, which may necessitate surgical exploration of bleeding source.
	Check HgB, Hct, and clotting studies on patient's arrival to ICU and q 2-4 h as indicated.	May reflect unstable postoperative protamine sulfate–heparin complex and reappearance of heparin activity.
	Administer blood and blood products as ordered.	To control bleeding and/or clotting disorders.
	Administer medications as ordered: protamine sulfate, micar.	Protamine sulfate reverses effect of heparin. Micar is used to treat fibrinolysis.
Anxiety related to actual or potential threat to biologic integrity, fear of dying, ICU environment	*Preoperative* Assess level of anxiety; report symptoms of acute, severe anxiety.	Acute, severe preoperative anxiety can be detrimental to outcome.
	Provide adequate instruction, allowing for questions and offering reassurance. Explain method of communication to be used after surgery while patient is intubated.	To allay fears and to ensure postoperative cooperation.

	Postoperative
	Implement measures that will reduce level of anxiety:
	  Orient patient to time, situation, and location.
	  Inform patient that surgery is over.
	  Assist with communication.
	  Anticipate needs if possible.
	  Allow family support and participation.
	  Provide reassurance of daily progress.
	  Encourage verbalization of fears and questions regarding surgery, recovery, and discharge.
	  Begin postoperative instruction.
		Combined effects of anesthesia, drugs, pain, ICU environment, and equipment contribute to limited recall by patient regarding preoperative information; therefore it is important to reorient frequently, explaining what is happening, until patient is fully awake.

Knowledge deficit	See Patient Teaching.	

5 EVALUATE

PATIENT OUTCOME	DATA INDICATING THAT OUTCOME IS REACHED
Hemodynamic and electromechanical stability is achievcd. Cardiac output is adequate.	Blood pressure, PAP, and CO/CI are within normal range. No dysrhythmia is present. ECG findings are within acceptable limits.
Oxygenation and lung perfusion are adequate.	Pa_{O_2} and Pc_{O_2} are within normal limits. No dyspnea or tachypnea is present. Lungs are clear on auscultation.
Patient maintains effective breathing pattern.	Patient is carrying out measures to improve ventilation: coughing, deep breathing, using incentive spirometer. Patient is afebrile; lungs are clear of atelectasis.
Fluid volume is balanced.	No signs of dyspnea or tachypnea; dry weight is maintained. Absence of S_3 and S_4 heart sounds; lung sounds are clear. No signs of interstitial fluid present on chest x-ray. JVD is decreased.
No infection is present.	Patient is afebrile.
No signs of bleeding are present.	HgB, Hct, clotting studies, and platelets are within normal limits; chest tube drainage is clear.
Anxiety is reduced.	Patient has no pain. Anxiety is absent or decreased. Patient demonstrates appropriate behavior patterns: asking questions and participating in self-care.
Patient has knowledge and understanding of primary cardiac disorder, surgical procedure performed, and discharge instructions.	Patient is able to describe specific action to take regarding diet, medications, and care of incision(s). Patient is able to describe activity allowances and limitations.

PATIENT TEACHING ■

1. Review the surgical procedure, emphasizing any associated precautions or complications.
2. Clarify what action(s) patient should take if symptoms of infection, bleeding, ventricular failure, or dysrhythmias develop.
3. Review any diet and fluid restrictions.
4. Review discharge medication, including purpose, dosages, side effects, and need for specific follow-up laboratory studies as indicated.
5. Discuss activity allowances or limitations. To increase activities gradually, instruct patient to rest regularly during day and rest between activities during first weeks after surgery. Instruct patient to avoid lifting heavy objects or performing isometric exercises and to restrict driving during first 4 to 6 weeks. Refer patient to cardiac rehabilitation for progressive ambulation.
6. Discuss the importance of avoiding fatigue and sitting for prolonged periods.
7. Discuss issues regarding resuming sexual activities, returning to work, and traveling.
8. Discuss care of incisions and symptoms of wound infection to report to physician.

CARDIAC TRANSPLANTATION

Cardiac transplantation has evolved rapidly during the past 30 years, but it was first performed in 1905, when Carrel and Guthrie transplanted the heart of one dog to another. Not until 1967, however, when Christian Barnard performed the first human cardiac transplantation, was serious interest stimulated. Because early survival rates were poor, transplantations continued to be performed on a limited basis. Since the introduction of the immunosuppressant agent cyclosporine in 1980, the number of centers performing heart transplantations has grown steadily.

By 1987 the medical centers throughout the world with active transplant programs numbered 134, 90 of which were located in the United States. One-year survival rates are reported to be 88%, and 5-year survival is 78%.

Infection and organ rejection continue to be the most common medical complications and the primary causes of death in long-term follow-up. However, as survival time increases, other medical problems are being identified, and these have contributed to the increased morbidity and mortality of patients over time.

Infection remains a major cause of morbidity and mortality for long-term, immunosuppressed transplant recipients, although the incidence and severity of infections decrease after the first year. The more common sites of infections in this population include the respiratory tract, urinary tract, mediastinum, and retina. The organisms typically involved in infections include bacteria (*Escherichia coli, Pseudomonas*), viruses (cytomegalovirus, herpes simplex, herpes zoster), and fungi (*Candida, Aspergillus, Cryptococcus*).

Rejection of the transplanted heart remains the major lifelong threat to the recipient. Cardiac rejection can occur as an acute episode or a chronic condition. The risk of acute rejection is highest in the first days and weeks after transplantation while immunosuppressant therapy is being adjusted. Although rejection rates decrease with each year of survival, the recipient is always at risk if therapy is interrupted or stopped. Immunosuppression is the only safeguard against acute rejection.

Graft atherosclerosis and chronic rejection have been reported to occur in approximately 35% to 40% of patients who survive 5 years after transplantation. The incidence among patients who had coronary artery disease (CAD) before receiving the transplant is similar to that among patients with pretransplant cardiomyopathy. Furthermore, because the donor heart has been denervated, patients who develop diffuse occlusive CAD do not have clinically apparent angina pectoris. Thus, if not monitored carefully, they can die suddenly or develop ventricular failure.

Malignancies, particularly lymphomas of the histiocytic type, have been reported.[75] Their occurrence is thought to be associated with immunosuppression therapy, particularly including antithymocyte globulin in addition to cyclosporine. Other reported malignancies include epithelial tumors of the skin and leukemia.

CARDIAC DONOR SELECTION CRITERIA

General

Imminent or established brain death (by two medical physicians)
Absence of systemic sepsis
No history of insulin-dependent diabetes
Absence of hepatitis, autoimmune disease
No history of IV drug or heavy alcohol use
No strong family history of heart disease

Specific

Age: males <55 yr; females <40 yr
No history of cardiac disease, no history of severe chest trauma
No history of prolonged cardiac arrest, no prolonged hypoxia
No history of prolonged hypotension, no prolonged use of dopamine
ECG: normal (nonspecific ST, T wave changes may be acceptable)
Laboratory values: normal WBC, creatinine phosphokinase–MB isoenzyme (CPK-MB); within normal limits—arterial blood gases, hemodynamic parameters
Echocardiogram: normal left and right ventricular (LV and RV) function

Other late complications associated with lifelong immunosuppression in long-term survivors include osteoporosis (18.2%), spinal disorders (8.8%), and visual problems (14.3%).[102]

The quality of life following cardiac transplantation has also been evaluated. One study reported that an average of 3.7 years after surgery, 89% of heart recipients perceived their quality of life as good to excellent, and 82% reported satisfaction with life as good to very satisfactory. Factors associated with negative life change were reported to be financial status, physical appearance, and sexual function. All recipients were bothered by the side effects associated with immunosuppression therapy, but these were found to have little impact on their evaluation of quality of life and life satisfaction.[102]

Immunosuppression. Increased understanding of immunosuppression and the introduction of various immunosuppressive agents have made organ transplantation a viable treatment modality. Since the late 1960s, a variety of nonselective immunosuppressive agents have been used in transplantations, but these were associated with impairment of the immune system, leaving the host vulnerable to various infections. With the introduction of cyclosporine A, morbidity and mortality figures were significantly reduced.

The primary goal of immunosuppressive therapy is to prevent rejection of the foreign graft (heart) while retaining the host's natural immune system, which protects the person from infections.

The immune system is a complex response mechanism. Its purpose is to destroy any tissue invasion or foreign material to maintain hemostasis.

Heart Transplant Procedures

Orthotopic: recipient's heart is excised, leaving the posterior walls of the atria, and is replaced with donor heart.

Heterotopic "piggyback": donor heart is placed in right chest adjacent to the recipient's heart. Anastomosis of the two hearts permits blood to pass through one or both hearts.

Patients with the following injuries who have documented brain death may be considered as potential heart donors:

Head trauma: motor vehicle accidents, gunshot to the head

Cerebrovascular results: subarachnoid hemorrhage, brain tumors, aneurysms, cerebral anoxia resulting from drug overdose, drowning

INDICATIONS

End-stage heart failure

CONTRAINDICATIONS

Absolute contraindications
  Pulmonary hypertension (PVR >6-8 wood units)
  Active infectious process
  Kidney failure or liver failure
  Severe peripheral vascular disease
  Active peptic ulcer disease
  Malignant or terminal systemic disease
  Emotional or psychologic instability
  Insulin-dependent diabetes
Relative contraindications
  Age: older than 65 years
  Lack of support systems
  Non-insulin-dependent diabetes
  History of drug and/or alcohol abuse

COMPLICATIONS

Infection
Organ rejection
Graft atherosclerosis

PREPROCEDURAL NURSING CARE

1. Follow preparation procedures similar to those for patient undergoing cardiac surgery (see page 215). Initiate immunosuppressive therapy as ordered. Begin reviewing drugs with patient.
2. Prepare skin: shave and clean with Betadine from chin to knees.

MEDICAL MANAGEMENT

GENERAL MANAGEMENT

ECG changes: Reflect lack of autonomic innervation of heart that occurs as result of denervation when donor heart is removed.

Heart rate: Resting heart rate generally higher (90-100 bpm); response to metabolic demands such as fever or exercise in a denervated patient is one in which heart rate changes gradually; as a result of these changes, response to drugs whose effect on the heart is mediated by autonomic nervous system is also altered.

Rhythm: Normal sinus but without respiratory variation.

P wave: Transplant procedure generally involves retaining posterior portion of recipient's atria, which includes sinoatrial (SA) node; therefore second P wave is sometimes visible.

Endomyocardial biopsy (EMB): Once a week for 1 month, then twice a week for 2 months; after first year, EMBs performed on an interval basis depending on recipient's clinical status.

Diet: Low saturated fat and cholesterol, moderate decrease in sodium intake (2 g sodium).

Laboratory studies: Regular monitoring to detect adverse reactions to immunosuppressive therapy—CBC, serum blood urea nitrogen (BUN) and creatinine, liver function (SGOT, SGPT, LDH), glucose, urinalysis. Serum cholesterol; triglycerides; high-, low-density lipoprotein (HDL, LDL); magnesium; potassium. Lymphocyte count; T-cell studies—while receiving ATG or OKT$_3$ (see Drug Therapy). Cyclosporine levels—radioimmunoassay (TDX/RIA) and high-performance liquid chromatography (HPLC).

General postoperative care of patient following a cardiac transplantation is similar to that for any patient following cardiac surgery (see page 216).

Strict reverse isolation is followed until all invasive lines are discontinued, then mask, gloves, and handwashing procedures are instituted.

DRUG THERAPY

Although a variety of immunosuppressant agents are available, maintenance immunosuppression protocols for cardiac transplant patients can include the following:

Cyclosporine (Sandimmune): Naturally occurring polypeptide antibiotic produced by fungi; inhibits T cell lymphocyte proliferation and activity, which is responsible for tissue graft rejection.

Usual dosage: 2-8 mg/kg/day PO; daily dose adjusted to maintain therapeutic levels (NOTE: therapeutic level dependent on biologic fluid, assay method).

Half-life: 18 to 40 h (average, 27).

Excretion: Metabolized by liver; excreted in bile and urine.

Side effects: Hirsutism, acne, fragile skin, gingival hyperplasia, fine hand tremor.

Adverse reaction: Nephrotoxicity, hypertension, hepatotoxicity, infection (viral, bacterial, and fungal), lymphoma.

Azathioprine (Imuran): Antimetabolite that produces immunosuppression by inhibiting purine and DNA synthesis.
Dosage: Adjusted to keep WBC above 4500.
Half-life: Approximately 3 h.
Excretion: Metabolized by liver; excreted in urine.
Side effects: Rash, bruising, nausea, vomiting, stomatitis, muscle wasting, arthralgia, fatigue, decreased libido, impotence.
Adverse reaction: Leukopenia, thrombocytopenia, anemia, hepatotoxicity, pancreatitis, jaundice.

MEDICAL MANAGEMENT—cont'd

Antithymocyte globulin (ATG): Reduces T lymphocytes; used to prevent rejection, or as an adjunct to immuno-suppression therapy during rejection episodes.
    Usual dosage: Rabbit ATG—2 mg/kg/day IM, adjusted according to circulating T lymphocytes (WBCs); equine ATG—15 mg/kg/day IV, adjusted according to circulating T lymphocytes (rosette count).
    Side effects: Localized pain and inflammation with IM injection; chills, fever, hypotension.
    Adverse reactions: Anaphylaxis.

Orthoclone (OKT$_3$, Ortho): New monoclonal antibody similar to ATG; reduces T cell function; used to prevent graft rejection.[123]
    Usual dosage: 5 mg IV push daily for 10-14 days; given in < 1 min.
    Side effects: fever, chills, dyspnea, chest pain, vomiting, wheezing, nausea, diarrhea, tremor.

Corticosteroids: Anti-inflammatory agents used to suppress both T and B lymphocyte function and to reverse capillary permeability, vasodilation, and edema; may be used as part of maintenance program to prevent rejection or as adjunct therapy when evidence of rejection present.

Prednisone (Meticorten, Deltasone): Used as part of maintenance therapy.
    Usual dosage: 0.1-0.2 mg/kg/day PO (NOTE: is increased with rejection).

Methylprednisone (Medrol, Depo-Medrol, Solu-Medrol): Used when evidence of rejection present.
    Usual dosage: 1 g/day for 3 days IV.
    Half-life: 3½ h.
    Side effects: cushingoid appearance, mood changes, GI distress, fragile skin, bruising, delayed wound healing.
    Adverse reactions: infection, diabetes, thrombocytopenia, pancreatitis.

Antihistamines and acetaminophen: Given before therapy to reduce incidence of side effects.

1   ASSESS

ASSESSMENT	OBSERVATIONS
Acute rejection	*Mild to early rejection:* generally no symptoms associated *Moderate rejection:* myocyte necrosis diagnosed on EMB; usually no clinical symptoms *Severe rejection:* shock state; weakness, fatigue, malaise; anorexia; nausea, vomiting; decreased urine output; weight gain; peripheral edema; distended neck veins; increased jugular venous pulsations and decreased perfusion—cool pale skin, diminished pulses, diaphoresis, confusion, restlessness; pulmonary venous congestion—DOE, cough, tachypnea; development of S_3, S_4 heart sounds; cardiac arrest
ECG	Using conventional immunosuppression: atrial dysrhythmias (e.g., PAC, atrial fibrillation, atrial flutter); with cyclosporine these ECG changes may not be seen
Chest x-ray	Increased C-T ratio (cardiomegaly)
Echocardiogram	Thickening of LV, decreased LV function, decreased contractility Decreased RV function possible in first year, but ejection fraction still > 60%

EMB	Changes in lymphocytes; finding varies according to degree of rejection:
	    Mild—occasional WBCs
	    Moderate—myocyte necrosis
	    Severe—extensive perivascular infiltration of lymphocytes, interstitial edema, myocyte necrosis
	Increased CPK-MB, SGOT, LDH

→ > >

ASSESSMENT	OBSERVATIONS
Infection	Usual signs and symptoms of infection often absent in immunosuppressed patient Fever: low grade; baseline temperature may be lower than before transplant, so elevation to 37.2° C (99° F) may be significant Malaise Cough: productive or nonproductive

2 DIAGNOSE

NURSING DIAGNOSIS	SUBJECTIVE FINDINGS	OBJECTIVE FINDINGS
Potential for injury (rejection) related to noncompliance with prescribed medical regimen	Reports confusion regarding drug therapy; unrealistic understanding regarding need for long-term therapy	Behavior of failure to adhere; failure to keep follow-up appointments Nontherapeutic cyclosporine levels Edema and weight gain
Potential for infection related to immunosuppressive drug therapy	Reports malaise	Laboratory values: lymphocytes and WBCs depressed T-cell numbers and function depressed Low-grade fever
Potential decreased cardiac output related to severe rejection	Reports fatigue, SOB, dizziness	Lethargy, elevated fever ECG—atrial, ventricular dysrhythmias Heart sounds—S_3, S_4; pericardial rub Jugular venous distention (JVD) Echocardiogram—decreased ejection fraction EMB—myocyte necrosis

Other related nursing diagnoses: Ineffective individual coping related to threat of disease process and inadequate coping resources; **Compromised family coping** related to knowledge deficit, increased multiple stressors that deplete family's coping resources

3 PLAN

Patient goals

1. Patient will demonstrate appropriate performance of prescribed behaviors and treatments in the prevention of organ rejection.
2. Patient will demonstrate understanding of appropriate countermeasures to prevent infection.
3. Patient will demonstrate stable CO.
4. Patient will demonstrate increased understanding of disorder and demonstrates skills necessary for home self-care management.

4 IMPLEMENT

NURSING DIAGNOSIS	NURSING INTERVENTIONS	RATIONALE
Potential for injury (rejection) related to noncompliance with prescribed medical regimen	Assess and evaluate patient for understanding and cognitive appraisal of prescribed lifelong therapy.	To identify misconceptions and cues that may indicate potential adherence problems.
	Encourage discussion regarding changes in life-style that have been positive or negative. Anticipate and allow questions regarding prescribed therapy.	By acknowledging patient's positive efforts, provider can help patient to explore alternative ways of dealing with negative ones. Reinforcing positive activities can also help to increase patient's sense of achievement and confidence.
	Encourage patient to have family member or friend accompany patient to clinic.	In addition to supportive role, family members or friends can help patient recall information given to patient.
Potential for infection related to immunosuppressive drug therapy	Assess and monitor for signs of infection (see Assess section): Take temperature q 4 h. Obtain cultures as indicated: sputum, throat, urine, any suspicious drainage sites in wounds. Obtain and assess CBC and chest x-ray as indicated. NOTE: Laboratory values may be altered because of steroids.	To detect signs of an infectious process; to begin appropriate medical therapy.
	Minimize or avoid use of invasive procedures: IV, indwelling catheters. Change IV tubings, bags, and dressings daily, using strict aseptic technique; discontinue as soon as possible.	Attention to potential ports of entry helps to decrease risk of nosocomial or bacterial infections.
	Avoid placing patient in room with other patient who is at risk for infection.	To avoid potential cross-contamination.
	Institute reverse isolation for staff and visitors as outlined.	To decrease potential new infection.
	Minimize number of visitors. Restrict visitors with signs of infections such as colds, herpes simplex.	Visitors may be unaware of risk they present to immunosuppressed patient.
Potential decreased cardiac output related to severe rejection	Assess and monitor for signs and symptoms of decreased CO and signs of rejection.	Early diagnosis of acute rejection is essential to reverse process.
	Auscultate heart sounds.	To assess changes in rhythm and development of gallop rhythm.
	Auscultate chest for lung sounds.	To assess for signs of increased pulmonary congestion.

→ > >

NURSING DIAGNOSIS	NURSING INTERVENTIONS	RATIONALE
	Weigh patient daily.	
	Prepare patient for EMB.	EMB confirms level of rejection.
	Administer immunosuppressive therapy as ordered.	Optimal immunosuppression is essential to prevent rejection.
Knowledge deficit	See Patient Teaching.	

5 EVALUATE

PATIENT OUTCOME	DATA INDICATING THAT OUTCOME IS REACHED
There are no signs of rejection on bi-opsy.	No new changes occur in EMB results. No clinical signs of rejection are present.
Patient is compliant with therapeutic regimen.	Serum drug levels are maintained. Patient keeps follow-up appointments and offers questions and concerns appropriately.
There is no infec-tion.	Patient maintains baseline temperature. No sign of infection exists: CBC, urinalysis, and cultures within normal limits.
CO is stable.	HR is 100-110 bpm; mean arterial pressure, 70-90 mm Hg; ejection fraction $>60\%$; ECG shows normal sinus rhythm. Skin is warm and dry; urine output >30 ml/hr.
Knowledge level is increased.	Patient verbalizes understanding of postoperative care, need for continuous follow-up, allowances and limitations, medications, and signs to report to physician.

PATIENT TEACHING

1. Discuss and review signs and symptoms of rejection. Emphasize the importance of keeping scheduled EMB appointments, since there are usually *no* signs of early rejection and appearance of symptoms is associated with moderate to severe rejection.
2. Discuss and review the need to take medications lifelong and the need to take them *exactly* as prescribed. Caution the patient *never to stop* taking medication. Notify the physician if a dose was skipped. Review medications, checking dosage, method of administration, and side effects.
3. Discuss signs and symptoms of infection to report: elevation of baseline temperature; early signs of sore throat, cold, or flu; and cuts and lesions that do not heal.
4. Discuss the need to reduce risk of infection by avoiding individuals with infections or contagious diseases, avoiding large crowds, and wearing a face mask when traveling in crowded areas.
5. Discuss the importance of lifelong follow-up: clinic visits, EMB appointments, and periodic stress tests, radionuclide studies, and cardiac catheterization.
6. Discuss activity allowances and limitations. Tell the patient to check with the physician before engaging in strenuous or competitive activities or sports.
7. Discuss importance of daily weighing and reporting more than 2 lb (0.9 kg) weight gain in 24 hours.

ARTERIAL REVASCULARIZATION

Arterial revascularization refers to any bypass procedure used to repair stenosed or occluded arteries. The bypass may be constructed from autologous vein (the saphenous being the most commonly used) or synthetic (Dacron and Polytetrafluoethylene [PTFE] being the two most frequently used materials).

Because atherosclerosis is a progressive disorder, surgery is palliative, providing relief from debilitating symptoms. Patients should be aware that unless they take an active role in modifying their risk factors, whatever relief they achieve from surgery will surely be short-lived.

AORTOILIAC DISEASE

Patients with disease of the distal aorta and iliofemoral arteries (also known as Leriche's syndrome) report claudication of the buttock, hip or thigh and, in males, impotence. Claudication of the larger, proximal muscles generally suggests aortoiliac disease, whereas calf claudication is the most common complaint with femoropopliteal disease.

Ischemic rest pain is not usually associated with aortoiliac disease unless it is accompanied by femoropopliteal disease or microembolization of atherosclerotic debris caused by an aneurysm or atherosclerotic plaque. The collateral circulation aids in providing adequate tissue perfusion to the lower extremities at rest. (Claudication reflects arterial insufficiency to contracting muscles. It is brought on by exercise [generally walking a predictable distance] and is relieved by rest.)[35]

FEMOROPOPLITEAL AND FEMOROTIBIAL DISEASE

Lesions of the superficial femoral artery and popliteal artery are the most common lesions seen in the lower extremity, with calf claudication being the most common symptom. The majority of arterial revascularization procedures done in the United States involve the femoropopiteal segment.

SURGICAL PROCEDURES

After evaluation is complete the surgical procedure is selected. Because atherosclerosis is a diffuse disease, there may be more than one area of stenosis. The procedure done is based on the location of the most hemodynamically significant lesion. First consideration is given to the condition of the inflow vessels, the aortoiliacs. If there is disease to these vessels, repair must be done before reconstruction is performed on the outflow vessels to the foot. This prevents thrombosis of a distal graft secondary to inadequate inflow.

TYPE OF DISEASE	SURGICAL PROCEDURE
Aortoiliac	Aortic-to-Femoral artery bypass graft
	Axillofemoral bypass graft (if the patient cannot tolerate an abdominal procedure)
	Femoral-to-Femoral artery bypass graft (if the patient cannot tolerate an abdominal operation and blood flow to the unaffected leg is adequate)
Femoropopliteal	Femoral-to-Popliteal bypass graft
Femorotibial	Femoral-to-Anterior Tibial artery bypass graft
	Femoral-to-Posterior Tibial artery bypass graft
	Femoral-to-Peroneal artery bypass graft

INDICATIONS

Proximal (aortoiliac) and distal (femoropopliteal and femorotibial) disease—performed when claudication becomes disabling, if rest pain is present, or there are ischemic ulcers

CONTRAINDICATIONS

May be based on individual patient situations

CAUTIONS

Caution should be taken with patients with confirmed or suspected coronary artery disease. A large percentage of patients presenting with symptoms of the peripheral arterial tree also have coronary disease, documented or undocumented. If cardiac or carotid disease becomes evident during diagnostic work-up, these problems need to be corrected before arterial reconstruction to decrease the possibility of postoperative MI or CVA.

COMPLICATIONS

Infection
Graft thrombosis
Myocardial infarction
Cerebral vascular accident

PREPROCEDURAL NURSING CARE

1. Initiate preoperative instruction for the patient and family. Include information about the operative procedure and postoperative care: routine postoperative procedures, whether it be in an intensive care unit or a post anesthesia care unit—monitoring of vital signs, vascular assessments, pulmonary care, and the equipment, which consists of ventilators, monitors, and urinary catheters. Also include information regarding pain management and family visiting guidelines. As ordered, instruct the patient to discontinue any antiplatelet medications 1 week before surgery. If the patient smokes or uses tobacco products, he should be instructed to stop.

2. Begin pulmonary preparation. Teach coughing and deep breathing techniques and use of incentive spirometer. Demonstrate how chest physical therapy will be performed.
3. Obtain baseline data: chest x-ray, ECG, laboratory work (CBC, electrolytes, serum chemistries, and urinalysis).
4. Obtain baseline information, vascular assessment, and height and weight information.
5. Deal with preoperative anxiety, offering reassurance and support.
6. Assist with insertion of a pulmonary artery catheter and radial artery catheter if indicated. Record baseline hemodynamic data.
7. Administer medications as ordered: antiarrhythmics and antihypertensives (usually continued until time of surgery); digoxin; preoperative sedation.

MEDICAL MANAGEMENT

DRUG THERAPY

Preoperative management: Pentoxifylline (Trental)—used for the treatment of intermittent claudication and occasionally for rest pain in those patients who are not surgical candidates. This drug is believed to improve capillary blood flow by making the red cells more "pliable," more able to "squeeze" through areas of stenoses, and better able to deliver more oxygen to the muscle and improve perfusion to the distal extremities. Pentoxifylline also prevents clotting of red cells and platelets. This drug is noted to be clinically effective if the patient has an increase in activity tolerance. It takes 4 to 8 weeks for therapeutic effectiveness to be noted. Pentoxifylline is administered three times a day in 400 mg dosages. Common side effects include headaches, nausea, and dizziness. Unfortunately, many patients do not tolerate the side effects, and use of the drug must be discontinued. In teaching patients about this drug they should understand that they **must** take it with meals and that it may take up to 8 weeks before they will notice a change in their exercise tolerance.

Calcium channel blockers

Antiplatelet agents

Postoperative management: Based on clinical symptoms, complications, and progress of the patient.

Antibiotics: Used for 24 to 48 hours postoperatively until invasive catheters are removed

Pain medications: Morphine sulfate, Percosett, epidural analgesia (bupivacaine and fentanyl delivered via epidural catheter first 3 to 4 days), dipyridamole, and ASA

1 ASSESS

ASSESSMENT	OBSERVATIONS
Vascular assessment	Normal operative leg is warm; capillary refill adequate; distal pulses are either palpable or audible by Doppler; ankle/brachial index is improved
Cardiac assessment	Complications: narrow pulse pressure, tachycardia, hypotension, increased PCWP, and increased PAP ECG: ischemic changes; atrial, ventricular dysrhythmias
Pain assessment	Infection: incision site—redness, drainage, odor Lab values; WBC $< 10,000/\mu L$

2 DIAGNOSE

NURSING DIAGNOSIS	SUBJECTIVE FINDINGS	OBJECTIVE FINDINGS
Pain related to surgical incision	Complains of pain	Elevated BP, tachycardia, tachypnea,
Potential altered tissue perfusion related to development of graft thromboses	Complains of increasing pain, numbness of the affected limb	Loss of pulses, decreased temperature, pallor of the affected limb, decreased ABI
Potential decreased cardiac output related to perioperative myocardial ischemia/infarction	Complains of chest pain	Hypertension, tachycardia, diaphoresis, ECG: ST, T wave changes
Potential for infection related to surgical intervention and graft placement (especially if synthetic)	Complains of increasing pain and tenderness around the incision site	Fever, increasing white count, erythema around the incision

3 PLAN

Patient goals

1. The patient will be free of pain.
2. The patient will demonstrate signs of increased perfusion—elevated temperature, palpable pulses, capillary refill within 2 to 3 seconds—in the immediate postoperative period. Should the graft thrombose it will be recognized and reported immediately.
3. The patient will maintain a stable CO. Complaints of chest pain and ECG changes will be investigated immediately.
4. The patient will remain free of infection. However, if an infectious process is suspected, it will be reported immediately.

→ > >

4 IMPLEMENT

NURSING DIAGNOSIS	NURSING INTERVENTIONS	RATIONALE
Pain related to incision	Administer analgesics as ordered.	Patient will tolerate increasing levels of activity if pain free.
	If patient is receiving epidural analgesics, ensure that the system is intact. Check the integrity of the catheter q 2-4 h. Assess the level of analgesia q 2-4 h.	System integrity must be maintained to assure therapeutic levels of analgesia. Patients tend to have very high levels of pain if the epidural medication is discontinued abruptly.
	Assist the patient with repositioning and relaxation techniques, which will help to decrease the pain.	Using relaxation techniques in conjunction with analgesia helps to decrease anxiety and positional discomfort.
Potential altered tissue perfusion related to graft thromboses	Assess the patency of the graft q 1 h for the first 24 h; q 2 h × 48 h, then q 4 h: assess color, temperature, pulses, sensation, and movement.	If the graft thromboses, pulses will be absent, the foot will rapidly become cold and pale. The patient will experience increased pain and difficulty moving the extremity.
	Maintain bed rest for 24-72 h; use pillow between knees when lying on side.	To avoid graft pressure.
Potential decreased cardiac output related to myocardial ischemia/infarction	Assess the components of cardiac output q 1-2 h in the perioperative period.	Because of the diffuse nature of vascular disease, it is essential to closely monitor these patients in the postoperative period.
	Assess and document the same q 4 h during recuperation.	These patients continue to be at risk as their exercise level increases in the postoperative period.
Potential for infection.	Observe for signs of impending sepsis: fever, shaking, and chills.	Gram positive organisms may present a febrile picture.
	Observe incision lines for edema, erythema, and drainage.	Early detection of an infectious process may prevent extension to synthetic grafts.
	Obtain cultures as ordered.	To identify the organisms so that appropriate antibiotics may be started.
	Remove invasive catheters as soon as possible.	To prevent nosocomial infection.
Knowledge deficit	See Preprocedural Nursing Care and Patient Teaching.	

5   EVALUATE

PATIENT OUTCOME	DATA INDICATING THAT OUTCOME IS REACHED
Patient is free of pain.	Good range of movement of the affected limb. Patient verbalizes pain relief.
Tissue perfusion remains improved; the graft remains patent.	The foot is warm with palpable pulses.
The patient maintains a stable CO without signs of myocardial compromise.	BP and HR are within normal limits. ECG is normal or at baseline.
There is no infection.	Patient is afebrile. Incision site is clean and free of drainage, with no signs of granulation.

PATIENT TEACHING

1. Discuss activity allowances and restrictions. Refer patient to a rehabilitative program for a program of progressive exercise.
2. Review discharge medication, including purpose, dosages, side effects, and need for specific follow-up laboratory studies as indicated.
3. Review nutritional program.
4. Discuss the importance of avoiding fatigue and sitting with legs dependent for prolonged periods of time.
5. Discuss care of incisions and symptoms of wound infection to report to the physician.
6. Assure that the patient has a follow-up appointment scheduled with the surgeon before discharge.
7. Discuss importance of modifying cardiovascular risk factors, especially importance of not smoking or using tobacco products.

PERCUTANEOUS TRANSLUMINAL CORONARY ANGIOPLASTY

Percutaneous transluminal coronary angioplasty (PTCA) is an invasive, nonsurgical, therapeutic procedure that restores patency of a coronary artery by compressing atheromatous plaques within the vessel. This results in an increase in coronary artery perfusion, thereby relieving myocardial ischemia. PTCA has evolved as an extension of peripheral balloon angioplasty. Intracoronary transluminal dilation, first developed by Andreas Gruentzig in 1977, has been used only on a highly selected population of patients with stable angina and in coronary arteries that had discrete, proximal, and noncalcified lesions. Since then, the selection criteria has widened because of equipment advances and modifica-

tions of guidewires and balloon catheters, operator experience, as well as perceived clinical indications. Current patient selection criteria focus primarily on accessibility of the lesion, its compressibility, and presence of single or multivessel disease. In 1979 the National Heart, Lung and Blood Institute[84] issued the following guidelines:

1. Stable angina with symptoms refractory to medical therapy
2. Single vessel coronary stenosis
3. Objective evidence of myocardial ischemia by exercise treadmill, thallium scintigraphy with exercise, or gated blood pool studies
4. Lesions suitable for successful angioplasty to be proximal, discrete, concentric, and noncalcified

Although these guidelines define the "ideal" situation for angioplasty, dramatic improvements in equipment and operator experience have surpassed these conservative guidelines. Multivessel angioplasty involving complex lesions is now routinely performed. Ongoing and future trials will address the medium- and long-term efficacy of angioplasty vs coronary artery bypass graft surgery in similar clinical settings.

The procedure, which is technically similar to a standard cardiac catheterization, involves passing a balloon-tipped catheter over a guidewire into a stenosed coronary artery, where the balloon is then inflated and deflated using a hand-held syringe or pressure-controlled device (Figures 6-3 to 6-4). Successful dilation is usually accompanied by reduction in the systolic gradient across the stenosis; however, the gradient may not be totally abolished, and the inflation/deflation cycle may be repeated several times until the previous angioplasty arteriogram demonstrates improved luminal diameter (Figure 6-5). Successful PTCA has been defined as an increase in lumen size of at least 20%. Given careful patient selection and physician experience, current studies indicate that primary success rates are being achieved in 85% to 90% of patients undergoing PTCA. Symptomatic relief is being achieved in 80%, and long-

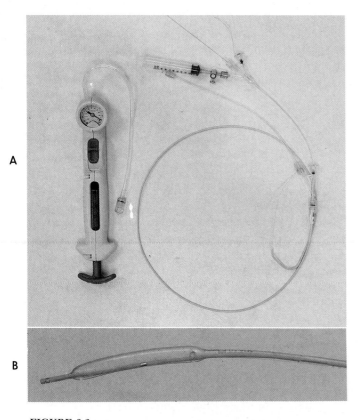

FIGURE 6-3
A, Pressure gun and balloon-tipped catheter used for PTCA.
B, Close-up of inflated balloon.

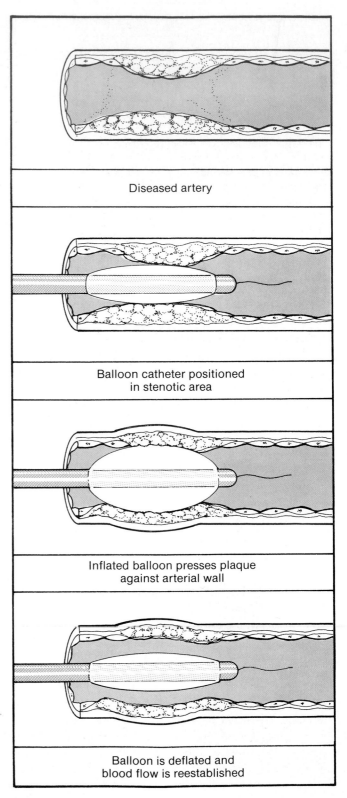

Diseased artery

Balloon catheter positioned
in stenotic area

Inflated balloon presses plaque
against arterial wall

Balloon is deflated and
blood flow is reestablished

FIGURE 6-4
Coronary angioplasty procedure.

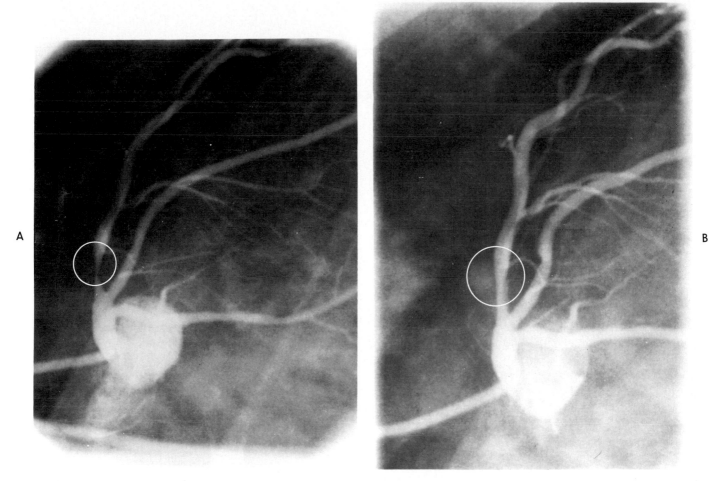

FIGURE 6-5
Coronary arteriograms. **A,** Before angioplasty. **B,** After angioplasty.

term follow-up shows continued lumen patency and symptomatic improvement from 6 months to 2 years. The recurrence rate, however, is currently 15% to 30%.[85] Adjunctive techniques such as atherectomy, laser therapy, and stents are being investigated as new methods in preventing restenosis following angioplasty.[70]

Catheters. The angioplasty procedure involves a two-catheter system. First, a guiding catheter is introduced percutaneously via the femoral artery. If the brachial artery is used, a cutdown is required. Once the guiding catheter is at the orifice of the stenosed coronary artery, a guidewire and balloon dilation catheter are inserted and advanced under fluoroscopy until the balloon "straddles" the lesion. The balloon is inflated and pressure applied at 5 to 10 atmospheres for 30 seconds to several minutes, depending on the patient's tol-

erance and degree of ischemia. Following angioplasty, the catheters are removed and a sheath left in place for continuous arterial blood pressure monitoring. Also, a venous sheath may be left in the femoral vein for infusion of fluid and medication.

Arteriograms. Pre- and postprocedure arteriograms are performed to allow evaluation of the results. Decisions can also be made regarding the need for further dilation.

INDICATIONS

Chronic stable angina
Unstable angina
Acute myocardial infarction
Clinical features that make bypass surgery unacceptable

CONTRAINDICATIONS

Left main CAD or left main equivalent
Coronary artery spasm

CRITERIA FOR SELECTION OF CANDIDATES

Complex coronary anatomic situations (distal disease)
Multivessel disease
Bifurcation lesions
Total occlusions
Diseased saphenous vein or internal mammary artery
  bypass grafts

COMPLICATIONS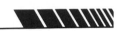

Failure to dilate coronary artery
Abrupt coronary occlusion
Myocardial infarction
Coronary artery dissection
Bleeding
Renal hypersensitivity to contrast material
Cannulated extremity:
  Ischemia
  Thrombosis formation

PREPROCEDURAL NURSING CARE

1. Initiate preprocedural instruction for patient and
   family.

   a. Instruct patient and family about purpose and in-
      dications for PTCA, its benefits, and associated
      risks.
   b. Describe procedure and that it is similar to car-
      diac catheterization (see page 273) and may last
      45 minutes to 1½ hours. Review sensations pa-
      tient will experience, such as groin and arm pres-
      sure during insertion of catheter and possible dis-
      comfort during balloon inflation.
   c. Stress importance of drinking fluids for first 6 to
      8 hours after procedure to wash out contrast ma-
      terial.
2. Obtain written informed consent for PTCA; ensure
   that it includes consent for emergency CABG,
   which has been reported to occur in 2% of patients.
   An operating room and cardiothoracic team is on
   standby.[85,172]
3. Obtain baseline data for PTCA and CABG: CBC, coagulation studies, electrolytes, BUN, creatinine;
   blood type and cross-match; ECG; chest x-ray; vital
   signs.
4. Perform skin preparation: both groin areas.
5. Permit nothing by mouth (NPO).
6. Establish patent intravenous line.
7. Administer medications as ordered.
8. Maintain NPO for at least 8 hours.
9. Administer preoperative sedation as ordered.

MEDICAL MANAGEMENT

GENERAL MANAGEMENT

During procedure: Intra-aortic balloon pump—Must be available on standby during procedure

Postprocedure: Cardiac monitoring—ECG pattern observed for rate; dysrhythmias and ST segment changes indicate signs of ischemia

  Bed rest— for first 6 hours after arterial and venous sheath removal and once hemostasis reestablished

  Laboratory studies—Careful monitoring of PTT, Hg; CPK; serum potassium and sodium; BUN and creatinine

  Diet—As ordered, force fluids for 24 h

  Intake and output—Record q 4-8 h

DRUG THERAPY

Preprocedure: Antiplatelets—aspirin, 325 mg BID; dipyridamole, 75 mg TID 48 h before procedure to decrease risk of platelet adhesion, which is thought to cause early restenosis following procedure

  Diphenhydramine—to reduce risk of allergic reaction

  Nitrates, calcium channel blockers—to reduce the risk of coronary arterial spasm

MEDICAL MANAGEMENT—cont'd

Beta blockers—held before procedure

During procedure: Heparin infusion—Continuous drip

Intracoronary nitroglycerin (100-300 mg) and/or sublingual nifedipine (10 mg) to prevent coronary artery spasm as catheter is introduced

Thrombolytic agents may also be administered during the procedure if thrombus present (see page 243 for details)

Postprocedure: Immediate:
Heparin infusion (800-1200 units/h): tapered doses given for 12-24 h to prevent coronary thrombosis from possible injury to the intimal lining of the vessel

Long-term:
Aspirin—Taken po for 6 mo; dose varies
Nitrates, calcium channel blockers—resumed while patient in hospital and continued 3-6 mo; dose varies
Dipyridamole—taken for 3 mo

1 ASSESS

ASSESSMENT	OBSERVATIONS
General complaints	Absence or presence of chest pain
ECG	Normal ST-T wave
Cannulated extremity	
Normal	Full pulses; skin color good, warm; patient able to move extremity without pain
Bleeding	Ecchymosis, hematoma, swelling
Ischemia	Diminished or absent pulses, numbness, pallor, pain
Arterial thrombosis formation	Diminished or absent pulses, pain, swelling, pallor
Failure to dilate coronary artery, abrupt occlusion, MI, coronary artery dissection	Chest pain, ST depression or elevation, hypotension, tachycardia, diaphoresis, ventricular dysrhythmias
Renal hypersensitivity to contrast material	Decreased urine output; increased circulating blood volume: JVD, dyspnea, crackles

→ > >

2 DIAGNOSE

NURSING DIAGNOSIS	SUBJECTIVE FINDINGS	OBJECTIVE FINDINGS
Anxiety (preoperative) related to perceived or actual threat to biologic integrity	Complains of irritability, palpitations, inability to sleep, restlessness, fear of the unknown	Tachycardia, diaphoresis; unrelaxed posture and facial expressions
Potential decreased cardiac output related to myocardial ischemia or electrical factors (dysrhythmias)	Reports chest pain, palpitations; skipped beats; dizziness	ECG—ST depression or elevation; Hypotension, tachycardia, bradycardia, diaphoresis, pallor, ventricular dysrhythmias
Potential altered peripheral tissue perfusion related to thrombus formation	Complains of numbness, pain, swelling involving affected extremity	Extremity pale, cold to touch; decreased absence of peripheral pulses; possible mottling of leg

Other related nursing diagnoses: Fluid volume deficit or Fluid volume excess related to renal sensitivity to contrast material

3 PLAN

Patient goals

1. Patient will demonstrate reduced anxiety level.
2. Patient will demonstrate stable CO and absence of complications.
3. Patient will demonstrate normal peripheral circulation.
4. Patient will demonstrate understanding of PTCA procedure.

4 IMPLEMENT

NURSING DIAGNOSIS	NURSING INTERVENTIONS	RATIONALE
Anxiety (preoperative) related to perceived or actual threat to biologic integrity	Assess level of anxiety, level of understanding associated with procedures.	To determine source of fears and identify any misconceptions regarding purpose and outcome of procedure.
	Provide explanations and description of procedure and sensations patient will experience. Provide opportunity for questions; assist patient to explore fears and discuss feelings.	Patient and family will be more at ease and comfortable, which will increase understanding.
	Provide patient with opportunity to meet with catheterization staff and visit laboratory and postangioplasty unit.	Being aware of what to expect, of the normal environment, and among staff faces provides patient with sense of comfort and assurance.

NURSING DIAGNOSIS	NURSING INTERVENTIONS	RATIONALE
	Provide patient opportunity to meet with patient who has had angioplasty procedure.	Provides added assurance of what to expect and lessens threat of being alone.
	Provide teaching materials/booklets on angioplasty.	Visual aids reinforce learning and understanding.
	Provide basic instruction on cardiac surgery in case emergency CABG is required.	Although the risk is small (<2% of patients require CABG), patient must have brief understanding of events following CABG.
Potential decreased cardiac output related to myocardial ischemia or electrical factors (dysrhythmias)	Assess for signs of diminished CO.	Any sign or symptom suggesting recurring myocardial ischemia my indicate reocclusion of coronary artery and/or MI; 50% of complications occur within first 24 h following PTCA.
	Monitor BP, HR, respiratory rate q 15 min immediately after procedure, decreasing frequency as clinical status stabilizes, then monitor vital signs q 4 h for 24 h.	Patient's vital signs and hemodynamic status must be closely assessed for any evidence of mechanical or electrical factors associated with altered CO.
	Monitor ECG observing for signs of ischemia or dysrhythmias; obtain 12-lead ECG with any episode of chest pain.	Altered coronary perfusion leads to ischemia and thus irritability of heart muscles. Dysrhythmias can occur as a result of ischemic tissue.
	Monitor urine output q 1 h or for every void if not catheterized. Report outputs < 30 ml/h or inability to void within first 4 h.	To detect beginning of renal failure caused by poor renal perfusion.
	Check peripheral perfusion: pulses, skin temperature, color.	Complications from catheterization site, such as thrombus or femoral artery aneurysm, can alter tissue perfusion of affected extremity.
	Auscultate heart sounds; note diminished or extra sounds. Auscultate lung sounds for presence of adventitious or diminished breath sounds.	To detect presence of LV heart failure.
	Administer medications as ordered: IV nitroglycerin, antiplatelets.	IV nitroglycerin decreases incidence of coronary artery spasm; antiplatelets given to reduce risk of restenosis, which is platelet mediated.
Potential altered peripheral tissue perfusion related to thrombus formation	Inspect cannulated extremity for ecchymosis, swelling, pain, warmth.	Reflects hematoma formation or bleeding.
	Assess pulses distal to site, noting any decrease in amplitude, q 15 min four times, decreasing frequency as ordered; note skin color, temperature.	Intravenous heparin has been been administered, which increases risk of bleeding and hematoma formation with excessive movements.

→ > >

NURSING DIAGNOSIS	NURSING INTERVENTIONS	RATIONALE
	Maintain bed rest in flat position until arterial and venous sheaths are removed, instructing patient to keep catheterized extremity immobile and extended.	Movements, which might stress abdominal and groin muscles, can disrupt protective hemostatic clot from forming.
	After sheaths are removed, maintain pressure over groin site with dressing, 5-10 lb (2.25-4.5 kg) sandbag, or compressor.	To decrease risk of bleeding and hematoma formation.
	Monitor coagulation laboratory studies, reporting prolonged PTT or abnormal results to physician.	Patient is receiving heparin, which alters PTT values.
	Administer antiplatelets as ordered.	To reduce risk of restenosis.
Knowledge deficit	See Preprocedural Nursing Care; Patient Teaching.	

5 EVALUATE

PATIENT OUTCOME	DATA INDICATING OUTCOME IS REACHED
Anxiety level is reduced.	Patient appears calm; patient/family state in own words purpose of procedure and general expectations postoperatively.
CO is maintained.	Chest pain is absent; ECG: no signs of ST changes, normal sinus rhythm; dysrhythmias absent. Negative cardiac enzyme results.
Tissue perfusion is maintained.	Pulses are full and bounding. AT cannulation site color is good; no signs of tenderness or swelling.
Knowledge level is increased.	Patient verbalizes understanding of purpose and rationale for procedure and self-care management following discharge; verbalizes understanding that PTCA is not cure and need to continue management and prevention of reocclusion by modifying risk factors such as stopping smoking, maintaining proper diet.

PATIENT TEACHING

1. Review explanation of procedure and postoperative results.
2. Instruct patient to report onset of chest pain, numbness, or excessive ecchymosis at insertion site.
3. Review and discuss need to modify and/or continue to modify coronary risk factors.
4. Discuss activity allowances and limitation: avoid strenuous activity, exercising, and heavy lifting 1 to 2 weeks after discharge; check with physician regarding driving and return to work.
5. Review medication: antiplatelets—discuss purpose, dosage, method of administration, and side effects.
6. Inform patient that it is frequently necessary to evaluate patency of coronary arteries, thus necessitating periodic treadmill testing.

THROMBOLYTIC THERAPY

We now know that long-term survival and prognosis following myocardial infarction (MI) depend on the degree to which ventricular function can be maintained. However, only in the past decade have investigators actively sought interventions that can retard the process of myocardial necrosis. Thrombolytic therapy, in the treatment of acute MI (AMI) has emerged from studies that examined the role of coronary thrombosis as the precipitating factor of MI.[34] Several investigators have demonstrated how clot lysis and reperfusion of an infarct-related vessel can reduce infarct size and preserve myocardial function.[81,82] One study demonstrated that in the acute stages (up to 6 hours) of MI, abrupt coronary occlusion, in the setting of an already narrowed coronary artery, is caused by an intracoronary thrombosis.[34] In this landmark study, total coronary occlusion resulting from intraluminal thrombosis occurred in 80% to 90% of patients with transmural infarctions. The study further showed that the incidence of coronary thrombosis decreased in patients who presented during 6 to 24 hours from the onset of chest pain.

Intracoronary infusion of thrombolytic agents has been demonstrated to achieve successful clot lysis, restore coronary blood flow, and limit myocardial ischemia.[138] The extent to which thrombolytic therapy is successful in salvaging myocardial function, however, is time dependent. One group found that the time from onset of clinical symptoms to initiation of intracoronary thrombolysis was the strongest predictor of achieving coronary reperfusion.[82] It is now generally accepted that thrombolytic therapy initiated within the first 4 to 6 hours to patients with an evolving AMI can reduce in-hospital and 1-year mortality rates.

Because early intervention is critical in effectively achieving clot lysis, IV administration of the thrombolytic agents has been advocated more recently. Its effectiveness has been found to be similar to that of intracoronary administration.[52]

Intracoronary thrombolysis is performed in the cardiac catheterization laboratory with selective angiography. Intravenous thrombolysis is performed in the emergency room or critical care unit; infusion is administered via peripheral vein. Depending on the patient's clinical status and if ischemia is present, PTCA may be performed immediately following reperfusion or before discharge. Postprocedural coronary arteriograms are performed before discharge or as indicated by clinical signs and symptoms.

Thrombolytic agents. Thrombogenesis, the result of a complex interplay of coagulation factors, involves platelet aggregation and adhesion. Prothrombin then converts to thrombin, which contributes to the conversion of fibrinogen to fibrin, which in turn stabilizes platelet aggregation, forming a hemostatic plug. The development of thrombolytic agents has been the key to the dissolution of the coronary thrombus. Lysis of thrombi results from two actions: (1) invasion of the site of injury by leukocytes and (2) activation of the fibrinolytic system. Normally the fibrinolytic system, which involves plasminogen activators, converts plasminogen, a circulating proenzyme, to plasmin. Plasmin, a proteolytic enzyme responsible for clot lysis, degrades fibrin into soluble fragments, which are then removed in the microcirculation. In the presence of large thrombi, this system cannot dissolve the large fibrin mass. However, the introduction of exogenous plasminogen activators produces more plasmin, which depletes circulating fibrinogen and promotes lysis. High titers of fibrinogen degradation products (FDPs) also are produced. In addition to the fibrinolytic process, exogenous plasminogen activators destroy coagulation factors V and VIII, causing a systemic lytic state that increases the potential risk of bleeding.

The following section briefly reviews approved and investigational fibrinolytic agents. Table 6-1 shows a comparison between tissue plasminogen activator (t-PA), streptokinase (SK), and urokinase (UK).

Streptokinase (Streptase, Kabikinase). SK, a synthetic protein, is derived from group C beta-hemolytic streptococci. It forms an activator complex with plasminogen to activate the fibrinolytic process. In addition, SK depletes fibrinogen levels and other coagulation factors, such as V and VIII, predisposing the patient to systemic bleeding. Furthermore, since SK is a bacterial protein with antigenicity when introduced into the body, it can produce a variety of allergic reactions.

Usual dosage: *Intracoronary*—25,000- to 50,000-unit bolus followed by a continuous infusion of 2000 to 4000 units/minute for 60 minutes (total dose, 150,000 to 500,000 units). The procedure is carried out in conjunction with angiography. Infusions are continued for 30 to 60 minutes after antegrade flow has been established.

Intravenous—continuous infusion of 750,000 to 1.5 million IU administered over 30 to 60 minutes. Infusion may be initiated in the emergency room or coronary care unit.

Half-life: Alpha and beta half-life is 18 minutes. Enzymatic action persists 18 to 80 minutes; enzymatic action on coagulation system persists for up to 18 to 24 hours.

> **EXAMPLE OF A CALCULATED STANDARD DOSE FOR T-PA**
>
> 100 mg: 1.0 mg/ml
> Lytic dose: 10 mg
> First hour: 50 mg
> Second hour: 20 mg
> Third hour: 20 mg
> **Total dose** 100 mg

Table 6-1 _____

COMPARISON OF THROMBOLYTIC AGENTS*

	t-PA	SK	UK
Binds to fibrin	Yes	No	No
Efficacy	70%-75%	40%-50%	Similar to SK
Bleeding risk	Yes	Yes	Yes
Systemic effect	Minimal (potentially greater at higher dose)	Severe	Severe
Resistance/allergic reaction	No	Yes	No
Hypotension on administration	No	Yes	No

*t-PA, Tissue plasminogen activator; SK, streptokinase; UK, urokinase.

Side effects: Bleeding and hypotension during rapid bolus infusion reported to occur in 15% of patients; allergic reaction—fever, flushing, rash, periorbital swelling, and bronchospasms.

Urokinase (Abbokinase). UK, a naturally occurring human proteolytic enzyme, is produced by the parenchymal cells of the kidney. It acts directly on circulating plasminogen to produce the fibrinolytic enzyme plasmin.

Usual dose*:

Intracoronary—10,000- to 30,000-unit bolus followed by a continuous infusion of 2000 to 24,000 units/minute. Infusion procedure must be performed in conjunction with coronary angiography.

Intravenous—10,000 to 20,000-unit bolus followed by a continuous infusion of 10,000 to 20,000 units/minute up to a total of 2 to 3 million units.

Half-life: 10 to 20 minutes; prolonged action on coagulation persists for up to 18 to 24 hours.

Side effects: None specified; may be administered rapidly either by bolus or infusion without side effects; bleeding occurs.

Tissue plasminogen activator (Activase). t-PA is a naturally occurring human enzyme present in the vascular endothelium, circulating blood, and human tissue. Unlike SK and UK, which activate plasminogen systemically, t-PA is a fibrin-specific agent. t-PA activates plasminogen only after plasminogen has bound to fibrin contained in the thrombus. Thus t-PA is a clot specific agent, producing relatively little circulating plasmin systemically, which does not deplete other clotting factors, thereby reducing the risk of bleeding.

*Drug dosages are not standardized; bolus and maintenance doses may have wide range.

Usual dose:

Intravenous

Standard dose—100 mg (concentration, 1.0 mg/ml); for patients less than 65 kg; for patients greater than 65 kg: 1.25 mg/kg over 3 hours

Lytic dose, first hour—60% of total dose, 10 mg of which (10%) is administered as an IV bolus

Maintenance dose—second hour, 20% of total dose; third hour, 20% of total dose

Intracoronary—at this time, no clinical trials have investigated the IC route.

Half-life: 5 to 7 minutes

Side effect: Bleeding

Investigational agents. Several thrombolytic agents are currently under investigation for use in the treatment of AMI. One is anisoylated plasminogen-SK activator complex (APSAC, Eminase), an SK-plasminogen activator that has been chemically modified by acylation.[80]

Another investigational agent is a single-chain UK plasminogen activator (SCU-PA), an inactive single-chain precursor to the active two-chain UK molecule. It is often referred to as Prourokinase and limits systemic plasmin production and its by-products.

INDICATIONS

Chest pain or equivalent lasting 15 min or longer

Recent onset (not to exceed 4-6 h) of chest pain unresponsive to conventional sublingual NTG therapy

ECG changes documenting acute myocardial injury: ST elevation with reciprocal changes; Q waves do not preclude the patient from receiving therapy

Patient <75 years of age

CONTRAINDICATIONS

Absolute
  Active internal bleeding
  History of cerebrovascular event
  Previous treatment with SK 6 months to 1 year (does not apply to t-PA)
  Intracranial neoplasm, aneurysm
Major relative
  Major surgery (within 10 days)
  Recent GI or GU bleeding
  Serious trauma
  Traumatic CPR
  Uncontrolled hypertension (>180 mm Hg systolic and/or >110 mm Hg diastolic)
Minor relative
  Left-sided heart thrombus
  Bacterial endocarditis
  Existing bleeding diathesis
  Pregnancy
  Advanced age (≥75 years)
  Diabetic hemorrhagic retinopathy

CAUTIONS

Current anticoagulant therapy
Acute pericarditis
Renal or liver disease

COMPLICATIONS

Bleeding and hemorrhage related to intravascular fibrinogenolysis (bleeding at puncture sites; gastrointestinal or, intracranial hemorrhage; hemopericardium)
Recurrent ischemia or infarction related to reocclusion—reported to occur in 20% to 40% of patients following successful recanalization

PREPROCEDURAL NURSING CARE

1. Initiate preprocedural explanation of procedure to patient and family.
   a. Instruct patient and family about purpose and indications for thrombolytic therapy, its benefits, and associated risks.
   b. Describe intracoronary procedure, that it is similar to cardiac catheterization (see page 273), and that the procedure may last from 1 to 2 hours. Review sensations to be experienced, such as pressure during insertion of catheter but no discomfort with infusion.
   c. Explain and review procedures and routines associated with procedure: monitoring in CCU, heart rhythm problems, and bleeding. Explain need for bed rest during and following administration and for frequent blood sampling to monitor clotting times.
   d. Instruct patient to inform nurse if chest pain develops.
2. Consents are required to perform cardiac catheterization, angioplasty, and CABG surgery.
3. Obtain baseline laboratory data to determine hemostatic status and degree of myocardial injury: CBC with platelets, PT, fibrinogen and fibrin split-product levels, CPK-MB, blood type and cross-match, electrolytes, BUN, creatinine.
4. Obtain diagnostic data such as 12-Lead ECG and chest x-ray; obtain vital signs and perform clinical assessment.
5. Administer medication as ordered; give IV lidocaine prophylactically.
6. Prepare for cardiac catheterization if indicated.
7. Establish at least two or three patent IV lines.

POTENTIAL BLEEDING SITES FOLLOWING THROMBOLYTIC INFUSION

Surface bleeding		Gastrointestinal	Genitourinary	Retroperitoneal	Intracranial
Source	**Symptom**				
Venous puncture sites	Mild to persistent oozing	Hematemesis	Hematuria	Low back pain	Headache
	Bleeding, hematoma	Tarry or bloody stools		Muscle weakness or numbness in lower extremities	Vomiting
Femoral artery catheter	Bleeding from gums	Gastritis			Disorientation
Gingiva	Bruising	Laboratory findings: presence of occult blood in stool, sputum			Mental confusion progressing to coma
Ecchymosis					Hemiplegia
					CVA
					Laboratory tests: CT scan, EEG, MRI

MEDICAL MANAGEMENT

GENERAL MANAGEMENT

Intra-arterial blood pressure: Used to observe for changes in BP and for drawing of blood sampling

Cardiac monitoring: ECG pattern observed for signs of reperfusion

Hemodynamic monitoring: PA, PCWP

Bed rest as ordered: Only after cardiac catheterization to prevent disruption of hemostatic clot at insertion site

Diet: As ordered

Laboratory studies (careful monitoring during and following thrombolysis): Serum fibrinogen levels—50 mg/dl lower following infusion of thrombolytic agent, returning to baseline within 24 h of completion of thrombolytic infusion

PTT, Hg, CPK-MB

DRUG THERAPY

During procedure: Thrombolysis

   Diphenhydramine (Benadryl)—50 mg IV given before SK infusion to reduce risk of allergic reaction (fever, rash)

   Heparin—5000- to 10,000-unit IV bolus followed by a continuous infusion to maintain PTT, 1.5 to 2 times control value; used to reduce risk of reocclusion immediately and after initial reperfusion

After procedure: Heparin—600 to 700 units continuous IV once PTT levels reach 2 times control value

1 ASSESS

ASSESSMENT	OBSERVATIONS
Preprocedure	
Myocardial ischemia	Chest discomfort: <4-6 h from onset of symptoms ECG: ST elevations of 0.1 mm, dysrhythmias Skin: clammy, diaphoretic Hypotension
Postprocedure	
Reperfusion of myo-cardium	Abrupt cessation of chest discomfort ECG: return of ST elevations to baseline Reperfusion dysrhythmias: sinus bradycardia, AV block with hypotension, accelerated idioventricular rhythm (AIVR), ventricular tachycardia Isoenzymes: early peaking of CPK-MB within 12 h from onset of symptoms
Bleeding/ hemorrhage	Surface bleeding: intermittent oozing from peripheral venous, arterial punctures; bleeding from femoral artery catheter site; gingival bleeding; ecchymosis GI: hematemesis, feces—positive for occult blood, tarry stools

ASSESSMENT	OBSERVATIONS
Reocclusion of coronary artery (ischemia/ infarction)	Chest pain ECG: ST-T wave changes, dysrhythmias Skin: cool, clammy, diaphoretic Hypotension, tachycardia, nausea

2 DIAGNOSE

NURSING DIAGNOSIS	SUBJECTIVE FINDINGS	OBJECTIVE FINDINGS
Potential fluid volume deficit related to bleeding/ hemorrhage secondary to thrombolysis-induced coagulopathy	Patient is restless; complains of thirst, low back pain, weakness	Surface bleeding Internal bleeding—hypotension, tachycardia, decreased urine output Skin—pale, cool Prolonged PTT; decreased HgB, Hct Fibrinogen level decreased
Potential decreased cardiac output related to reperfusion dysrhythmias	Complains of palpitations, skipped beats, dizziness, lightheadedness	Hypotension ECG—inferior wall and posterior wall MI: bradycardia, 1st- and 2nd-degree AV heart block Anterior wall MI: ventricular tachycardia or fibrillation AIVR
Potential for pain (chest) related to reocclusion of coronary artery	Complains of recurrent chest pain, difficulty breathing, nausea	Skin—cool, clammy, diaphoretic HR—tachycardia, irregular pulse ECG—ST segment elevation/depression: 　Anterior V_1, V_4 　Lateral V_5, V_6I, AVL 　Inferior 2, 3, AVF 　Posterior V_1-V_3 (reciprocal changes) 　Dysrhythmias—PVCs

3 PLAN

Patient goals

1. Patient will show no signs of bleeding or hemodynamic changes as a result of fluid volume deficit (blood loss).
2. Patient will demonstrate stable CO.
3. Patient will experience and verbalize relief of ischemic chest pain.
4. Patient will verbalize knowledge and understanding regarding early recognition of recurrent ischemic symptoms and anticipated bleeding and bruising associated with therapy.

→ > >

4 IMPLEMENT

NURSING DIAGNOSIS	NURSING INTERVENTIONS	RATIONALE
Potential fluid volume deficit related to bleeding/ hemorrhage secondary to thrombolysis-induced coagulopathy	Assess for signs and symptoms of surface or internal bleeding.	Surface bleeding is often superficial, but continuous oozing can lead to intravascular volume deficit. Internal bleeding occurs from dissolution of protective hemostatic clot. Early detection minimizes complications caused by blood loss.
	Monitor BP, HR, respiration frequently according to protocol during first hour, decreasing frequency as condition stabilizes.	To detect early sign of internal bleeding. Risk of bleeding depends on thrombolytic agent used. Effect may extend to 48 h after procedure.
	Inspect puncture sites every 15 min; apply manual pressure when removing catheters, following venipunctures.	To detect hematoma; to control superficial bleeding.
	Implement measures that prevent disruption of vascular integrity: avoid use of venous or arterial punctures, IM injections; nonelectric razors. Instruct patient to avoid vigorous toothbrushing. Avoid removing arterial or venous lines during first 24-48 h or as indicated by agents used. Use heparin lock for IV access, blood sampling.	Disruption or injury to vascular integrity can lead to bleeding because of temporary inability to form protective hemostatic clot at site of tissue or vascular injury.
	Monitor PTT values until hemostasis has been reestablished.	To evaluate hemostatic parameters. PTT reflects coagulation status. PTT that extends beyond 100 sec (>1.5-2 times control), should be considered risk for internal bleeding.
Potential decreased cardiac output related to reperfusion dysrhythmias	Assess and record changes in ECG tracing during and following thrombolytic therapy to detect appearance of reperfusion dysrhythmias.	Reestablished blood flow to ischemic myocardium is often accompanied by what are termed *reperfusion dysrhythmias.*
	Assess and monitor BP, HR, respiration, and hemodynamic response to reperfusion dysrhythmias. Notify physician promptly of any signs of decreased CO.	CO may not be compromised by some reperfusion dysrhythmias, but careful assessment and documentation of hemodynamic response to dysrhythmia is essential before initiation of antiarrhythmic therapy.
	Administer antiarrhythmic medications as ordered; keep medications and defibrillator at bedside.	To facilitate quick, definitive treatment of dysrhythmias.
Potential for pain (chest) related to reocclusion of coronary artery	Assess and monitor chest pain, noting patient's verbal, nonverbal expressions; compare with preprocedural chest pain complaints.	Chest pain following perfusion period may represent reinfarction of salvaged myocardium caused by reocclusion. Risk of reocclusion is within first 24 h after successful thrombolysis.

NURSING DIAGNOSIS	NURSING INTERVENTIONS	RATIONALE
	Obtain 12-Lead ECG; compare with baseline ECG taken immediately after successful thrombolysis. Report any changes immediately.	To detect onset or recurrent myocardial ischemia, which indicates rethrombosis of coronary artery and increased risk of reinfarction.
	Maintain bed rest.	To reduce myocardial O_2 demand.
	Prepare patient for possible cardiac catheterization, repeat thrombolysis, or PTCA or CABG.	Depending on findings, patient may undergo any of these procedures on emergent basis.
Knowledge deficit	See Preprocedural Nursing Care; Patient Teaching.	

5   EVALUATE

PATIENT OUTCOME	DATA INDICATING THAT OUTCOME IS REACHED
No evidence of bleeding; hemostasis is reestablished.	Coagulation studies are within acceptable limits. No overt or covert signs of bleeding; no hematoma, petechiae are present. Vital signs are within normal limits. Patient is alert and oriented.
CO is maintained.	ECG remains stable; absence of uncontrollable dysrhythmia. Vital signs are stable.
Comfort level is achieved.	Patient verbalizes absence of chest discomfort or pain. Patient is able to resume activity level without complaints of pain.
Knowledge level is increased.	Patient verbalizes understanding of procedure, rationale, anticipated risks, and understanding of signs and symptoms to report.

PATIENT TEACHING

1. Review explanation of procedure and postprocedural results.
2. Instruct patient to report any signs of bleeding: bruising, bleeding gums, hematuria, tarry stools.
3. Instruct patient to report pain relief or new onset of pain.
4. Discuss activity allowances and limitations.
5. Discuss need to modify and/or continue to modify coronary risk factors.
6. Discuss importance of continued follow-up and that coronary angiography may be necessary to evaluate the patency of coronary arteries.
7. Review medications, discussing dosage, method of administration, and side effects.

PACEMAKERS

Pacemakers are battery-operated generators that initiate and control the heart rate by delivering an electrical impulse via an electrode to the myocardium. Implantation of myocardial electrodes is initiated when a patient has symptomatic AV block. However, since the development of pacemakers in 1960, their use has expanded to include treatment of symptomatic bradyarrhythmias from other causes and to control (overdrive suppression) refractory tachyarrhythmias (Figure 6-6).

Pacemaker implantation may be performed for temporary or long-term pacing. Temporary cardiac pacing is most often used for hemodynamic or life-support purposes. Therapeutically the indications for use include prophylactic pacing for complete heart block, symptomatic bradyarrhythmias, particularly in the setting of acute MI, as well as an emergency measure for malfunction of an implanted permanent pacemaker.[103] In addition to controlling heart rate, temporary pacing is being used increasingly in the electrophysiologic laboratory to evaluate cardiac dysrhythmias as well as to interrupt tachycardias.

Permanent cardiac pacing is indicated in the continuous presence of symptomatic bradyarrhythmias.

Today, pacing systems are classified according to a universal code that uses a three-letter designation for the mode of pacing and the chambers to be sensed and paced. The first letter describes the chamber that will be paced: the atrium (A), ventricle (V), or both (dual) chambers (D). The second letter represents the chamber that will be sensed: atrium (A), ventricle (V), dual (D), or none (0). The third letter reflects the mode that will be used: triggered (T), inhibited (I), or both (D).

For example:

> *For VVI:*
> V The pacemaker will pace the ventricle.
> V The pacemaker will sense the ventricle.
> I The pacemaker will inhibit pacing when the patient's own impulse is sensed.

There are three types of pacemakers: (1) asynchronous or fixed rate, in which rate and rhythm of pacemaker beats are unaffected by spontaneous beats; (2) demand pacing or standby pacing, which discharges (fires) only when spontaneous beats drop below a preset minimum rate; and (3) synchronous pacemakers, in which a sensing circuit is used to detect atrial and ventricular activity.

The method of implantation depends on whether pacing will be temporary or permanent:

Transvenous approach (endocardial)—most frequently used technique for temporary pacing; catheter electrode is passed into right ventricle via a peripheral vein (brachial, femoral, subclavian, or internal jugular). Electrode is then connected to external battery-operated pulse generator that can be set manually for direct or demand pacing mode (Figure 6-7).

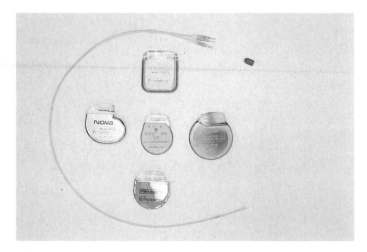

FIGURE 6-6
Various types of permanent pulse generators with pacing electrode.

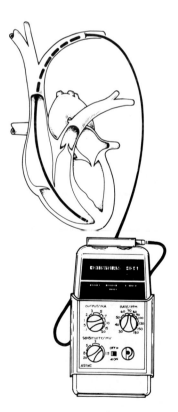

FIGURE 6-7
Temporary external pacemaker unit. Transvenous approach. (From Tucker et al.)[176]

Transthoracic approach—used primarily after open heart surgery or in emergencies; catheter is passed directly into heart through chest wall.

Permanent transvenous pacing—most frequently used procedure for insertion of permanent pacemakers; catheter electrode is passed into right ventricle via a cutdown method into the cephalic vein or by percutaneous method into the subclavian or an internal or external jugular vein. The catheter electrode is then attached to a small, sealed, battery-operated pulse generator that is planted subcutaneously in the shoulder or upper left quadrant (Figure 6-8).

Epicardial pacing—performed less frequently; electrode is sutured to epicardial surface of right ventricle; procedure requires a thoracotomy.

Pacemaker unit. The pulse generator is a self-contained device consisting of an electronic circuit and a power source of lithium batteries that is hermetically sealed to protect the unit from the biologic environment. Lithium-powered pacemakers can last from 5 to 8 years before a battery charge is required.

Pulse generators use either unipolar or bipolar leads, and most generators are programmable to both. With unipolar leads the electrode (negative terminal) is at the distal tip of the catheter, touching the endocardium or myocardium. With a bipolar lead two electrodes are located at the distal tip of the catheter. Current flows from the pulse generator to the distal electrodes into the heart, where it stimulates myocardial contraction.

A pacemaker magnet is used to test pacemaker function. The sensing mechanism can be deactivated by placing the magnet over the pulse generator. The pacing rate can be higher, lower, or constant, based on the type of magnet used.

INDICATIONS

Bradyarrhythmias
Acquired AV block
  Complete heart block (third degree): intermittent, persistent
  Mobitz type II (second degree): intermittent, persistent
  Mobitz type I (first degree): only when symptoms present
Congenital complete AV block
Atrial fibrillation with slow ventricular response
Sick sinus syndrome
  Sinus arrest
  Sinus bradycardia when symptoms present
  Bradycardia-tachycardia (brady-tachy) syndrome
AV block associated with MI
Carotid sinus syndrome
Refractory tachyarrhythmias
Supraventricular tachyarrhythmias (SVTs)
  Sinus tachycardia
  Atrial tachycardia
  Atrial fibrillation
  Junctional tachycardia
  Ventricular tachycardia
Prophylaxis for cardiac surgery

CONTRAINDICATIONS

Active infections
Possibly in presence of atrial fibrillation or any poorly controlled SVT

CAUTION
Safety from electrical hazards

COMPLICATIONS

Infection and pressure necrosis of pocket site of pulse generator
Pacemaker system failure
  Head wire break
  Pulse generator malfunction
  Catheter dislodgement/misplacement
Ventricular perforation leading to:
  Stimulation of diaphragm and hiccough
  Cardiac tamponade
Thrombosis and embolism

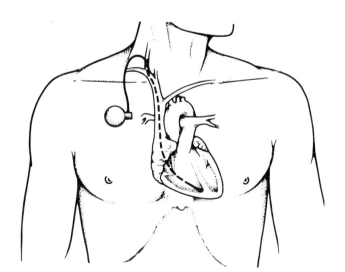

FIGURE 6-8
Permanent pacemaker. (From Tucker et al.)[176]

PREPROCEDURAL NURSING CARE

1. Initiate preoperative instruction for patient/family, including the purpose and indications for pacemaker implantation, benefits, and associated risks. Provide information regarding type and mode of pacemaker used, method of insertion, and that procedure is done under local anesthesia. Stress postoperative care, including need for routine 24-hour ECG monitoring and need to restrict activities for 4 to 6 hours.
2. Obtain written informed consent.
3. Teach passive ROM exercises to be done postoperatively.
4. Perform skin preparation.
5. Obtain baseline assessment data: underlying ECG rhythm, heart rate, pulse, respirations, blood pressure, and level of consciousness.
6. Permit nothing by mouth.
7. Initiate IV line.
8. Check functioning of external generator, including battery (for temporary unit).
9. Administer preprocedural medication.

MEDICAL MANAGEMENT

GENERAL MANAGEMENT

After procedure: Physical activity—bed rest for 8 h after implantation, keeping arm below level of shoulder; range of motion (ROM) exercises to affected extremity when ordered after third postoperative day

Avoidance of excessive extension or abduction of arm closest to insertion site

12-Lead ECG with and without use of magnet testing

Cardiac monitoring—ECG pattern—patient's underlying rate, signs of pacing or nonpacing, dysrhythmias (Figure 6-9)

Diet—as ordered

Chest x-ray—to check position of electrodes

DRUG THERAPY:

Preoperative and intraoperative—mild sedation, tranquilizers 30 min before procedure; local anesthesia for temporary and long-term transvenous pacing; general anesthesia for transthoracic approach

Postprocedure—analgesics

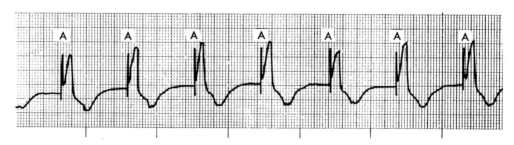

FIGURE 6-9
ECG strip showing paced beat. (From Andreoli, K., et al.)[6]

1 ASSESS

ASSESSMENT	OBSERVATIONS
Pacemaker function	Pacemaker unit: location of pulse generator, type of pacemaker, selected rate, preprogrammed time intervals (if dual chamber) Pacemaker failure: Clinical symptoms—syncope, hypotension, bradycardia, pallor, SOB ECG rhythm—loss of pacemaker artifact, change in paced QRS complex, decreased amplitude of pacemaker artifact, competition between patient's underlying rhythm and paced beats, dysrhythmias Catheter dislodgement—change in QRS configuration, loss of artifact on ECG, failure to sense, hiccoughs, muscle twitching in chest or abdomen
Incisional site	Infection: redness, discoloration, pain, swelling, heat; fluid collection, drainage; skin breakdown; elevated temperature
Cardiac dysrhythmias	Premature ventricular beats, sustained ventricular tachycardia; patient complains of palpitations

2 DIAGNOSE

NURSING DIAGNOSIS	SUBJECTIVE FINDINGS	OBJECTIVE FINDINGS
Anxiety related to perceived and/or actual change in health status and role functioning	Apprehension; verbalizes uncertainty, fear of dying; expresses concern regarding changes in life-style that may be necessary because of pacemaker	Insomnia, worried appearance, focus on self
Decreased cardiac output related to pacemaker failure and perforation of ventricle	Reports lightheadedness, dizziness	Decreased mentation, syncope Decreased BP, bradycardia Irregular rhythm, decreased amplitude of pulse SOB, pallor cardiac tamponade
Pain related to incision and to physical immobility of affected arm	Complains of stiffness, pain when moving shoulder or arm on operative site Requests pain medication	Guarded or withdrawal of arm/shoulder on operative site; crying; grimacing on movement Irritability Limited ROM

Other related nursing diagnoses: Potential for infection related to incision site; **Potential for injury** related to microshocks

→ 〉 〉

3 PLAN

Patient goals

1. Patient will demonstrate reduced anxiety level.
2. Patient will demonstrate electromechanical stability and maintenance of CO.
3. Patient will verbalize absence of discomfort and will demonstrate full ROM of affected arm.
4. Patient will demonstrate increased level of understanding of procedure and skills necessary for self-maintenance.

4 IMPLEMENT

NURSING DIAGNOSIS	NURSING INTERVENTIONS	RATIONALE
Anxiety related to perceived and/or actual change in health status and role functioning	Assess level of anxiety, level of understanding, and fears associated with pacemaker implantation.	Many expressed concerns of patients with pacemaker have focused on need for permanent life-support system, fear of dying from pacemaker failure, and need to alter life-style.
	Provide explanation and rationale for pacemaker, gauging reactions of patient. Initiate patient education program. Anticipate and allow questions from patient regarding changes in life-style, cautions, and concerns over pacemaker management.	Permitting patients to question and discuss fears and concerns increases their understanding of living with pacemaker, thus reducing anxiety level.
Decreased cardiac output related to pacemaker failure and perforation of ventricle	Assess patient and pacemaker unit for proper functioning of pacemaker unit: capturing, sensing.	To assess for signs of pacemaker failure and postoperative complications.
	Place patient on cardiac monitor: check rhythm strip, noting pacemaker function and rate on admission to unit and following any changes in parameters.	To evaluate pacemaker functioning.
	Assess for signs of dysrhythmias.	Postoperative dysrhythmias may occur as result of ventricular irritability from insertion of stiff catheter.
	Monitor vital signs q 4 h after insertion.	To detect any signs of compromised cardiac function that may reflect onset of pacemaker failure or ventricular perforations.
Pain related to incision and to physical immobility of affected arm	Assess quality and source of pain.	To determine if pain is related to immobility or onset of infectious process at incision site.
	Administer pain medication as ordered.	To alleviate pain, which will permit exercises.
	Encourage ROM exercises to affected shoulder as ordered.	To avoid stiffness of extremity with restricted movement.
Knowledge deficit	See Preprocedural Nursing Care; Patient Teaching.	

5 EVALUATE

PATIENT OUTCOME	DATA INDICATING THAT OUTCOME IS REACHED
Anxiety level is reduced.	Patient appears calm and relaxed; verbalizes concerns and fears associated with self-care and management of pacemaker; actively participates in instruction; reports restful sleep.
Pacemaker functions properly.	Patient is normotensive and without dizziness, syncope, palpitations, chest pain, SOB, or fatigue. HR is acceptable. Temporary pacemaker fires at preset rate, sensing mechanism is visualized, and pacemaker artifact is visualized on ECG. Permanent pacemaker fires at preset rate, and pacemaker artifact is visualized on ECG.
Patient is free of pain.	Incisional site is clean with no swelling or redness. Patient verbalizes comfort; has full ROM of affected arm and shoulder.
Knowledge level is increased.	Patient verbalizes understanding and rationale for procedure of self-care management, signs of pacemaker failure and actions to take; demonstrates pulse taking and skin care management.

PATIENT TEACHING

1. Instruct patient/family about purpose, rationale, and basic function of permanent pacemaker.
2. Describe type of pacemaker and pacemaker's set rate. Instruct patient on pulse rate and rhythm checking, emphasizing that pulse rate monitoring in lithium pacemakers must be done once a week or when patient is feeling symptomatic.
3. Describe signs and symptoms of pacemaker failure, including dizziness, weakness, lightheadedness, or drop in pacemaker's set rate. Discuss actions to take if pacemaker malfunction is suspected, including calling for pacemaker check via transtelephonic monitoring and notifying physician or pacemaker clinic.
4. Describe activity allowances and limitations: avoid traveling and driving for first 4 weeks following insertion. With exception of competitive contact sports, which can increase risk of lead dislodgment, patients should be encouraged to resume normal daily activities and recreational interests.
5. Discuss need to avoid and protect against electrical hazards from high-output electrical generators, such as diathermy motors, welding equipment, or radar. Most household electrical devices (e.g., microwaves, blow dryers) are considered safe, but review symptoms that may reflect electromagnetic interference and what action to take if symptoms occur.
6. Explain need for continued medical follow-up and for periodic battery replacements; refer patient to pacemaker clinic where available.

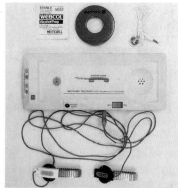

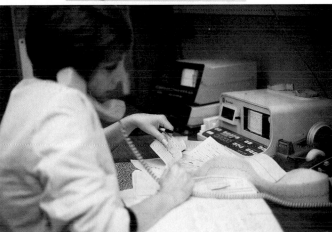

FIGURE 6-10
A, Telephone ECG transmitter equipment allows patient to have periodic evaluation of heart rate and rhythm. **B,** Pacemaker transmission clinic. Technician monitors ECG strip as it is transmitted via the telephone.

7. Describe use of telephone transmitters where available (Figure 6-10).
8. Explain signs and symptoms of wound or pocket infection, and instruct patient or family to report to physician if fever or drainage develops.
9. Stress need to protect pacemaker site: avoid constricting clothing and direct contact or blows to site; contact sports are usually contraindicated.

10. Explain need to carry identification card.
11. Women in their reproductive years should be reassured that pregnancy is not contraindicated. They should, however, inform their physician of desired pregnancy before conception to check pacemaker program and adaptation to rate changes typically associated with pregnancy.

AUTOMATIC IMPLANTABLE CARDIOVERTER-DEFIBRILLATOR

The automatic implantable cardioverter-defibrillator (AICD) is a self-contained automatic system capable of identifying and treating life-threatening ventricular dysrhythmias. Originally designed to correct ventricular fibrillation (VF), the current generation of AICD units can identify and treat ventricular tachycardia (VT).[112]

Surgically implanted, the device, a battery-operated pulse generator with two-lead electrodes, continuously monitors and analyzes patient's heart rate and waveform configuration. In the presence of ventricular tachycardia and ventricular fibrillation, electrical countershock is delivered via two transcardiac electrodes directly to the heart. One catheter electrode is positioned in the superior vena cava, while the second may be a ventricular patch lead made of titanium mesh that is placed on the pericardium or myocardium during surgery.[20]

Surgical approach for implantation is determined by various clinical circumstances, such as whether the patient has had previous chest surgery or will also undergo corrective cardiac surgery.[135] The surgical approaches used for AICD implantation include:

Thoracotomy: for patients who previously underwent cardiac surgery and may have scar tissue around the heart

Median sternotomy (most frequently used approach): for patients undergoing concomitant cardiac surgery, such as antiarrhythmic surgery or CABG

Subxiphoid: incision made below the xiphoid process, entering the pericardial space anteriorly

Subcostal: similar to thoracotomy, but involves a smaller incision and shorter recovery time

Pulse generator: has two modes, inactive and active; if left in active mode, electrical shock delivered within 10 to 35 seconds after AICD senses a tachyarrhythmia.

INDICATIONS

Survivors of sudden cardiac death not associated with acute MI and whose dysrhythmias are not controlled with antiarrhythmic therapy

Patients who have had more than one cardiac arrest, but whose dysrhythmia cannot be induced during electrophysiologic testing

Patients with sustained VT not controlled with conventional antiarrhythmics

CONTRAINDICATIONS

Uncontrollable congestive heart failure

Severe psychologic fear about device

Patient with history of severe chronic obstructive pulmonary disease (COPD)

Use of unipolar pacemakers

NMR procedure; may damage AICD

CAUTION

Safety from strong magnetic fields should be ensured; can cause AICD device to activate or deactivate

COMPLICATIONS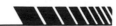

False-positive shocks reported to occur in 71% of patients with AICD implants

Lead migration into the vena cava, lead fracture

Infections involving pocket holding pulse generator

Pneumothorax

Death: operative mortality (2% to 3%); recurrent sudden cardiac death caused by ventricular dysrhythmias

PREPROCEDURAL NURSING CARE

1. Initiate preoperative instruction for patient/family, including information about AICD device, its benefits and risks, implantation procedure, and postoperative care. Include discussion regarding surgical approaches that may be used (thoracotomy, median sternotomy, subxiphoid and subcostal approaches). Explain that because device is large, tight-fitting clothing may be uncomfortable. Discuss routine postoperative procedures and equipment of ICU, where patients receiving implants will stay for 24 to 48 hours postoperatively.
2. Obtain written informed consent.
3. Obtain baseline data as ordered: ECG—baseline rhythm, vital signs; laboratory work—CBC, blood type and cross-match, electrolytes, PT, PTT; chest x-rays.
4. Perform skin preparation: chest and abdomen.
5. Permit nothing by mouth.
6. Deal with preoperative anxiety and fears of discomfort associated with shocks and/or malfunction of device.

MEDICAL MANAGEMENT

GENERAL MANAGEMENT

Postprocedure: General management of patient following implantation of AICD is similar to that for any cardiac surgical patient (see page 216).

Continuous ECG monitoring—observe for inappropriate shocks during sinus or patient's preestablished rhythm; observe for dysrhythmias

Hemodynamic monitoring—may be required until patient stabilizes

Diet—as ordered

IV therapy—as ordered

Physical activity—level determined by clinical status and postprocedural exercise stress test

NOTE: Patients with permanent pacemakers must be monitored for possible interaction between both devices (AICD, pacemaker).

DRUG THERAPY

Antiarrhythmics: Must be carefully selected to avoid interfering with defibrillation threshold; for example, amiodarone increases threshold

Lidocaine to control ventricular dysrhythmia

Beta blockers to control rapid sinus rhythms

---

1 ASSESS

ASSESSMENT	OBSERVATIONS
ECG	Appropriate discharge for VT/VF
	Transient episodes of supraventricular dysrhythmias, nonsustained ventricular tachycardia

ASSESSMENT	OBSERVATIONS
Malfunction of AICD	Failure to sense and discharge; sudden cardiac death
Infection of pulse generator pocket site	Redness, swelling, heat; fluid collection or drainage; skin irritation or breakdown; elevated temperature
Postoperative complications	
Atelectasis	Elevated temperature, decreased or absent breath sounds over affected area, tachypnea, SOB
Pericarditis	Chest discomfort, pericardial friction rub

2 DIAGNOSE

NURSING DIAGNOSIS	SUBJECTIVE FINDINGS	OBJECTIVE FINDINGS
Potential decreased cardiac output related to recurrent ventricular dysrhythmias	Reports palpitations, dizziness, syncope	Unpalpable BP ECG: VT, VF, asystole
Fear related to anticipated shock and to possible death	Minor—verbalizes fear, helplessness, panic Major—verbalizes dread, apprehension	Increased alertness Sympathetic stimulation—increased HR, BP Insomnia, lack of concentration, emotional outburst, crying
Activity intolerance related to functional limitations and prolonged immobility	Complains of fatigue, weakness; verbalizes difficulty in performing task	History of bed rest/immobility Pallor, vertigo, increased HR

Other related nursing diagnoses: Body image disturbance related to perceived changes in body structure and function; **Sexual dysfunction** related to perceived limitations imposed by AICD device and/or fear of inducing dysrhythmias

3 PLAN

Patient goals

1. Patient will demonstrate electromechanical stability.
2. Patient will experience increase in psychologic comfort.
3. Patient will exhibit greater physical endurance to increased levels of activities.
4. Patient will demonstrate increased knowledge and skills to support self-care during and following hospital stay.

4 IMPLEMENT

NURSING DIAGNOSIS	NURSING INTERVENTIONS	RATIONALE
Potential decreased cardiac output related to recurrent ventricular dysrhythmia	Monitor HR and rhythm, BP, and level of consciousness.	To detect any signs of recurrent VT/VF, presence of unsustained ventricular dysrhythmias, or supraventricular tachycardia.
	Determine if AICD is in active or inactive mode.	Postoperative device may be left in inactive mode because common postoperative dysrhythmias such as sinus tachycardia can trigger defibrillation of device.
	Administer medications as ordered: antiarrhythmics.	Indicated if patient is having nonsustained VT, which can trigger device.
	In presence of sustained VT/VF:	
	Active mode—assess AICD function.	Device delivers electrical shock in 10-35 sec; if dysrhythmias not terminated, device will recharge and deliver three more shocks at higher energy levels.
	Inactive mode—initiate external cardioversion/defibrillation. (External cardioversion/defibrillation will not harm AICD device.)	To terminate life-threatening dysrhythmias.
	Prepare for discharge: Electrophysiologic (EP) study as ordered. During procedure, AICD may be activated.	To test adequacy of AICD device's ability to terminate dysrhythmia; to permit patient to experience "shock" while awake and in controlled setting.
Fear related to anticipated shock and to possible death	Assess level of understanding, encouraging patient to verbalize subjective feelings and perceptions of AICD.	Fear, aroused when perceived external threat present, is predominant emotion expressed by patients.
	Provide information to correct distorted perception; assist patient to identify source(s) of fear.	Understanding and sense of adequately dealing with danger can reduce level of fear.
	Assist patient to cope with fear(s); review strategies to cope with unpredictability of dysrhythmias and discomfort from shocks. Offer brief description of shock, what additional symptoms may accompany shock. Review signs and symptoms of battery failure or device malfunction and interventions to take if suspected.	Most common fears associated with AICD units include fear of shocks and battery failure, which leads to self-imposed decreased level of activity and social interaction and onset of depression.
	Refer to AICD support groups.	Use of support groups helps to provide information, reassurance, and emotional support in nonthreatening atmosphere of sharing.

→ 〉 〉 〉

NURSING DIAGNOSIS	NURSING INTERVENTIONS	RATIONALE
Activity intolerance related to functional limitations and prolonged immobility	Assess patient's tolerance/intolerance to activities of daily living (ADLs); determine if intolerance related to progressive heart disease vs perceived fear of AICD device.	Because of prolonged immobilization before implant, patients are deconditioned and may be hesitant to increase activity levels.
	Encourage patient to engage in exercise activities as tolerated. Refer to monitored exercise program.	Structured exercise programs can assist in providing patient with security in engaging in routine activities and in increasing endurance level.
	Develop activity plan that includes discussion of activity and allowance.	Based on precomplaint history, each activity must be individualized.
Knowledge deficit	See Preprocedural Nursing Care; Patient Teaching.	

5 EVALUATE

PATIENT OUTCOME	DATA INDICATING THAT OUTCOME IS REACHED
AICD unit functions properly.	Patient demonstrates no further episode of syncope, cardiac arrest; AICD unit shows appropriate discharge response during magnet testing.
Fear level is reduced.	Patient is able to verbalize specific fears and concerns regarding AICD unit. Patient verbalizes comfort with AICD unit, asking appropriate questions regarding home maintenance of AICD and home monitoring. Patient actively participates in patient teaching activities.
Activity level is increased.	Patient is able to resume ADLs and participates in exercise as allowed. HR $\leq$120 bpm during exercise (or within 20 bpm of resting HR if taking beta blockers). BP within 20 mm Hg of baseline range.
Knowledge level is increased, and self-care management skills are demonstrated.	Patient verbalizes understanding of AICD unit, its functioning, follow-up care, activity allowances and limitations, frequency of follow-up contact with physician, signs and symptoms to report; demonstrates proper method of keeping diary, pulse taking, skin care, use of magnets, and how to inactivate AICD.

PATIENT TEACHING

1. Instruct patient/family about purpose and basic function of AICD device. Include discussion about benefits and limitations.
2. Describe the AICD device, discussing signs and symptoms of defibrillation discharge.
3. Describe signs and symptoms of AICD malfunction (e.g., inappropriate shocks, loss of consciousness) and need to notify physician if suspected.
4. Explain need for regular follow-up magnet testing to predict end of generator life. Describe use of transtelephonic system if available.
5. Explain signs and symptoms of wound or pocket infection, and instruct patient or family to report to physician if fever or drainage develops.
6. Instruct patient regarding need to protect implantation site; avoid constricting clothing such as belts and girdles.
7. Describe activity allowances and limitations. State that most former activities may be resumed; that driving is permitted within 4 to 6 weeks after implantation unless patient bothered by neurologic symptoms and/or continues to have syncope after

AICD implantation; and that sexual activity can be resumed without danger to patient or partner.

8. Discuss need to avoid strong magnetic fields that may activate or deactivate AICD unit (e.g., areas around radio- or television-transmitting towers, use of diathermy motors). Instruct patient not to touch spark plugs of running motor (e.g., lawn mowers, cars).

9. Assure patient that normal household appliances (e.g., microwave ovens, hair dryers) will not interfere with AICD unit.

10. Assure patient that routine contact with another person (e.g., during sexual contact) will not activate unit and that if discharged during physical contact, slight muscular contraction may be felt by other person, but discharge will not harm individual.

11. Explain need to carry AICD identification card and wear Medic-Alert bracelet at all times.

12. Encourage family members to be certified in CPR.

13. Instruct patient in cough CPR.

CHAPTER 7

Patient Teaching Guides

Patient education has always been an important part of the nursing process. In today's hospitals, teaching patients about their disease and treatment poses a great challenge as diagnostic and treatment modalities become increasingly complex. Hospitalized patients often confront an array of threatening-looking equipment, and many procedures are based on technology that is unfamiliar to the general public.

Cost-control measures have mandated shorter hospital stays, so less time is available for patient teaching. This is contrary to basic principles of learning, which stress that learning is best accomplished by presenting information in small doses and reinforcing it through repetition. Unfortunately, this teaching method takes time, a luxury that is seldom available in today's hospital setting.

To compound the problem, the shorter hospital stays mean that patients are being discharged "quicker and sicker." They are often expected to continue treatments at home that, until a few years ago, were provided in the hospital. They may have to learn skilled techniques such as wound care or how to operate "high-tech" self-testing or monitoring equipment at home. Consequently, the nurse is faced with teaching patients more information, more quickly so they can manage at home.

Written materials can help reinforce patient teaching and encourage compliance. This chapter provides teaching handouts that can be photocopied and given to patients or their caregivers. Although handouts do not replace direct teaching, they provide basic information on procedures and guidelines for home care.

The handouts are designed to be used in combination, according to the patient's needs. For example, a patient scheduled to have a percutaneous transluminal coronary angioplasty (PTCA) can be given Angioplasty, along with the Cardiac Catheterization and Coronary Artery Disease handouts. The patient who has had an uncomplicated myocardial infarction might receive Recovering from a Heart Attack, Diet Guidelines for a Healthy Heart, Starting Your Exercise Program, and Counting Your Pulse. Someone who has just been diagnosed with hypertension might benefit from High Blood Pressure, Cardiovascular Disease Risk Factors, and Diet Guidelines for a Healthy Heart.

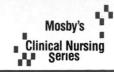

Cardiovascular Disease Risk Factors

Many deaths from cardiovascular disease are preventable. In addition, for people who already have been diagnosed with cardiovascular disease, the risk of death and further complications can be reduced. Research has uncovered several factors that contribute to heart attacks and strokes. The more risk factors a person has, the greater the chance of developing cardiovascular disease. Although some risk factors cannot be changed, you can modify others with your doctor's help, and still others can be eliminated altogether. The following checklists can help you determine your risk.

Major risk factors that cannot be changed

Heredity. A tendency toward heart disease runs in families. If one or both parents had cardiovascular disease, one's chances of developing it are higher.

Race. For reasons presently unknown, blacks have a much greater risk of developing high blood pressure than whites; twice as many have moderately high blood pressure, and three times as many have extremely high blood pressure. As a result, their risk of heart disease is greater.

Sex. Men have a higher risk of heart attack and stroke than women. During the childbearing years, women produce hormones that keep blood cholesterol levels low. Male hormones have the opposite effect—they raise blood cholesterol. However, women lose this protection after menopause or surgical removal of the ovaries, and women over age 55 have a 10 times greater risk than younger women. In recent years, however, more women under age 40 have developed coronary artery disease and high blood pressure. This probably results from the use of oral contraceptives and increased smoking.

Age. Fifty-five percent of heart attacks occur in people age 65 or older.

Major risk factors that can be changed

Smoking. Smokers have more than twice as many heart attacks as nonsmokers. Sudden cardiac death occurs two to four times more frequently in smokers. Peripheral vascular disease (narrowing of the blood vessels in the arms and legs) is almost exclusively a disease of smokers. When people stop smoking, the risk of heart disease drops rapidly, and 10 years after quitting, their risk of death from cardiovascular disease is about the same as for people who never smoked.

High Blood Pressure. High blood pressure makes the heart work harder, causing it to enlarge and become weaker over time. This can lead to stroke, heart attack, kidney failure, and congestive heart failure. For some people, high blood pressure can be controlled by a low-salt diet, weight reduction, and regular exercise. Other people also require medication to lower their blood pressure.

Blood Cholesterol Levels. A cholesterol level between 200 and 240 mg/dl increases the risk of heart disease. A cholesterol level greater than 240 mg/dl doubles the risk of coronary artery disease. The American Heart Association Diet, which is low in cholesterol and other fats, is recommended for anyone with a level of 200 or higher. Medication may also be necessary.

Other risk factors

Diabetes. Diabetes increases the risk of heart attack because it raises blood cholesterol levels. In addition, people who develop diabetes in midlife are often overweight, which is an additional risk factor.

Obesity. Excess weight forces the heart to work harder. People who are overweight are more prone to high blood pressure and high blood cholesterol levels. Obesity is defined as 30% or more over your ideal weight.

Physical inactivity. Researchers have found that people who seldom exercise do not recover as well from heart attacks. Although it is not clear if lack of exercise alone is a risk factor for developing heart disease, in combination with other risk factors, such as overweight, the risk is higher.

Stress. Excessive emotional stress over a prolonged period appears to increase the risk of heart disease. Stress can increase other existing risk factors, such as overeating, smoking, and high blood pressure.

Oral contraceptives. Birth control pills can worsen other risk factors. They raise blood cholesterol levels and increase blood pressure, so women who already have these problems should not take oral contraceptives. Smokers who take "the pill" run the risk of developing dangerous blood clots (thrombosis).

Alcohol. Heavy drinking can cause high blood pressure and lead to heart failure. Alcohol should be consumed only in moderate amounts—2 ounces of liquor a day or less.

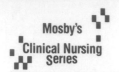
Coronary Artery Disease

The heart is the hardest working muscle in the body. Every day it beats an average of 100,000 times and pumps about 2000 gallons of blood throughout the body. To handle this enormous amount of work, the heart muscle requires a continuous supply of oxygen and other nutrients from the blood. To get enough nourishment, the heart muscle has its own circulation, the right and left coronary arteries.

The coronary arteries form a network of blood vessels on the outside of the heart. If these arteries become narrowed, the heart muscle is deprived of some of its blood supply, which eventually damages the heart muscle. This is referred to as a heart attack, or **myocardial infarction.**

What causes coronary artery disease?

Cholesterol and other material can collect on artery walls, causing the arteries to narrow. This condition, called **atherosclerosis,** prevents the passage of normal amounts of blood through the arteries. As a result, two events can occur: (1) these deposits build up over time until they clog the artery so that little or no blood can pass; or (2) blood cells cling to the rough deposits, forming a clot **(thrombus).** The thrombus may grow until it completely blocks the artery, or it can break away and travel to a smaller artery, where it lodges, completely closing off circulation.

How serious is coronary artery disease?

Coronary artery disease (CAD) is very serious. Although it begins so gradually you don't notice any change, eventually it can cause chest pain (angina) or heart attack.

Angina is a burning, squeezing, or crushing sensation in the chest lasting from a few seconds to 15 minutes. It is caused by a temporary lack of oxygen to the heart muscle. The symptoms of angina can also be very similar to those of a heart attack—the pain may radiate to the arm, jaw, shoulder, or neck. Physical exertion, emotional stress, exposure to extremes of hot or cold, or overeating can prompt an angina attack. The pain usually goes away when the aggravating activity is stopped.

Heart attacks occur when the coronary artery becomes completely blocked. When the blockage is caused by a blood clot, this is called a **coronary thrombosis.** Lack of oxygen to a portion of the heart muscle causes the tissue to die. If a large area is deprived of oxygen, the heart ceases to beat, and death

results. It's important to know the symptoms of a heart attack and act promptly. Call the emergency rescue service immediately if any of the following symptoms occurs:

Severe pressure, fullness, squeezing, or pain in the center of the chest that lasts 15 minutes or longer and is not relieved by rest or taking a nitroglycerin tablet, if prescribed

Pain spreading to the shoulders, neck, or arms

Dizziness, fainting, sweating, nausea, or shortness of breath that accompanies chest pain

How is it diagnosed?

Some people have no idea they have coronary artery disease until they have a heart attack; others have the warning symptoms of angina. Sometimes coronary artery disease is diagnosed from an abnormal electrocardiogram (ECG) during a routine physical examination.

Several tests are used to diagnose coronary artery disease. **Blood tests** are done to determine the blood cholesterol level. An **electrocardiogram (ECG)** provides some basic information on the heart's performance. An **exercise stress test** shows how the heart reacts to exertion. This consists of an ECG while exercising on a treadmill or exercise bicycle.

Nuclear studies, such as a **thallium scan,** show how well the blood supply is distributed to the heart muscle. This involves injecting a small amount of radioactive material into a vein and taking motion pictures with a specialized x-ray scanner.

Cardiac catheterization gives the most complete information on coronary artery disease. This procedure allows the doctor to make a series of x-ray films called a **coronary angiogram,** which shows the number and exact location of the blockages.

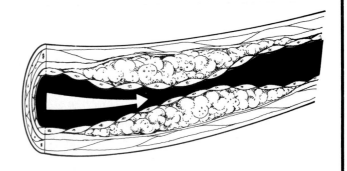

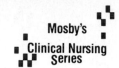
Treatment of coronary artery disease

The treatment of coronary artery disease depends on the severity of the blockages. However, all patients are advised to adopt a low-cholesterol, low-fat diet, exercise regularly, quit smoking, lose excess weight, and eliminate caffeine. Alcohol can be consumed in moderation, but no more than two drinks a day. A walking or jogging program can help lower the blood cholesterol level, reduce high blood pressure, and control weight. Many people with coronary artery disease have high blood pressure and should also be on a low-salt diet. Medication may be necessary to control high blood pressure or high blood cholesterol levels.

Nitroglycerin is prescribed to prevent or treat angina. This medication acts rapidly, usually within 5 minutes, to relax the blood vessels and increase the blood supply to the heart. Nitroglycerin is available in several forms. The tablets and spray are used when an angina attack starts or before exercise is begun to prevent an attack. People who are troubled with several episodes every day may need to wear nitroglycerin skin patches to prevent attacks.

If drug therapy fails to relieve angina or the blockages are severe, your doctor may decide on more aggressive treatment. **Percutaneous transluminal coronary angioplasty (PTCA),** also called **balloon angioplasty,** is a procedure to reopen the blocked arteries. A thin tube called a catheter is inserted into an artery in the arm or leg and then guided to the obstructed coronary artery. The balloon on the tip of the catheter is inflated to press the blockage against the artery wall.

Coronary bypass surgery is another procedure used to correct severe blockages. Veins from other parts of the body are grafted onto the diseased coronary artery above and below the blockage. This graft restores blood circulation to the damaged area.

No cure presently exists for coronary artery disease. Even if you have PTCA or bypass surgery, blockages can recur. To prevent this, you must make a commitment to a "healthy heart lifestyle." This means continuing to follow the diet your doctor recommends, keeping your blood cholesterol levels and blood pressure under control, giving up smoking, adhering to your exercise program, and returning for checkups as often as your doctor recommends.

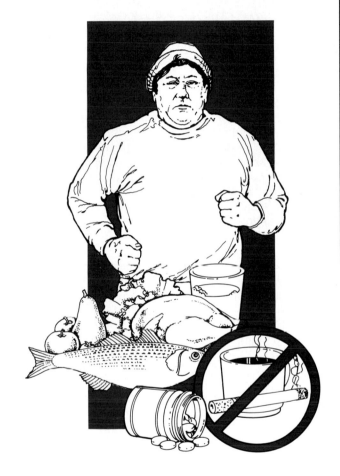

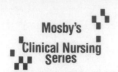
Recovering from a Heart Attack

Rehabilitation after a heart attack begins in the hospital, but it continues for 3 months after the patient goes home. For many people, rehabilitation means making some permanent changes toward leading a healthier life. These include not smoking; losing weight if you are overweight; eating a healthy low-cholesterol, low-fat diet; and avoiding stress. Your doctor will prescribe an exercise program to encourage healing. If you also have high blood pressure, a low-sodium diet may be recommended.

Many people do not require any medications after a heart attack. However, drugs may be prescribed for other conditions that may be related, such as angina, high blood pressure, high blood cholesterol level, or irregular heart beats (dysrhythmias). Since some studies report that aspirin reduces the chance of heart attacks, your doctor may recommend that you take aspirin. If medications are prescribed, take them exactly as ordered. Do not take any other medications, not even over-the-counter drugs, without first consulting your doctor.

A heart attack is a frightening event. Many people believe that because they survived this life-threatening experience, they have been given a second chance at life. As a result, they learn to slow down and do things they enjoy. You, too, may find yourself thinking about your life-style and making some important changes during the rehabilitation period.

Activity

Your first week at home should be quiet—no visitors, no work, and no telephone calls. During the first 2 or 3 weeks after leaving the hospital, socializing should be limited to a few brief visits with friends in your home. Usually after the third week, you can begin to go out for short visits.

About 6 to 8 weeks after a heart attack marks the next phase of your recovery—the gradual return to normal activity. You can usually begin driving for short distances, but avoid heavy traffic or other stressful situations. If your job is not physically demanding, your doctor may allow you to start back to work for 1 or 2 hours a day. By adding an hour or two each week, you will be working full time by the end of a month. However, you should limit yourself to no more than 8 hours a day for at least 6 months, and you should not take on any additional responsibilities.

If your job is physically demanding, it may be 3 to 4 months before you can resume work full time. It may be advisable to make a job change, particularly if your work involves heavy lifting, long hours, or considerable stress. Heavy lifting or pushing is not permitted. Avoid picking up anything that weighs more than 10 pounds.

A graduated walking program is an important part of recovery for most patients. Your doctor will prescribe a home exercise program, just as he or she prescribes any other treatment.

Sexual activity

Many heart attack patients and their spouses worry that sexual activity will bring on another heart attack. Actually, a heart attack during or after sexual intercourse occurs no more often than after any other normal activity. Sexual activity can be resumed once healing is under way. For most patients, this means refraining from sexual intercourse for at least 2 to 4 weeks after leaving the hospital. However, this depends on the severity of your heart attack, so ask your doctor.

A few heart attack patients experience chest pain (angina) during intercourse. Changing positions so that less tension is placed on the chest muscles may relieve this problem. Lying side-by-side with your partner or lying on the bottom with your partner on top may be more comfortable. Your doctor may recommend taking nitroglycerin beforehand.

Smoking

Nicotine causes the blood vessels to constrict, slows the healing process, and may cause chest pain. Smoking or chewing tobacco places an extra workload on the heart, forcing the heart to pump harder. It also interferes with the blood's ability to deliver oxygen to the body's tissues, especially the myocardium. If you were a smoker at the time of your heart attack, here's some good news: since you have not been allowed to smoke while you were in the hospital, you already have a headstart on giving it up for good. **Don't start again.**

Symptoms to report

Notify your doctor if you have any symptoms that could mean heart distress. These include chest pain that is not relieved by rest or taking a nitroglycerin tablet, rapid heartbeats, shortness of breath, extreme fatigue, dizziness, lightheadedness, or fainting.

PATIENT TEACHING GUIDE

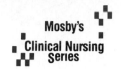

Mosby's
Clinical Nursing
Series

High Blood Pressure

Most people are surprised to learn they have **hypertension** (high blood pressure). "But I feel just fine!" they say, and often think that it can't be very serious as long as they don't have symptoms. Unfortunately, that's why high blood pressure is so dangerous—you can have it for years without knowing it, but all the time it is making your heart work hard and raising your chances of heart attack and stroke. For this reason, high blood pressure has earned the title of "The Silent Killer."

What is blood pressure?

Every time your heart beats, it pumps out about 5 ounces of blood, less than a cup. But because the blood must travel through about 12,400 miles of blood vessels, the heart pumps with a great deal of force. This produces a high-pressure wave of blood through your arteries. Normally, the arteries are elastic and expand with each heartbeat. When the heart relaxes between beats, the arteries also relax, and the pressure is lower.

What do the numbers mean?

Blood pressure readings are always given as two numbers, for example, 120 over 82 (written as 120/82). The first number (the **systolic blood pressure**) is always higher and measures the pressure during the heartbeat. The lower second number **(diastolic blood pressure)** is the pressure in the arteries while the heart is relaxed.

These two numbers tell much about how hard your heart is working and the condition of your blood vessels. The harder it is for blood to flow through your arteries, the higher both the systolic and the diastolic readings will be.

How is high blood pressure defined?

Your blood pressure changes constantly to adjust your circulation to your activities. It increases during exercise and decreases during sleep. However, during rest a normal reading is a systolic blood pressure less than 140 and a diastolic pressure less than 90.

A person is diagnosed as having high blood pressure if the blood pressure stays at 140/90 or more. The doctor usually will not make this diagnosis until you have been checked more than once and your blood pressure is high each time.

People over age 65 often have systolic pressures between 140 and 155, even when the diastolic pressure is normal. Systolic high blood pressure is caused by **arteriosclerosis,** or hardening of the arteries.

How does high blood pressure cause damage?

As part of the normal aging process, the arteries harden and become less elastic. But high blood pressure speeds this process up, so that a person age 40 may have arteries closer to those of a 65-year-old person. The arteries no longer "cooperate" by expanding when blood pumps through them. This raises the pressure inside the arteries. Your heart is forced to work harder and harder to pump that 5 ounces of blood. Over a long period, the heart enlarges and the blood vessels to the brain and kidneys become damaged. This combination of heart enlargement and damaged blood vessels greatly increases the risk of heart attack, stroke, and kidney failure.

What causes high blood pressure?

About 90% of people with high blood pressure have **essential hypertension**, meaning that the cause is unknown. It can strike anyone, regardless of age, sex, race, economic status, or background. However, your chances of developing high blood pressure increase if you have a family history of hypertension or you are black, a man over age 35, a woman past menopause, are overweight, or are sensitive to salt.

For unknown reasons, blacks develop high blood pressure much more often than whites, and the disease tends to be more severe. It is estimated that one in every three blacks over age 18 years has high blood pressure. Other factors that seem to be related to high blood pressure are heavy alcohol consumption and lack of physical activity.

Women also have some special risks. Oral contraceptives can cause high blood pressure in susceptible women. If you are a woman with a strong family history of high blood pressure, have your doctor take your blood pressure before prescribing birth control pills, and then have it checked every 6 months as long as you take them. High blood pressure can develop suddenly during the last 3 months of pregnancy, endangering both mother and child if not treated. Prenatal care is important so that any blood pressure problems can be detected. After menopause, the chance of developing high blood pressure increases, even in women who have had normal blood pressure all their lives.

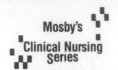
Controlling your blood pressure

At present there is no cure for high blood pressure, but it can be controlled to reduce the chances of developing problems. This takes a team effort, and you are the most important member of the team. Mild or moderate high blood pressure can often be controlled successfully by a low-salt diet, exercise, and weight loss.

Sodium (salt) causes your body to retain fluids, which can put extra strain on the heart and make the blood vessels narrow. For this reason, low-sodium diets are recommended to reduce the amount of retained water, which then helps to lower the blood pressure. Foods that are high in potassium and calcium also help lower blood pressure.

A moderate amount of regular exercise has several benefits. It improves your overall physical conditioning, helps with weight loss by burning extra colories, reduces blood cholesterol, and may have a more direct effect on lowering your blood pressure.

Maintaining yourself at the right weight for your height and bone structure is important. Extra fat makes your heart work harder. A low-fat, low-calorie diet has the further advantage of reducing your blood cholesterol levels and delaying the beginning of arterioscleroisi. People with high blood pressure can consume moderate amounts of alcohol (about two drinks per day), but a heavy intake of alcohol raises blood pressure. If you are on a weight reduction diet, keep in mind that alcohol is high in calories.

Although high blood pressure is not caused by "bad nerves," prolonged stress does increase blood pressure. Learning to relax and taking time out to do things you enjoy should be part of your blood pressure control program.

Medication

Medication is necessary if you have severe high blood pressure or high blood pressure that is not controlled by diet, exercise, and weight reduction. Diuretics (water pills) are often prescribed to eliminate the excess sodium form your body. If diuretic therapy is not effective in bringing your blood pressure down, your doctor will add other medication to the treatment program.

Several different types of antihypertensive drugs are available: nerve blockers, beta blockers, blood vessel dilators, hormone inhibitors, and calcium channel blockers. Each type of drug works differently, but basically they control blood pressure by relaxing and opening up narrowed blood vessels. Since everyone is different, your doctor may have to try more than one drug to find the most effective medication with the fewest side effects. When your doctor prescribes an antihypertensive drug, ask about the type and possible side effects.

Be sure to keep appointments with your doctor. Several visits may be necessary to determine exactly the right drug and dosage. Once your blood pressure is under control, you will need to see your doctor only about three or four times a year.

Remember: diuretics and antihypertensive medications lower your blood pressure only while you are taking them. You cannot stop taking the drug, even after your blood pressure is lowered.

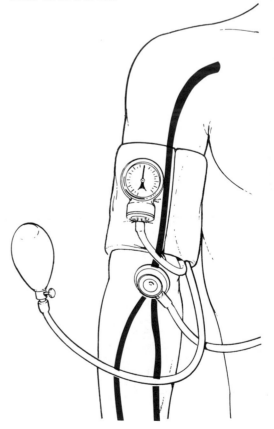

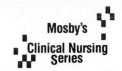
Heart Failure

The term **heart failure** describes a condition in which the heart muscle is unable to pump the blood properly throughout the circulation. Heart failure can occur as the result of almost any type of heart disease in which the heart muscle has been weakened or damaged, such as after a heart attack. The signs and symptoms of heart failure also can occur if damage has occurred to any of the heart valves or if the heart muscle has been weakened or damaged by an infection. Whatever the cause, the problem is the same: the heart is unable to pump the blood properly, and thus blood begins to back up. To compensate for this problem, the heart must work harder and harder and beat faster. If nothing is done to help the heart, the muscle becomes progressively weaker. However, with careful control of diet and the proper medications, the heart can be helped to pump more efficiently and not work as hard.

Types of heart failure

The two types of heart failure are left-sided and right-sided heart failure. When the *left ventricle* is not pumping properly, blood and fluid begin to back up into the lungs. This causes symptoms of shortness of breath, a dry hacking cough, an inability to lie flat so that several pillows are needed to sleep at night, night awakenings with spells of breathlessness, and a feeling of needing fresh air. When the *right ventricle* is not pumping properly, blood and fluid begin to back up into the general circulation. This causes a weight gain, swelling of the feet and ankles, and in more severe cases swelling of the abdomen. Left-sided heart failure and right-sided heart failure can occur alone or at the same time. When both ventricles are affected, the term **congestive heart failure** is used.

These symptoms occur because the heart muscle is not working as well and thus the blood entering the heart is not being pumped out in the usual amount. As a result, less blood goes to the kidneys. The kidneys automatically respond to this decrease in blood by retaining the salt and water that normally would be removed in the urine. Unfortunately, this extra salt and water only add to the amount of blood the heart must pump, making it necessary for the heart to work even harder. Over time, the heart can become enlarged.

Diagnosing heart failure

The diagnosis of heart failure is made primarily from the patient's symptoms. However, several tests can help the doctor confirm the presence of extra fluid in the body and determine how well the heart muscle is working.

The easiest test to determine if fluid is present in the lung is the **chest x-ray,** or **roentgenogram.** It can also tell the doctor if the heart is becoming enlarged. The **electrocardiogram (ECG)** is done to determine if the heartbeat is regular or has developed irregular beats, which you might feel as palpitations. Other special tests, called **nuclear studies,** are like x-rays. These tests, which use a small amount of radioactive material that is injected into the vein, show how well the heart muscle is working. They are painless and can be done on an outpatient basis.

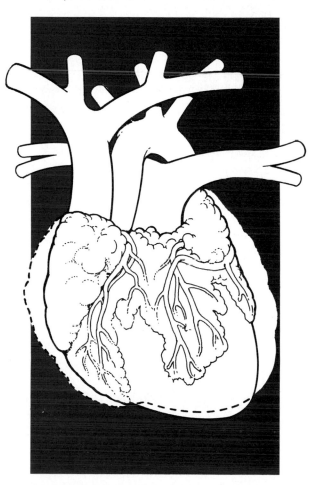

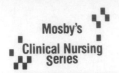
Treating Heart Failure

The goal of treatment for heart failure is to help the heart muscle pump stronger and work less. This is done primarily by removing any excess fluid. The simplest way to achieve this is to decrease the intake of salt. Salt, or sodium, is a mineral normally found in the body. It is also found in many foods, including table salt. Although important in the diet, too much sodium causes your body to retain fluid. This added fluid increases the amount of blood your heart must pump. Therefore the best way to decrease the amount of sodium in the body is to avoid salt in the diet. Your doctor can tell you how much salt you can have in your diet, but in general you should avoid cooking with salt, or only lightly salt food, and should not add salt to your food. You should also learn to read labels carefully to avoid foods that contain sodium. A nurse can give you a chart of prepared food items with their sodium content.

Medications are the second way to help your heart pump stronger. First, your doctor may order diuretics. These are pills that make your kidneys release the excess fluid in your body. You will notice that you urinate more frequently when you first start taking the pills, but once the excess fluid is removed, urine output returns to normal. Potassium pills or syrups are usually given with diuretics because potassium is also flushed out with the fluid, and your body needs this mineral. Bananas and tomatoes also are good sources of potassium.

Second, your doctor may order certain pills that make your heart muscle stronger. One pill frequently prescribed is **digitalis (digoxin),** but others are available, and the nurse can review these in detail. Your doctor may also prescribe pills to make your heartbeat regular. Because heart failure is complex, you may find that you are taking several different pills. So it is important that you take them exactly as your doctor has ordered and that you understand *what pills you are supposed to take, how many or the correct dosage, and when to take them.* For some patients, it is easier to make a calender to keep track of medications. Your nurse can help you do this.

Another way to help your heart is to rest. Set aside at least one rest period every day. When you sit, prop your feet up to help the circulation to your feet and to keep the swelling down. Avoid working long days, and more importantly, avoid becoming overtired. Space periods of heavy activity with rest, even if this means just sitting down for a few minutes.

You should also avoid extreme temperatures. Try to stay in a comfortable environment. In hot or smoggy weather, rest during the hottest part of the day, and if possible try to stay where there is a fan or air conditioner. In cold weather, dress warmly and wrap a scarf over your nose and mouth to warm the air you breathe.

Points to remember

1. Contact your doctor or nurse if you develop any of the following symptoms:
   Unusual shortness of breath
   Overtired after little exertion, such as walking
   Shortness of breath after awakening suddenly
   Shortness of breath during or following sexual intercourse
   Persistent dry cough
   Sudden weight gain of 2 pounds or more in 1 day; swelling of feet and ankles
   Very weak or dizzy, nauseated, loss of appetite, or palpitations
2. Weigh yourself every day, nude or with the same clothing, preferably when you first wake up, but after you urinated. A weight gain of more than 2 pounds in 24 hours is probably fluid retention, not a calorie weight gain.
3. Do not smoke or use tobacco. Nicotine use robs your heart of vital oxygen that is carried in the blood. Nicotine also can contribute to development of an irregular heart rate.

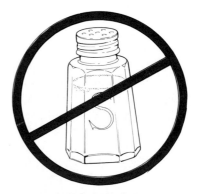

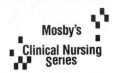
Mitral Valve Prolapse

Mitral valve prolapse (MVP) is a condition that affects both men and women, but more often occurs in women. It is believed that 1 in 20 persons has MVP. The cause is unknown, and it is not usually serious. Most people do not have any symptoms and are surprised when their doctor diagnoses this condition.

How your heart and valves work

Your heart is a pump with four chambers. The top two chambers **(atria)** are the filling chambers, and the bottom two **(ventricles)** are the pumping chambers. To control the flow of blood through the heart, you also have four valves that open and close. The valves work to keep the flow of blood going in one direction. Normally, when blood returns to the heart, it enters the right atrium and goes through the tricuspid valve into the right ventricle, then through the pulmonic valve into the lungs. Here oxygen is put back into the blood and carbon dioxide is removed. The blood returns to the heart, this time entering the left atrium. When the left atrium fills, the mitral valve opens and blood flows into the left ventricle. From here, it is pumped through the aortic valve and back into the circulation.

The **mitral valve** has two flaps, or leaflets, that open and close. These leaflets are attached to the wall of the heart by thin cords of muscle. This arrangement makes the mitral valve look somewhat like a parachute. When the left atrium is full, the leaflets are forced open to let blood flow into the left ventricle. Once the left ventricle is full, the leaflets are forced closed so that blood does not leak back into the atrium. The cords keep the leaflets from "ballooning" up into the atrium.

What is MVP?

In MVP, one (or sometimes both) leaflet(s) enlarges and some of its cords are too long. Every time the heart beats, part of the leaflet balloons up into the atrium. In some cases a small amount of blood leaks back into the left atrium, which can cause what is called a *murmur*. MVP may also cause a clicking sound. Your doctor hears this sound with a stethoscope. Some people have only a click, and some have both a click and a murmur.

To confirm the diagnosis of MVP, your doctor may order an **echocardiogram,** which is a simple, painless test that uses high-frequency sound waves. These waves produce a picture of your heart valves.

How is it treated?

Most people with MVP have no symptoms and do not need treatment. If you have a definite murmur from a leaky valve, you may need to take antibiotics any time you have surgery or dental treatment. This precaution prevents infection, which could spread to the mitral valve. If your doctor says you need preventive antibiotics, be sure to inform your dentist and any other doctor of this before you have surgery or dental work.

A few people have chest pain (angina) or irregular heartbeats with their MVP. Medication is prescribed to control these symptoms.

Most people with MVP lead active lives without any restrictions. However, ask your doctor about the safest level of activity for you.

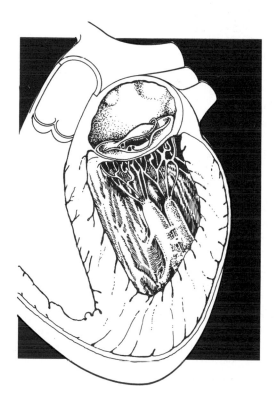

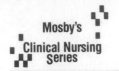
Endocarditis

What is endocarditis?

Endocarditis is an infection of the inner wall of the heart. It starts out as a usually harmless infection called **bacteremia,** which is caused by various bacteria. These bacteria enter your body like any other infection, through cuts, food you eat, and especially dental work and poor oral hygiene. Your body usually controls these infections, but bacteremia that grows out of control can turn into endocarditis. This happens more easily if you already have heart disease.

In endocarditis, bacterial growth gathers around your heart valves, interfering with blood flow. The growth can break off and form blood clots, which can travel to other parts of your body and can block blood flow and cause serious problems. Endocarditis can permanently damage the tissue and valves in your heart.

How is endocarditis treated?

Since endocarditis can be so serious, you will be kept in the hospital until the infection is gone, often as long as a month or more. You will be given some medicine to fight the infection, mainly antibiotics, which are introduced right into your blood system through a vein. Blood tests will be taken to identify the bacteria, so the best antibiotic can be chosen. You will probably get aspirin to relieve flu-like aches and fever, and you may get other medicine to dissolve clots. More blood tests will be taken from time to time to make sure the medicine is working.

You should rest, so your heart can rest. You should eat well to help your body heal. This is especially important because you may not have much of an appetite.

After you recover. . .

Once you've have endocarditis, you will always be at risk for getting it again. You should make some minor changes of habit to help make sure you don't get it again.

The best way to prevent endocarditis from coming back is to control the bacteria entering your body, especially during medical and dental procedures, when you have a cut, and anytime your body is directly exposed to the outside world. *Whenever you visit your doctor or dentist, make sure you tell them you have had en-*

docarditis. If they will be doing anything that puts them in direct contact with your blood or might break your skin, they should give you antibiotics beforehand, and you should remind them. Take these simple precautions:

1. See your doctor regularly for follow-up care of your heart.
2. Remind your physician to give you antibiotics if you will have blood tests, surgery, and any internal examinations whatsoever.
3. See your doctor immediately if you think you have any kind of infection, especially infections of the sinuses, throat, lungs, bladder, kidney, vagina, or skin.
4. Visit your dentist every 6 months for preventive care.
5. Make sure your dentist knows you have had endocarditis and make sure you take antibiotics whenever you have a tooth pulled, whenever the dentist works on your gums, and when you have your teeth cleaned.
6. Practice good oral hygiene and brush your teeth after meals.
7. Never use unwaxed dental floss, since this can more easily cut your blood-rich gums.
8. Always see your dentist immediately if you have a toothache or think you might be getting an abscess.

Always, always take your complete prescription of antibiotics, even after you feel better.

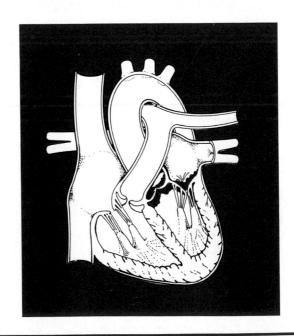

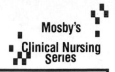
Cardiac Catheterization

You may have had other tests already and wonder why cardiac catheterization is necessary. Athough other tests can reveal a problem, this procedure allows your doctor to pinpoint it.

How safe is catheterization?

Cardiac catheterization is a very safe procedure. Complications are so rare that it may be done on an outpatient basis. As with any medical procedure, though, there are risks. Your doctor will discuss these with you.

How it's done

Cardiac catheterization is performed by a specially trained team of technicians, nurses, and doctors. A long, thin, flexible tube, a catheter, is inserted into a blood vessel in the arm or leg. A special type of x-ray screen, called a **fluoroscope,** shows the blood vessels and the heart so the doctor can guide the catheter into the correct position.

Heart pressures are measured inside the heart chambers. Samples of blood are taken through the catheter. Other tests depend on your particular problems.

X-ray studies are usually made during cardiac catheterization. Dye is injected through the catheter into different areas of the heart. One type, the **coronary angiogram,** shows blood flow through the coronary arteries to locate blockages. A **ventriculogram** shows the size and pumping action of the heart muscle, as well as the opening and closing of the heart valves.

The electrical conduction system can also be tested to pinpoint the cause of irregular heartbeats and test how well the drugs are working to correct them.

What to expect

If done in a hospital, you will usually be admitted a day before the procedure. If you are allergic to shellfish or have ever had a reaction to x-ray dye, be sure to tell your doctor. The area where the catheter is inserted, usually the arm or the groin area, is shaved. You are not allowed to have anything to eat or drink 6 to 12 hours before the procedure.

Most people are a little nervous to learn that they will be awake during the procedure to follow the doctor's instructions. However, you should experience little discomfort. You are given a sedative before the procedure to help you relax. You will be monitored throughout the procedure.

Some procedure rooms may use tables that move from side to side while the x-rays are taken. In other rooms the table remains in one position while the camera moves around you. In either case, you are securely strapped to the table.

The area where the catheter is inserted is shaved and disinfected, and your arm or leg is strapped down. Sterile towels are placed over you to prevent infection. You usually cannot see what is occurring. After a local numbing medicine is injected, a small incision is made for the insertion of the catheter.

As the catheter is inserted, you will feel a slight pressure. At times during the procedure, the doctor may ask you to hold your breath, cough, and breathe deeply. You may also be asked to breathe oxygen.

When the x-ray dye is injected, you will experience a flushing sensation and nausea, but this will disappear quickly.

Medications may also be given during cardiac catheterization. Nitroglycerin is sometimes used to dilate the coronary arteries. If your heart's electrical conduction system is tested, you may be given drugs to speed up or slow down your heat.

Cardiac catheterization takes between 1 to 4 hours, depending on how many tests are performed. After the catheter is removed, the incision is closed with a few stitches.

After the procedure

Following cardiac catheterization, you will be on complete bed rest for 6 to 8 hours. Nurses will check your pulse, blood pressure, and incision from time to time. You will drink plenty of liquids to help flush the dye out of your system. You may eat a regular diet unless your doctor instructs otherwise.

Most people can resume a normal routine the following day. However, this depends on your physical condition. Your doctor will discuss with you how much physical activity is safe.

The incision will be sore for several days. Call your doctor if it bleeds or shows signs of infection—swelling, pain, fever, or drainage.

The stitches are removed about a week later. You will have a small lump in the area, but this will gradually disappear. The incision scar should be almost invisible in a few months.

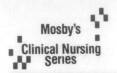

Angioplasty

Fatty deposits (plaques) that have accumulated on the inside of the coronary arteries can narrow these passages considerably, causing blood flow to the heart to be dangerously reduced. Providing adequate circulation to the heart muscle is important to prevent a heart attack. Percutaneous transluminal coronary angioplasty (PTCA) and bypass surgery are two procedures that can improve the blood supply. They are performed on people who have chest pain (angina) and sometimes on those who have had a heart attack.

Who is a candidate for PTCA?

Angioplasty is not for everyone with coronary artery disease. Whether you are a good candidate for this procedure depends on the severity of your coronary artery disease and the overall functioning of your heart. Your doctor will perform a cardiac catheterization to obtain a coronary angiogram. These x-ray studies show the number and exact location of blockages. Only after a complete evaluation is done can he or she decide whether you should have angioplasty or bypass surgery.

What is PTCA?

Ballon angioplasty, also known as percutaneous transluminal coronary angioplasty PTCA, is done during cardiac catheterization. A thin, plastic tube, called a catheter, is inserted into a blood vessel in either the right groin or the right arm. Once it is positioned into the coronary artery near the narrowed portion, a smaller catheter with a deflated balloon at its tip is threaded through the cardiac catheter. When the balloon catheter reaches the narrowed portion, the balloon is inflated to flatten the fatty deposit against the artery wall. The balloon may be inflated and deflated several times.

The procedure is monitored on an x-ray screen that magnifies the images so the doctor can observe when the artery is open sufficiently. Once the artery is opened and blood is flowing more freely through the vessel, the balloon catheter is removed.

You can expect the recovery period to be similar to that following cardiac catheterization. However, you may be kept in the hospital for 1 or 2 days after PTCA to ensure no complications develop.

How safe is PTCA?

PTCA is a very safe procedure with few complications. Occasionally, emergency bypass surgery is necessary. For this reason, PTCA is performed with a heart surgery team standing by. However, this occurs in less than 5% of people who have PTCA.

How effective is PTCA?

The dilated portion of the artery narrows again in about 30% of people who have PTCA. When this happens, the patient is reevaluated to determine whether PTCA should be repeated or bypass surgery performed.

Home instruction

You will be sent home with certain medications to prevent the formation of blood clots, which helps keep the newly opened arteries open. It is important that you take these drugs as prescribed.

Your doctor will give you specific instructions on when you can return to work, resume driving, and engage in sexual activity. In general, you should avoid any heavy lifting or demanding work for at least the first week. You may feel soreness over the groin area. If you begin to experience a return of chest pain, it is important that you notify your doctor.

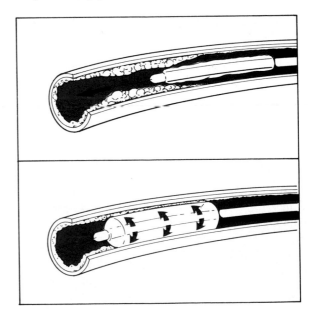

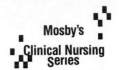

Coronary Artery Bypass Surgery

In coronary artery disease, the blood vessels that nourish the heart muscle become narrowed or completely blocked, causing the amount of blood flow through them to decrease. When blood flow becomes severely reduced, there is risk of heart attack. The purpose of coronary artery bypass surgery is to improve the blood supply to an area of the heart that has been deprived of adequate circulation.

How bypass surgery is done

Coronary bypass surgery is actually two surgeries performed at the same time. One incision is made in the leg to remove a vein. This vein is used as a graft, or conduit, to create a new coronary artery. Another incision is made in the chest to allow the surgeon to reach the heart.

One end of the vein graft is sewn in the side of the aorta, the large artery of the heart. The other end of the graft is sewn below the area of the blocked coronary artery. This vein actually detours the blood around the obstruction to restore good blood flow to the area.

Sometimes more than one coronary artery is blocked, and it is necessary to insert more than one graft. The terms **double bypass, triple bypass,** and **quadruple bypass** indicate how many grafts are required.

The graft is usually taken from the saphenous vein in the leg or an internal mammary vein. These two veins are used because they are long enough. Since the legs and arms have numerous other blood vessels, these veins are not missed and circulation is still good after surgery. The length and number of incisions depend on how many bypasses are needed.

Coronary artery bypass surgery generally takes from 3 to 6 hours, again depending on how many bypasses are needed.

What to expect

Most patients are admitted to the hospital 1 or 3 days before coronary artery bypass surgery. Your body is shaved to help reduce the risk of infection. After midnight on the day before surgery, you receive nothing by mouth. About an hour before surgery, you are given medication to make you sleepy and relaxed. Once you are in the operating room, you receive an anesthetic that puts you to sleep.

After you are asleep, a breathing tube is put into your mouth and a drainage tube in your bladder.

After the surgery, you will spend 1 to 2 days in the intensive care unit so you can be monitored closely. Don't be alarmed by the tubes and wires—everyone is connected to all types of equipment after heart surgery. Equipment in this case includes an electrocardiogram (ECG) to monitor your heart, chest tubes to drain fluid from around your heart, a breathing tube to help you breathe, a urinary catheter to drain urine from your bladder, and an intravenous (IV) tube in your arm. Each is removed as you become more awake.

Because of the breathing tube, you won't be able to talk. A nurse will show you other ways of communicating. This tube can usually be removed within 24 hours, as soon as the effects of anesthesia have passed and you can breathe on your own.

For the first few days, most patients experience moderate pain and soreness from the surgical incisions. Inform the nurse of this, and you will receive medication to make you more comfortable.

Once the breathing tube is out, you will start deep breathing and coughing exercises and using a breathing instrument. Doing these exercises helps clear your lungs and prevents any infection such as pneumonia. Because you are sore, this may be uncomfortable at first, but this is a very important part of your quick recovery. Coughing does not disturb the stitches or bypass graft.

You will probably start getting out of bed the day after surgery. This may be very tiring at first, but your strength will improve and you'll find that each day you can walk farther with less fatigue.

Standing or walking may produce a burning sensation in the leg where the graft was taken. Your ankle may also swell. Elastic support stockings helps decrease the swelling. Foot and ankle exercises and walking also helps the circulation in your legs and hastens the healing process. These symptoms gradually disappear.

A slight fever is not unusual after bypass surgery. You will be given aspirin or an aspirin substitute for 3 or 4 days until your temperature returns to normal.

Today most surgeons use stitches that dissolve by themselves. If you have regular stitches or staples, they are removed from your chest about a week after surgery, and a few days later the ones from the leg can be removed.

The usual hospital stay after bypass surgery is 1 to 2 weeks.

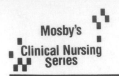
Going home after coronary artery bypass surgery

Almost everyone feels weak when they first return home, regardless of the surgery performed. By gradually increasing your activity every day, your strength will soon return. Your doctor will probably prescribe an exercise program of walking. Try to maintain a good balance between activity and rest. Space your activities with rest periods to avoid fatigue. Avoid lifting objects heavier than 25 to 30 pounds until your incisions have completely healed. When you feel stronger, you can resume your normal activities, such as driving a car, visiting friends, and climbing stairs. You can also resume sexual activity. Your doctor will advise you when it is safe to resume these activities. Most people receive no extreme diet restrictions, but in general you should limit the sodium in your diet. Alcohol can affect the heart; therefore you should limit alcohol consumption to 1 or 2 drinks per day.

By the time you leave the hospital, your incisions are healing well. Wash the areas daily with mild soap and water. Examine the incisions to ensure no signs of infection are present: increased redness, swelling, or drainage. The incisions heal completely in about 6 weeks.

Most people who have jobs that are not physically demanding can return to work 4 to 6 weeks after bypass surgery. If your job requires considerable physical activity or heavy work, you may need to wait longer.

You should expect to feel some emotional letdown while you are recovering at home, and it may be a trying period for both you and your family. People often feel frustrated when their progress seems too slow. They become bored, irritable, and depressed. The best way to combat this is to discuss your feelings with your family, friends, or doctor. As your strength returns and you are able to do more, these feelings will gradually disappear.

Remember to report any signs that your incisions are infected: increased redness, swelling, or drainage. Call your doctor if any of the following symptoms occur: fever, chills, increased fatigue, shortness of breath, swelling of the legs or feet, sudden or excessive weight gain, a change in your heart rate or rhythm, or any other symptoms that worry you.

Staying healthy

To keep your new veins from developing blockages, you may need to make some permanent changes in your life-style to keep your blood cholesterol levels, blood pressure, and weight under control through diet and exercise. Medication may also be necessary to lower your blood pressure or cholesterol levels.

You must not smoke or use tobacco products. Tobacco causes the blood vessels to narrow and the heart to work harder. If you smoked before your bypass surgery, don't start again. You have already made it through the toughest part of quitting while you were in the hospital and weren't allowed to smoke.

Do not take any medications unless they are prescribed by your doctor. This includes any medications you took before your bypass surgery, unless your doctor tells you to continue taking them. Don't take any nonprescription (over-the-counter) drugs, even aspirin, until you check with your doctor first.

If you have any questions, be sure to ask. Today the risks associated with coronary artery bypass surgery are very small, and by taking proper care of yourself, you should return to a healthy, normal life-style very soon.

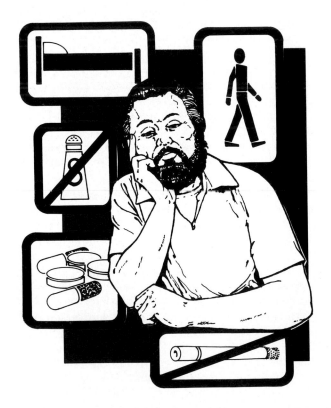

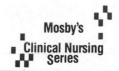

Pacemakers

An artificial pacemaker is a battery-operated device that is programmed to keep the heart beating at a certain rate. It is inserted by placing a special wire (catheter) into the right side of the heart and attaching the wire to a small, metal-covered battery that is placed just under the skin in the upper chest or sometimes in the abdomen. Insertion causes little discomfort and is done with the patient awake. The stitches are removed about a week later.

Types of pacemakers. Today many different types of pacemakers are available, but the two major types are **demand** and **fixed rate. Demand pacemakers** are set to generate a beat only when they sense that the natural heartbeat is too slow. When the heart is beating normally, the demand pacemaker is "on standby." Most often the demand pacemaker is set for 60 or 70 beats per minute; if your natural heartbeat slows below this number the demand pacemaker is activated. **Fixed-rate pacemakers** are set to beat at a certain rate. They are working all the time and will not turn off.

Pacemaker batteries have to be changed. How often depends on the type of battery, the usual time being every 5 years. Changing the battery is a simple procedure that usually does not require an overnight hospital stay. You or your doctor may begin to detect certain warning signs that the battery needs to be checked. Therefore, you must check your heart rate twice a day—morning and evening, after you have rested for a few minutes. Also check your pulse if you have shortness of breath, dizziness or fainting, chest pain, weakness, sweating, palpitations, or prolonged hiccoughing. Keep a diary of your heart rate and take it along at each visit to your doctor.

Your pacemaker and your pulse (check one)

___ Your doctor has inserted a demand pacemaker. It will begin to work automatically whenever your pulse falls below ___ beats per minute. Although your pulse may increase with exercise, it should not be above ___ beats per minute while you are resting.

___ Your doctor has installed a fixed-rate pacemaker. It will keep your pulse rate at ___ beats per minute all the time. The beats should be regular. If your pulse is five beats faster or slower than the fixed rate, call your doctor.

General care

For the first month after insertion, watch the incision site for signs of infection (pain, tenderness, swelling, redness, or drainage). Daily showers are permitted. Gently wash the area using soap and water. You may feel sore and stiff for a week or so. Gently exercising your arm, neck, and shoulders should help relax the muscles. Your doctor will tell you when you can return to work, drive a car, and exercise.

Having a pacemaker does not limit your physical activities. Most people say they can actually do more without becoming tired. Walking, playing golf, and swimming are good activities, but check with your doctor about the amount of exercise best for you. The only restrictions are to avoid contact sports and any isometric activities such as lifting weights. Having a pacemaker has no effect on sexual activity.

Pacemaker precautions

1. Avoid tight-fitting clothing over the pacemaker area, which can cause irritation.
2. When you visit another doctor or dentist, be sure to tell them you have a pacemaker, since some electrical medical equipment may interfere with your pacemaker, or you may need antibiotics to prevent infection.
3. Because of possible electrical interference with pacemakers, you must take certain precautions when handling electrical equipment. Read instructions carefully for warning labels. Do not place any electrical device directly over your pacemaker. You can safely use ordinary electrical household appliances as long as they are grounded and in good working order. Most newer microwave ovens now have special shielding. Avoid use of electrical tools (such as large shop tools) or gasoline engines (lawn mowers, snowmobiles) unless they are properly grounded. Do not lean over running engines and motors.
4. You can safely operate a car, gas lawn mower, or boat as long as you don't position your pacemaker directly over the engines.
5. Avoid television-transmitting and radar stations.
6. Carry a pacemaker identification card. This lists your doctor's name, hospital, type of pacemaker, and date of implantation. The pacemaker manufacturer should send you a card. You can also wear Medic-Alert jewelry.
7. When traveling by plane, inform airport personnel that you are wearing a pacemaker before you go through metal detectors.

Notify your doctor immediately if any of the following symptoms occur:

Pulse rate faster or slower than normal, chest pain, shortness of breath, dizziness or fainting, swelling of the legs and ankles, prolonged hiccoughing (more than 2 hours), elevated temperature, or drainage from the incision.

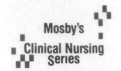
Counting Your Pulse

Your pulse is the beat of your heart. You can feel it in several parts of your body, including the inside of your wrist or the carotid artery, which is high in your neck.

Counting your pulse is the best way you can monitor your own heart rate. By counting your pulse, you know how many times your heart beats in 1 minute and how regular the beats are.

You may need to count your pulse for several reasons: (1) you may have an irregular heartbeat; (2) you may be taking a special drug to control irregular heartbeats, and you need to be sure it is working; (3) you may have a pacemaker; or (4) you may need to check your heart rate as part of an exercise program.

How to take your pulse

To count accurately, you need a clock or a watch with a second hand. You can use the pulse on your wrist or your neck, whichever is easiest for you.

To find the pulse on your wrist, press the fingertips of your index and middle fingers on the inside of your wrist (the thumb side). Do not use your thumb. If you have trouble finding this pulse, move your fingertips around until you locate it.

To find the pulse in your neck, press your fingertips in the area just under the jawbone, alongside your Adam's apple.

If you have trouble finding either pulse, try varying the amount of pressure. You can miss the pulse by pressing too lightly, but pressing too hard can obscure the pulse. Once you've found your pulse, it will be easy the next time.

Taking your pulse while resting

Your resting pulse can be taken almost any time, except after exercising, eating a large meal, or taking prescribed drugs that control heart rate.

Sit quietly for 2 minutes and relax. Find your pulse, look at the second hand on your watch or clock, and begin counting.

If you have an irregular heartbeat, you must count for exactly 60 seconds. For example, if you counted 77 pulse beats in 1 minute, this is your heart rate. Otherwise, you can count for 30 seconds and multiply by 2. For example, 41 pulses × 2 = 82.

Take your resting pulse as often as your doctor instructs.

Taking your pulse after exercising

Your pulse rate during exercise can tell you whether you are getting the most benefits from your exercise program. Your doctor will give you a "target heart rate." This is how fast your heart should beat after exercising. If your pulse rate is lower than your target heart rate, you need to exercise harder next time. If your pulse rate is higher than your target rate, you must take it easier next time.

As soon as you stop exercising, locate your pulse and look at the second hand on your watch or clock. Count the beats for 6 seconds and add a zero. For example, if you counted 12, your heart rate is 120.

You should not count your exercising rate for a full minute. Because your heart slows down quickly when you stop exercising, counting for a full minute gives a lower rate.

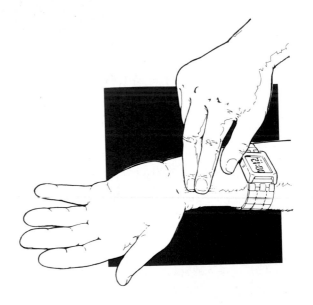

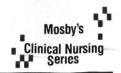

Diet Guidelines For A Healthy Heart

These guidelines offer a brief summary of three diets for a healthy heart. If your doctor has prescribed one of these diets for you, you need more complete information. The American Heart Association has free pamphlets available that explain the low-cholesterol and low-sodium diets in detail.

Read the labels

Labels on packaged foods make it easier to select healthier products, but you must understand how to interpret them. If the product makes any nutritional claim, the label lists two categories of information. **"Nutritional Information per Serving"** lists the amount of calories, protein, carbohydrates, fat, and sodium (salt) in one serving. It also tells you how much is considered *one* serving, which can be confusing. For example, one normal serving of milk is 1 cup, or 8 ounces. If you pour milk into a tall drinking glass, however, you may have 10 to 16 ounces.

The second category is **"Percentage of U.S. Recommended Daily Allowances (U.S. RDA)"** for protein, vitamins, and minerals in each serving. Remember that these numbers are percentages, so if the label on a milk carton says "Protein 20," this means that 1 cup provides 20% of the protein you need each day.

Packaged foods that don't claim to provide nutrition don't have these labels, but they do list the ingredients. The largest quantity is listed first and the smallest amount last. For example, a jar of sweet pickles lists the ingredients as "Cucumbers, water, corn syrup, vinegar, peppers, salt, natural and artificial flavors, preservatives, and articifial coloring." This tells you cucumbers are the main ingredient, water the next highest ingredient, and so forth.

Of course, fresh meats, fish and seafood, fruits, and vegetables do not carry labels. You need to learn which ones are the best for your diet and which ones to avoid.

Low-cholesterol diet

The average American consumes a large amount of cholesterol every day: men about 500 milligrams (mg) and women about 320 mg. A low-cholesterol diet limits cholesterol intake to less than 300 mg a day. To manage this, only 30% (or less) of the total calories you eat every day should come from fat. In addition, most of this fat should come from **polyunsaturated fat**, the "good" fat that helps lower blood cholesterol.

How can you tell the difference between "good" and "bad" fat? Polyunsaturated oil is usually liquid and comes from vegetables such as corn, cottonseed, soybean, sunflower, and safflower. Peanut, canola, and olive oil are **monounsaturated fats** that are neutral and do not add cholesterol. The "bad" fats are **saturated fats,** which harden at room temperature and are found in meat, dairy products made from whole milk or cream, solid and hydrogenated shortening, coconut oil, palm oil, and cocoa butter.

Here are some tips for avoiding too much saturated fat:

1. Eat less meat. Adults need about 5-7 ounces of meat, poultry, fish, or seafood a day.
2. Avoid "prime grade" or heavily marbled meats, corned beef, pastrami, regular ground beef, frankfurters, sausage, bacon, lunch meat, goose, duck, or organ meats. Select very lean cuts of meat. Trim skin off chicken and turkey.
3. Avoid fried meat, chicken, fish, or seafood. Use a rack to drain off fat when broiling, baking, or roasting.
4. Eat no more than two whole eggs (yolks and whites) per week. (Egg whites are allowed, since they contain little cholesterol.)
5. Avoid dairy products containing more than 1% milk fat, such as butter, sour cream, cream cheese, creamed cottage cheese, and most natural and processed cheeses. Select milk products that contain only up to 1% milk fat. Use polyunsaturated margarine.
6. Avoid packaged foods or bakery items that contain egg yolks, whole milk, saturated fats, cream sauces, or butter. Select only those that have a low-cholesterol rating.
7. Avoid cashews, coconut, pistachios, and macadamia nuts. Most other types of vegetables, fruits, nuts, and seeds are low in cholesterol.

Low-sodium diet

The average American consumes about 1 to 2 teaspoons of salt every day, 6 to 18 grams, and most of this salt is added at the table. Your body needs only about 0.5 gram of salt a day. Since most foods that come from animals (meat, poultry, fish, eggs, milk) are naturally high in sodium, your body's requirements are easily met without adding salt to your food.

What is the difference between salt and sodium? Sodium keeps the right amount of water in your body, so some is necessary for good health. However, too much sodium causes water retention, which raises your blood pressure.

It may take a little time to get used to a low-sodium diet, particularly if you are accustomed to eating highly salted foods. Start by eliminating salt from the table. Use spices and herbs that contain no sodium to add flavor, and try some of the new salt substitutes that contain no sodium.

Many packaged and processed foods are now marketed as low sodium, including cheeses, luncheon meats, canned and packaged food, and even snacks such as potato chips. However, beware if the package reads "reduced sodium"; the sodium content may still be too high. If you are not sure of a product, read the ingredients carefully and look for the words "salt, sodium, soda, baking powder, monosodium glutamate (MSG), and disodium phosphate." If you are still in doubt, don't eat it.

Here are some tips for eliminating the "hidden" sodium from your diet:

1. Avoid cured or smoked meat, poultry, or fish. These include ham, bacon, corned beef, regular luncheon meats, sausage, commercially frozen fish, canned fish packed in oil or brine, and canned shellfish.
2. Avoid frozen, canned, and dehydrated main-dish foods such as pizza, TV dinners, spaghetti, chili, stews, and soups.
3. Avoid canned vegetables and vegetable juices.
4. Avoid cheese, buttermilk, and cocoa mixes.
5. Avoid commercial sauces (catsup, chili sauce, steak sauce, soy sauce), mayonnaise, salad dressing, olives, pickles, meat tenderizers, and seasoning salts.

Low-calorie diet

Losing weight (or keeping weight off) is an important part of controlling blood pressure and reducing blood cholesterol levels. Your doctor, a dietitian, or a nutritionist can advise you about calories, since this depends on your how active you are, your height, and your physical condition.

The low-cholesterol diet is an excellent basis for a weight loss program. Fats are high in calories, and the low-cholesterol diet is essentially a low-fat diet. For example, 1 cup of whole milk contains 150 calories, but the same amount of skim milk has only 86 calories. Also, because it emphasizes fresh fruits and vegetables and discourages processed foods, the low-cholesterol diet is nutritionally well balanced.

Weight loss should be gradual. Remember: it probably took you several years to put the pounds on, so expect it to take several months to lose them.

Here are some other tips for helping you lose weight:

1. Divide your daily calorie allowance into several small meals a day, instead of eating one or two large meals.
2. For between-meal snacks, choose high-fiber, low-calorie foods such as apples or celery. High-fiber foods make your stomach feel full quicker.
3. For between-meal hunger pangs, fool your stomach with a glass of ice water, hot tea, or calorie-free soda.
4. If you eat when you're bored, busy yourself to take your mind off food. Change your activity—do something you enjoy, take a walk, or take a shower.
5. If you eat when you are "blue," try the "buddy system" with a dieting friend. Agree to call each other for help whenever you're tempted to indulge.
6. Regular exercise that burns calories (walking, jogging, swimming, etc.) is the magic ingredient in many people's exercise programs. Check with your doctor first about the safest program for you.
7. "Too good to be true" weight loss programs are just that—they are either worthless or dangerous. Follow a diet that has been medically recommended and skip the "fad" diets.

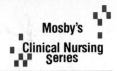
Starting Your Exercise Program

If you are recovering from heart surgery or a heart attack, your doctor has probably prescribed a daily graduated walking program to help your recovery. This program is also good if you have not exercised in a long time, and your doctor recommends walking to help control your blood pressure or reduce your chances of cardiovascular disease.

Daily exercise may be one of the best gifts you can give yourself. It improves circulation, lowers blood pressure, helps in a weight control program, and strengthens your muscles. It can also help you sleep better, feel more energetic, and increase your sense of well-being.

General guidelines

1. If you are recovering from heart surgery or a heart attack, have someone with you for the first several weeks.
2. Wait at least 2 hours after eating.
3. Wear comfortable rubber-soled walking shoes and loose clothing.
4. Avoid extreme heat or cold. Don't exercise if the temperature is over 85° F (particularly if the humidity is over 75%) or under 20° F. During bad weather, walk in a covered shopping mall or gym.
5. Always begin with a 5-minute warm-up of stretching and slow walking.
6. Adopt a steady, rhythmic pace and keep it up. If you have attacks of leg cramps (claudication), you may need to alternate walking with rest periods.
7. Watch for signs of overexertion. Stop walking if any of these symptoms occurs: chest pain (angina), palpitations, irregular heartbeat, dizziness or lightheadedness, shortness of breath for more than 10 minutes, nausea or vomiting, extreme fatigue, pale or splotchy skin, or "cold sweat." Call your doctor if these symptoms persist.
8. Cool down with light activity for 5 minutes; for example, if you are walking fast, slow down to a stroll.

Graduated walking program

Graduated walking programs are designed to slowly increase the time, distance, and walking pace. Because they begin very slowly, you may be tempted to skip ahead if you feel the schedule is "too easy." Don't. The graduated schedule allows your heart time to adjust to increasing amounts of work. Skipping ahead may overwork your heart. Carry out the program just as your doctor orders. If you develop symptoms of overexertion, return to the previous week's schedule until you are ready to progress.

You must know the exact distance to determine how fast you should walk. You can measure the distance on your car odometer. If you find you walk the distance in less time than the schedule specifies, slow your pace down next time. If it takes longer, you need to walk a little faster.

As soon as you stop walking, take your pulse. Your heart rate should not exceed the upper limit of the target heart rate set by your doctor. For many people, this is less than 115 beats per minute.

FIRST 9 WEEKS

Week	Walking time	Distance
1	5 minutes	¼ mile
2	5 minutes	¼ mile
3	10 minutes	½ mile
4	10 minutes	½ mile
5	15 minutes	¾ mile
6	15 minutes	¾ mile
7	20 minutes	1 mile
8	20 minutes	1½ miles
9	30 minutes	2 miles

At this point, you are ready to extend your walking time. Because the exercise will be sustained for a longer time, your pace will need to be a little slower the first few weeks. By week 12, your walking speed will increase to a brisk walk.

WEEKS 10 to 12

Week	Walking Time	Distance
10	40 minutes	2 miles
11	40 minutes	2 miles
12	60 minutes	3 miles

You must continue with an exercise program after week 12. You should continue your walking program, join a medically supervised walk-jog program, or add another form of exercise to your program such as bicycling. Follow your doctor's advice about the best program for you.

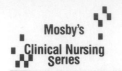

Anticoagulant Therapy

How to take the medication

If your doctor has given you a prescription for an anticoagulant, this is to pevent clots from forming in your blood. It is important to take the medication exactly as ordered, since too much of the drug can cause bleeding and too little can cause clotting. For this reason, you must have blood tests done periodically to ensure your blood is clotting properly. If it is not, your doctor will change the dosage. Here are important guidelines for taking your medication:

1. Take your anticoagulant at the same time of day. If you are supposed to take it on alternate days, marking a calendar can help.
2. If you forget to take a dose, do not double up next time. Just take the next dose as scheduled. If you miss two doses, call your doctor.
3. Keep your appointments for blood tests.
4. Refill your prescription 1 week ahead so you don't run out.
5. Keep anticoagulants away from heat and cold.

Helping the medication work

Your diet, health, and other drugs can also affect the way anticoagulants work in your body. For this reason, follow these guidelines:

1. Eat only normal amounts of green leafy vegetables (spinach, broccoli, etc.). These foods have a high content of vitamin K, which helps your blood clot. However, too much vitamin K can interfere with the anticoagulant.
2. If you drink alcohol, limit the amount to one drink per day. Excessive alcohol can affect blood clotting.
3. **Do not take aspirin** or any drugs containing aspirin. Check with your doctor or pharmacist before taking over-the-counter drugs to be sure they do not contain aspirin or other substances that might affect blood clotting.
4. Do not take any supplements that contain vitamin K. If you take multivitamins or other supplements, check with your doctor or pharmacist to ensure they are safe.
5. Many prescription drugs can interfere with anticoagulants. Take other prescription medications only as prescribed by your doctor.
6. If you develop diarrhea, vomiting, or fever that lasts longer than 24 hours, call your doctor.

Safety first

While you are taking anticoagulant medication, your blood will clot more slowly if you are injured. Therefore, you should take precautions against even minor cuts and bruises. In addition, you must be alert for signs that you may be bleeding internally. The following safety measures will help prevent problems:

1. Use a toothbrush with soft bristles.
2. Avoid putting toothpicks or other sharp objects in your mouth.
3. Protect your feet from injury. Don't walk barefoot, and don't trim corns or calluses yourself. See a podiatrist if necessary.
4. Inform all doctors (for example, dentist, gynecologist) that you are taking anticoagulants *before* receiving any treatment.
5. Avoid using cutting tools or other sharp objects that could result in injury.
6. Avoid rough sports.
7. Protect yourself from falling. Put a nonskid mat in your bathtub or shower, remove hazardous throw rugs, and wear low-heeled shoes with nonslip soles.
8. If you cut yourself, keep pressure on the injury for 10 minutes. If the bleeding doesn't stop, call your doctor immediately.
9. If you are bruised, draw a line around the margin. If the bruise enlarges, call your doctor.
10. Check urine and stools daily. Call the doctor if you see pink or red urine or black stools.
11. Call your doctor if you suddenly develop excessive nosebleeds, bleeding gums, purplish or reddish spots on your skin, unusual vaginal bleeding or excessive menstrual flow, or bleeding hemorrhoids.
12. Carry either an identification card or a Medic-Alert bracelet at all times. It should include the name of the anticoagulant you're taking and your doctor's name and phone number.
13. If you are planning a long trip, inform your doctor so he or she can arrange for the blood tests to be done while you are away.

FOR WOMEN: Coumadin is a drug that crosses the placenta and can cause serious birth defects. Therefore you should take precautions to avoid pregnancy while on this drug. If you suspect that you are pregnant, notify your doctor **immediately.**

CHAPTER 8

Cardiovascular Drugs

ANTIARRHYTHMIC AGENTS

ELECTROPHYSIOLOGIC CLASSIFICATION OF ANTIARRHYTHMIC AGENTS

Class I Agents: Membrane-Stabilizing Agents/Sodium-Channel Blockers

Class IA	Class IB	Class IC
Quinidine	Lidocaine	Flecainide
Procainamide	Mexiletine	Encainide
Disopyramide	Aprindine	Propafenone
	Phenytoin	
	Tocainide	

The major electrophysiologic action of these drugs is to block sodium channels in the membrane, thereby depressing fast inward sodium currents. This is the so-called "local anesthetic effect." Conduction velocity is slowed, and phase 4 is suppressed. The subclasses differ primarily in their effects on repolarization.

Class II Agents: Beta-adrenergic Blocking Agents

Propranolol
Acebutolol
Metoprolol
Pindolol

Class II agents work primarily by blocking sympathetic stimulation (beta-receptors), a major contributing factor in the development of dysrhythmia. Beta-blockers are used mainly for controlling HTN and for other purposes, such as controlling angina supraventricular dysrhythmia. Although all these agents have antiarrhythmic effects, propranolol is the agent of choice.

Class III Agents: (No specific name given to this class)

Amiodarone
Bretylium

Class III agents prolong all phases of the action potential. These agents have a low disrhythmogenic potential and little to no effect on inotropic activity. Bretylium and amiodarone belong to this classification.

Class IV Agents: Calcium-Channel Blockers

Diltiazem
Verapamil
Bepridil

These agents block the slow (calcium) channels. In contrast with class I agents, they have very little effect on the sodium channels in therapeutic concentrations. Both the SA and AV nodes are slow-response fibers that are activated by calcium channels. Calcium-channel blockers suppress the automaticity of the SA node, depress conduction velocity, and prolong the effective refractory period of the AV node.

CLASS IA ANTIARRHYTHMIC AGENTS
Quinidine

Quinidine slows phase 0 of the action potential and depresses spontaneous phase 4 diastolic depolarization, leaving the resting membrane potential unaltered. Quinidine lengthens the effective refractory period in the atria, ventricles, His-Purkinje system, and accessory pathways.

Indications: Reentrant, as well as ectopic atrial and ventricular tachyarrhythmias.

Usual dosage: PO loading: 12 mg/kg; **Maintenance:** 6 mg/kg q 6 h (longer intervals with SR products), **IV:** 0.3-0.4 mg/kg/min (gluconate solution given slowly).

Precautions/contraindications: ECG: widened QRS, prolonged QT, decreased ST segment, AV block, bradycardia.

Side effects/adverse reactions: CV: Hypotension; **GI:** Nausea, vomiting, diarrhea; **Blood:** Hemolytic anemia, thrombocytopenia; **CNS:** Headaches, tinnitus, dizziness; **Miscellaneous:** Drug fever, SLE-like syndrome, hepatotoxicity, hepatitis, jaundice.

Pharmacokinetics: Onset of action: 15 min with peak activity in 2-4 h; **Plasma half-life:** 7-9 h; **Therapeutic blood level:** 2-5 μg/ml; **Route of elimination;** metabolized in liver; small amount excreted in urine.

Interactions: Increases effect of warfarin sodium and concentration of digoxin.

Nursing considerations: Administer with food and observe patient for diarrhea. Negative inotropic effect may lead to hypotension (especially with IV route). Continuously monitor BP during and immediately after IV administration. Monitor ECG for prolonged QT intervals. Monitor serum potassium levels and watch for torsades de pointes, advanced AV block. For patients with poor compliance, slow-release oral preparations are available (Quindex Extentabs, Drug Tabs, Cardioquin).

Procainamide (Pronestyl)

Procainamide has electrophysiologic properties similar to those of quinidine in that they both are class I agents; however, procainamide does not prolong the QT interval to the same extent as quinidine does, and it is safer to use intravenously than quinidine.

Indications: Acute management of ventricular tachycardia unresponsive to lidocaine, control of premature ventricular complexes, and long-term control of atrial fibrillation.

Usual dosage: PO: 375-500 mg q 4-6 h; **IM:** 250-500 mg q 3-6 h, **IV:** 100 mg bolus at a rate of 25-50 mg/min q 5 min. Up to 1 g over the first hour. **Maintenance:** 2-4 mg/min.

Precautions/contraindications: Severe heart block, SVT. Use with caution in pregnancy and lactation.

Side effects/adverse reactions: ECG: widened QRS, prolonged QT interval, AV block; **CV:** hypotension, CHF; **GI:** dyspepsia, nausea, vomiting, anorexia; **Blood:** agranulocytosis, thrombocytopenia; **CNS:** dizziness, confusion, depression; **Miscellaneous:** SLE-like syndrome, rash, fever, joint pain.

Pharmacokinetics: Peak action: 2-4 h; **Plasma half-life:** 2-5 h (6-8 h with procainamide SR); **Therapeutic blood levels:** 4-10 μg/ml, **NAPA:** 2-22mg/ml; **Route of elimination:** metabolized in the liver, 30%-60% excreted unchanged in the urine.

Interactions: Potentiates effect of diuretics and hypotensive agents. Amiodarone and cimetidine increase concentration of procainamide.

Nursing considerations: Discontinue drug use if the following have occurred: (1) QRS widened by >50%; (2) hypotension; (3) 1 g total has been given (IV route).

During IV administration of loading dose, monitor BP q 5 min. Monitor serum potassium levels. Monitor ECG for prolonged QT intervals and observe for torsades de pointes and AV block. Metabolite of procainamide is NAPA. Both procainamide (30-60%) and NAPA (85%) are cleared by the kidney. Monitor plasma levels of both procainamide and NAPA and decrease dose in renal failure.

Slow-release preparations: procainamide SR 500-1000 mg q 6 h.

Disopyramide (Norpace)

Disopyramide has electrophysiologic properties similar to quinidine, but disopyramide has more vagolytic action and negative inotropic effects. These effects are a major drawback to the use of disopyramide in patients with poor LV function. It is most effective in preventing recurrent atrial fibrillation or recurrent atrial dysrhythmias in patients *without* a history of CHF or in patients with ventricular dysrhythmia.

Indications: Suppresses or prevents ventricular ectopy, atrial dysrhythmias in patients with MVP.

Usual dosage: Loading: 4 mg/kg; **Maintenance:** 100-200 mg q 6 h.

Precautions/contraindications: Should be avoided in patients with glaucoma or urinary retention.

Side effects/adverse reactions: Increased QRS and QT intervals—bradycardia, heart blocks; **CV:** CHF, hypotension; **GI:** nausea, vomiting, diarrhea, bloating; **CNS:** nervousness, dizziness, fatigue, headache, depression.

Pharmacokinetics: Peak action: 2-4 h; **Plasma half-life:** 6-8 h; **Therapeutic blood levels:** 2-6 mg/ml; **Route of elimination:** metabolized in the liver, 40%-60% excreted in the urine.

Interactions: Increases effects of oral anticoagulants.

Nursing considerations: Assess patient for signs and symptoms of CHF. Observe for urinary retention, edema, constipation, dry mouth (due to anticholinergic effects).

As with quinidine-type drugs (quinidine, procainamide), patients with atrial fibrillation/flutter should be digitalized first to increase effective refractory period of the AV junction.

CLASS IB ANTIARRHYTHMIC AGENTS
Lidocaine (Xylocaine)

Lidocaine's major electrophysiologic action is depression of spontaneous phase 4 diastolic depolarization.

This depression causes a decrease in automaticity of ectopic ventricular pacemakers and raises the ventricular fibrillation threshold. Lidocaine is more effective in the presence of a normal serum potassium level; therefore, if hypokalemia is present, it should be corrected to obtain lidocaine's maximum effect.

Indications: Is the standard parenteral agent for suppression of ventricular dysrhythmias associated with AMI and cardiac surgery.

Usual dosage: 1-2 mg/kg (50-100 mg) by IV bolus followed by 1-4 mg/min. Repeat ½ initial dose 10-15 min after bolus and infusion.

Precautions/contraindications: Contraindicated in patients with known hypersensitivity to local anesthetics of the amide type or with Stokes-Adams syndrome, severe SA, AVF, or intraventricular block.

Side effects/adverse reactions: ECG: sinus arrest, AV block, asystole; **CV:** hypotension; **CNS:** restlessness, dizziness, irritability, confusion, seizures, tinnitus, double vision.

Pharmacokinetics: Onset of action: 45-90 sec; **Plasma half-life:** 2 h; **Therapeutic blood levels:** 1.4-6.0 μg/ml; **Route of elimination:** rapidly metabolized in liver and excreted in urine.

Interactions: Cimetidine and beta blockers may increase the concentration of lidocaine.

Nursing considerations: Obtain baseline BP, HR, and ECG intervals and increase HR (using atropine, pacing) in patient with sinus bradycardia before administering lidocaine, because of the potential ECG side effects. Assess neurologic status for lidocaine toxicity (CNS side effects). (Cimetidine and beta-blockers increase the concentration of lidocaine; elimination of lidocaine is decreased with liver disease and CHF). Record weight daily in kilograms since the dosage of lidocaine is weight-related.

Mexiletine (Mexitil)

Mexiletine is a local anesthetic agent whose electrophysiologic properties resemble those of lidocaine. It is not effective in the control of supraventricular tachyarrhythmias. It has been reported that mexiletine has no significant effect on LV contractility.

Indications: Used in management of chronic ventricular dysrhythmia after MI.

Usual dosage: PO loading: 400 mg; **Maintenance:** 200-300 mg q 6-8 h; **Maximum:** 1200 mg/day.

Precautions/contraindications: Contraindicated in patients with cardiogenic shock, bradycardia, AV block, severe heart failure. Caution in patients with liver failure.

Side effects/adverse reactions: ECG: bradycardia; **CV:** hypotension, palpitations, syncope; **GI:** nausea, vomiting, diarrhea; **CNS:** tremor, ataxia, dizziness, blurred vision, confusion, headache, seizures; **Miscellaneous:** Liver enzymes increase greater than three times baseline with or without liver damage.

Pharmacokinetics: Onset of action: IV < 5 min; 1-2 h; **Plasma half-life:** 9-10 h, **Therapeutic blood levels:** 0.5-2.0 μg/ml; **Route of elimination:** metabolized in the liver and about 20% excreted unchanged in the urine.

Interactions: Phenytoin, Rifampin, and smoking may decrease concentration.

Nursing considerations: OK with food and antacids. Monitor liver function tests.

Aprindine (Fibocil)

Aprindine is an antiarrhythmic agent which has a depressant effect on all levels of cardiac conduction, including SA, AV, and His-Purkinje fibers. It also depresses the antegrade transmission of impulses through the accessory pathway of pre-excitation syndromes. Aprindine exerts mild negative inotropic activity. The rare but serious side effects (agranulocytosis and hepatotoxicity) are a distinct drawback.

Indications: Indicated in the treatment of ventricular dysrhythmias of diverse etiologies. Aprindine may also be effective in the treatment of supraventricular tachycardias such as Wolff-Parkinson-White (WPW) syndrome.

Usual dosage: Loading: 200-400 mg; **Maintenance:** 100-200mg daily; **IV:** 20-25 mg q 2 min up to 150 mg.

Precautions/contraindications: None.

Side effects/adverse reactions: ECG: bradycardia; increase in PR and QT intervals; **CNS:** dizziness, tremors, hallucinations, ataxia, diplopia; **Blood:** agranulocytosis; **Liver:** hepatotoxicity.

Pharmacokinetics: Plasma half-life: 22 h, **Therapeutic blood levels:** 1.2 μg/ml; **Route of elimination:** metabolized by the liver, excreted in the urine.

Interactions: None.

Nursing considerations: Monitor CBC and bilirubin weekly.

Phenytoin (Dilantin)

Phenytoin depresses automaticity. Like lidocaine, it appears to selectively affect ischemic myocardium with little or no effect on conduction in normal tissue.

Indications: Indicated in the treatment of digitalis-induced ventricular dysrhythmias, dysrhythmias of MVP not responding to propranolol, and for the prevention of ventricular dysrhythmias after surgery for congenital heart disease.

Usual dosage: IV: 100 mg over 2 min. Repeat q 5 min to 1 g maximum.

Precautions/contraindications: Caution in patients with liver and renal disease. Contraindicated in pregnancy and psychiatric disease.

Side effects/adverse reactions: ECG: decreased PR and QT intervals; **CV:** hypotension; **GI:** nausea, vomiting, anorexia; **CNS:** tremor, ataxia, dizziness, blurred vision, confusion, headache, seizures; **Blood:** decreased platelets, WBCs; **Miscellaneous:** rash, gingival hyperplasia.

Pharmacokinetics: Onset of action: slow and variable; **Plasma half-life:** 24 h; **Therapeutic blood levels:** 10-18 µg/ml; **Route of elimination:** metabolized by liver, excreted in the urine.

Interactions: Decreased effects of this drug with chronic alcohol use and CNS depressants.

Nursing considerations: Administer IV at less than 50 mg/min. Dilute with normal saline only. Avoid IM injections because absorption is inconsistent and tissue necrosis may occur. Monitor CBCs. Take oral dose with food to avoid GI upset.

Tocainide (Tonocard)

Tocainide exhibits pharmacologic and electrophysiologic actions similar to lidocaine and is referred to as "oral lidocaine." It produces no significant myocardial depression and has no effect on conduction through the AV node and His-Purkinje system. This agent decreases the effective refractory period and shortens the action potential duration.

Indications: To control serious ventricular dysrhythmias resistant to quinidine, procainamide, and propranolol.

Usual dosage: Loading: 400-600 mg q 4-6 h; **maintenance:** 400-600 mg q 8 h; **Maximum:** 2400 mg.

Precautions/contraindications: Caution in patients with renal failure for severe hepatic impairment. Caution in pregnancy.

Side effects/adverse reactions: ECG: slight decrease in QT interval, tachycardia, bradycardia, asystole; **CV:** hypotension, pericarditis; **GI:** nausea, vomiting, diarrhea; **Blood:** aplastic anemia; **CNS:** tremor, headache, dizziness, ataxia, confusion, nystagmus; **Pulmonary:** pleurisy/fibrosis fever, dyspnea, cough, chest infiltrates; **Miscellaneous:** rash, arthralgia.

Pharmacokinetics: Onset of action: 1.5 h; **Plasma half-life:** 13.5 h; **Therapeutic blood levels:** 3.5-7.0 µg/ml; **Route of elimination:** metabolized in liver, about 40% excreted unchanged in the urine.

Interactions: Allopurinol may increase tocainide concentration.

Nursing considerations: OK with food (may decrease side effects). Monitor blood counts. Assess for pulmonary signs and symptoms.

CLASS IC ANTIARRHYTHMIC AGENTS
Flecainide (Tambocor)

Flecainide shares some of the electrophysiologic properties of quinidine (class IA) and lidocaine (class IB). The major drawback to flecainide is its proarrhythmic effect, which occurs mainly in patients with heart failure, low ejection fraction, and a history of MI and/or an episode of cardiac arrest.

Indications: Management and suppression of PVCs and complex refractory ventricular dysrhythmias. It is also indicated in dysrhythmias associated with Wolff-Parkinson-White syndrome.

Usual dosage: PO loading: 100 mg bid; **Maintenance:** 100-200 mg bid; **Maximum:** 600 mg/day.

Precautions/contraindications: Caution in patients with renal and hepatic failure, CHF, AV block, and sinus bradycardia. Negative inotropic effect may cause or worsen CHF.

Side effects/adverse reactions: ECG: increase in PR, QRS, and QT intervals—bradycardia, tachycardia, ventricular dysrhythmias; **CV:** CHF; **GI:** nausea, vomiting, dyspepsia, anorexia; **CNS:** dizziness, visual changes, headache, tremor, fatigue; **Blood:** decreased blood counts (WBCs, platelets).

Pharmacokinetics: Plasma half-life: 12-27 h; **Therapeutic blood levels:** 400-800 mg/ml; **Route of elimination:** extensively metabolized, renal 10%-50% unchanged in urine.

Interactions: Flecainide may increase concentration of digoxin. Amiodarone may increase flecainide levels. Small increases in both flecainide and propranolol plasma levels are seen during coadministration.

Nursing considerations: Monitor for dysrhythmias (proarrhythmic effect). OK to take with food and antacids. Observe for postural hypotension.

Encainide (Enkade)

Encainide is effective in suppressing life-threatening and complex ventricular dysrhythmia. Encainide affects primarily conduction in the His-Purkinje system. Encainide interferes with sodium entry into cardiac cells through the fast sodium channel, shortens the action-potential duration, and elevates the ventricular fibrillation threshold. Aggravation of dysrhythmias (proarrhythmic effect) is the most serious side effect encountered with encainide.

Indications: Complex refractory ventricular dysrhythmia.

Usual dosage: Loading: 25 mg tid for 48 h; **Maintenance:** 50 mg tid; **Maximum:** 300 mg daily.

Precautions/contraindications: Contraindicated in 2-3 degree AV block.

Side effects/adverse reactions: ECG: increase in PR, QRS, and QT intervals; ventricular dysrhythmias; **CNS:** headache, tremor, blurred vision, paresthesia; **Skin:** urticarial skin rash; **GI:** nausea, vomiting, dyspepsia; **Liver:** elevated values on liver-function test; **Miscellaneous:** metallic taste.

Pharmacokinetics: Plasma half-life: 3-4 h; **Therapeutic blood levels:** > 100 mg/ml; **Route of elimination:** metabolized in liver and excreted in urine.

Interactions: Cimetidine increases plasma concentrations of encainide (reduce dosage of encainide).

Nursing considerations: Monitor for dysrhythmis (proarrhythmic effect). Preexisting hypokalemia or hyperkalemia should be corrected before administration. Dosages of encainide should be adjusted gradually, allowing 3-5 days between dosing increments.

Propafenone (Rythmonorm)

Propafenone is an investigational agent and a potent antiarrhythmic. In addition to sharing the electrophysiologic properties of other Class I antiarrhythmic agents, propafenone has weak effects similar to beta-adrenergic blocking agents, as well as calcium antagonists. Propafenone exerts a mild negative inotropic effect and should be used cautiously in patients with poor LV contractility.

Indications: Suppression of symptomatic ventricular dysrhythmias, including frequent unifocal or multifocal premature ventricular contractions, couplets, and ventricular tachycardia.

Usual dosage: 300-900 mg/day.

Precautions/contraindications: Caution in patients with poor LV contractility, liver and/or renal disease, and severe obstructive pulmonary disease.

Side effects/adverse reactions: ECG: slight increase in PR interval and QRS duration, bradycardia, SA block; **CV:** hypotension, CHF, **GI:** nausea, vomiting.

Pharmacokinetics: Plasma half-life: 3 h, chronic administration (6-7 h); **Therapeutic blood levels:** 0.5-2.0 μg/ml, **Route of elimination:** metabolized in the liver and excreted in urine/feces.

Interactions: Increases serum digoxin levels by about 35% during concomitant administration; may potentiate the effects of warfarin sodium.

Nursing considerations: Monitor for signs and symptoms of decreased LV function. Administration with food results in increased bioavailability, thus an increase in maximum plasma levels.

CLASS II ANTIARRHYTHMIC AGENTS: BETA-ADRENERGIC BLOCKING AGENTS

Beta-blocking agents are used to control dysrhythmias that are induced or exacerbated by increased sympathetic activity through increased levels of catecholamines as can happen in myocardial ischemia. Beta-blockers increase VT threshold significantly. They may be given prophylactically to survivors of AMIs, as they have been found to reduce the incidence of sudden death in the first year or two after the acute event.[130] (See page 289 for specific information on beta-blockers.) Indications include inappropriate sinus tachycardia, paroxysmal atrial tachycardia provoked by emotion and exercise, chronic ventricular dysrhythmias in absence of heart failure, and dysrhythmias in MVP.

CLASS III ANTIARRHYTHMIC AGENTS
Amiodarone (Cordarone)

Amiodarone lengthens the effective refractory period by prolonging the action potential of atrial and ventricular tissues. Unlike other antiarrhythmic agents, amiodarone has three distinct properties: (1) a wide spectrum of antiarrhythmic activity against both supraventricular and ventricular tachyarrhythmias, (2) a wide margin of safety with little or no negative inotropic effect, and (3) a long and variable elimination half-life. In addition, amiodarone has a mild vasodilator effect. The side effects and long half-life are the major drawbacks to using amiodarone.

Indications: Atrial and ventricular dysrhythmias.

Usual dosage: PO loading: 800-1600 mg/day for 1-3 wks; **Adjustment:** 600-800 mg/day for 3-4 wks; **Maintenance:** 200-400 mg/day; **IV:** 5 mg/kg over 5 min.

Precautions/contraindications: None.

Side effects/adverse reactions: ECG: increased QRS and QT intervals, SA arrest, bradycardia; **CV:** hypotension; **Eye:** corneal microdeposits, blue-green halos, photosensitivity; **CNS:** peripheral neuropathy, tremors, insomnia; **Skin:** photosensitivity, blue-gray pigmentation to sun-exposed areas; **Pulmonary:** pulmonary alveolitis; **GI:** nausea, vomiting, constipation; hepatotoxicity; endocrine hyperthyroidism or hypothyroidism.

Pharmacokinetics: Plasma half-life: 20-110 days; **Therapeutic blood levels:** 0.6 to 2.8 μg/ml; **Route of elimination:** liver.

Interactions: If given concurrently with beta-blockers or calcium-channel blockers, may produce bradycardia, hypotension, or sinus arrest.

Nursing considerations: Patient should avoid prolonged exposure to sun and use protective clothing and sun screens. Monitor thyroid and hepatic function. If patient is receiving concurrent beta-blockers and/or calcium blockers, may produce bradycardiac, hypotension, or sinus arrest. Monitor vital signs, pulmonary status.

Bretylium (Bretylol, Bretylan)

Bretylium, a sympathetic ganglion-blocking agent, depresses norepinephrine release and produces sympathetic blockade by preventing the release of the neurotransmitter norepinephrine. Similar to beta-adrenergic blocking agents, bretylium has an adrenergic blocking effect. However, this effect is by prolongation of all phases of the action potential simultaneously rather than by prolongation of one specific phase.

Indications: Acute management of life-threatening ventricular tachycardia, ventricular fibrillation; used as a second line drug in conjunction with cardioversion.

Usual dosage: IV: bolus 5-10 mg/kg followed by infusion of 1-2 mg/min.

Precautions/contraindications: Contraindicated in digitalis toxicity and pulmonary hypertension. Caution in renal disease and pregnancy.

Side effects/adverse reactions: ECG: increase in QRS, QT intervals; **CV:** transient HTN followed by postural hypotension; **CNS:** dizziness, syncope; **Miscellaneous:** necrosis/muscle atrophy with IM injections.

Pharmacokinetics: Plasma half-life: 5-10 h, **Therapeutic blood levels:** 0.5-1.5 µg/ml; **Route of elimination:** excreted in urine.

Interactions: Toxicity: digitalis. Incompatible with all medication in solution or syringe.

Nursing considerations: When giving second bolus of bretylium, repeat 10-15 min after initial bolus and administer slowly. Initial sympathomimetic effect may cause an increase in ventricular dysrhythmias, HR, and BP. This increase is a transient effect, lasting about 30 min. For IMs, inject deep and rotate sites to prevent necrosis.

CLASS IV ANTIARRHYTHMIC AGENTS: CALCIUM-CHANNEL BLOCKERS

Calcium-channel blockers are agents that selectively depress the myocardial slow channels. Slow, inward currents of calcium ions are distinguished from the fast, inward sodium currents by their electrophysiologic and pharmacologic characteristics. Cells in which slow channels predominate, in the absence of fast inward sodium currents, are characteristically found in the SA and AV nodes. Verapamil, nifedipine, diltiazem, and bepridil are examples of class IV agents that increase AV conduction and refractoriness. See page 293 for specific information on these drugs.

BETA-ADRENERGIC BLOCKING AGENTS

Adrenergic receptors within the sympathetic division of the autonomic nervous system are divided into alpha-receptors and beta-receptors. The alpha-receptors reside primarily in the resistance vessels of the skin, mucosa, intestine, and kidney. Stimulation of alpha-receptors causes contraction of the vascular musculature and may produce vasoconstriction of these vascular beds.

The beta-receptors cause a relaxation of the vascular musculature and an increase in HR, conduction velocity, and contractility. Beta-receptors can be subdivided into beta 1 and beta 2 receptors. Beta 1 receptors are located throughout the body but are concentrated heavily in the heart and to a lesser degree in the intestine and the renin-secreting tissue of the kidney, adipose tissue, eye, and other organs. Beta 2 receptors are found primarily in bronchial and vascular smooth muscle and to a lesser degree in the heart, uterus, and insulin-secreting tissue of the pancreas. Stimulation of beta 2 receptors causes bronchodilation and vasodilation of vascular smooth muscle.

Mechanism of Action

Beta-adrenergic blockers either block beta 1 and beta 2 receptors or block beta 1 receptor sites selectively. Structurally they resemble the sympathetic catecholamines, norepinephrine and epinephrine.

Beta-blockers are competitive inhibitors; their action depends on the ratio of beta-blocker concentration to catecholamine concentration at beta-adrenergic sites. Beta-blockers reduce myocardial oxygen needs by (1) slowing HR (negative chronotropic effect), (2) lowering systolic blood pressure, and (3) decreasing myocardial contractility (negative inotropic effect).

The mechanism of antiarrhythmic effect is through the depression of phase 4 depolarization. Beta-blockers also decrease conduction velocity through the AV node and decrease myocardial automaticity. A decrease in myocardial contractility occurs with blockade of beta 1 receptors. This decrease is a result of blocking the receptor-operated channel for calcium entry inside the myocardial cell. In addition beta-blockade may produce coronary-artery vasoconstriction. The vasoconstrictive action of beta-blockade could be detrimental if coronary artery spasm is present. Therefore nitrates and beta-blockers usually are given together for their pharmacologic complementary effects. See the table on page 289 for effects of both stimulation and blockade of beta-adrenergic receptors.

EFFECT OF STIMULATION AND BLOCKADE OF BETA-ADRENERGIC RECEPTORS

	Beta 1 Receptors	Beta 2 Receptors
Stimulation	Increased HR Increased conduction velocity Increased myocardial contractility	Vasodilation of vascular bed and bronchial smooth muscle
Blockade	Decreased HR Decreased conduction velocity Decreased myocardial contractility • Depression of Phase 4 • Diastolic depolarization • Reduced rate pressure • Product on exercise Decreased MVo_2	Vasoconstriction of vascular bed and bronchial smooth muscle

Pharmacologic Properties of Beta-Adrenergic Blockers

Beta-blocking agents have unique pharmacologic properties. Each property influences the site of action, pharmacokinetics, and potential side effects of each beta-blocker. Understanding these properties facilitates selection of the appropriate beta-adrenergic blocker for a specific patient.

I. Beta-Adrenergic receptor selectivity
   a. Cardioselectivity—drugs that inhibit or block beta 1 receptors, with less inhibition of beta 2 receptors. They are associated with less bronchospasm and therefore are safer to use in patients with pulmonary disease. They are also less likely to compromise peripheral vascular circulation and are safer to use with diabetic patients.
   b. Non-cardioselectivity—drugs that block both beta 1 and beta 2 receptors. As beta 2 blockers, these agents may reduce secretion of insulin in response to glucose administration and may impair diabetic patients' carbohydrate tolerance. Similarly they may induce or exacerbate bronchospasm, particularly in asthmatic patients. They may increase PVR and induce or exacerbate peripheral vascular disease.

II. Intrinsic sympathomimetic activity (ISA)
   Beta-blockers that stimulate as well as block the beta-adrenergic receptors. This is referred to as partial agonist activity. ISA blockers are associated with a lower incidence of bradycardia.

III. Lipophilicity
   The ability of the drug to cross the blood-brain barrier. Beta-blockers with strong lipid solubility (lipophilic) reach high concentrations in the brain and are metabolized in the liver. This can result in vivid dreams, fatigue, weakness, and depression.
   Low lipid solubility (hydrophilic), which leads to decreased concentrations in the brain, is mainly excreted by the kidneys and has a decreased potential for CNS side effects.

IV. Bioavailability
   That fraction (percentage) of the dose administered that reaches the systemic circulation. IV dosage forms are considered to have 100% bioavailability.

V. Effects on renin
   All beta-blockers cause a decrease in plasma renin activity. Noncardioselective agents may have a greater effect. Beta-blockers with high ISA cause less decrease in renin activity.

Indications

Cardiac indications:
HTN, angina (control post-MI), reduce incidence of reinfarction and death following AMI, dysrhythmias (supraventricular, ventricular dysrhythmias), HCM, MVP syndrome.

Non-cardiac indications:
Migraine, glaucoma (applied topically), thyrotoxicosis, anxiety states.

Contraindications

Most contraindications listed apply to use of *non-selective* beta-blocking agents, which block both beta 1 and beta 2 receptors. To avoid complications such as those related to pulmonary disease or those that mask symptoms associated with diabetes, the drug of choice should be a cardioselective agent that blocks primarily beta 1 receptors.

Pulmonary
Absolute: Severe asthma or bronchospasm

Relative: Mild asthma or bronchospasm or chronic airways disease. Use agents with cardioselectivity, plus beta 2 stimulants (by inhalation). High ISA also protects, but there is loss of sensitivity to beta 2 stimulation.

Cardiac
Absolute: Symptomatic bradycardia, low CO, LV failure (except for some cardiomyopathies), high-degree heart block, AMI unless monitored.

Relative: Treated heart failure, cardiomegaly without clinical failure, Prinzmetal's angina (unopposed alpha-spasm), high doses of other agents depressing conduction (verapamil, digitalis, antiarrhythmic agents). In angina avoid sudden withdrawal. Danger in unreliable patient.

Central nervous system
Absolute: Severe depression (avoid propranolol).

Relative: For vivid dreams avoid highly lipid-soluble agents (propranolol, alprenolol) and pindolol, avoid evening dose, or try atenolol. For hallucinations change from propranolol. For fatigue (all agents) try change of agent. For migraine avoid selective agent. Psychotropic drugs (with adrenergic augmentation) may adversely interact with beta-blockers.

Peripheral vascular
Absolute: Gangrene, skin necrosis, severe or worsening claudication.

Relative: Cold extremities, absent pulses, Raynaud's phenomenon. Avoid nonselective agents without ISA (propranolol, nadolol). Prefer high-ISA (pindolol, oxprenolol) or cardioselectivity.

Diabetes mellitus
Relative: For insulin-requiring diabetes, nonselective agents decrease reaction to hypoglycemia. Use selective agents—atenolol, metoprolol (acebutolol more doubtful). Beta-blockers may increase blood sugar by 1.0-1.5 mmole/L. Adjust control accordingly.

Renal failure
Relative: In general, renal blood flow falls. Reduce doses of all beta-blockers except pindolol.

Liver disease
Relative: Avoid agents that require high hepatic clearance (propranolol, alprenolol, oxprenolol, timolol, acebutolol, metoprolol). Prefer agents with low clearance (atenolol, nadolol, or pindolol). If plasma proteins are low, reduce dose of highly bound agents.

Pregnancy HTN
Avoid unless treatment essential, but beta-blockers may be better than methyldopa. Avoid thiazide diuretics.

Surgical operations
Beta-blockade may be maintained throughout, provided indication is not trivial; otherwise, stop 24-48 h beforehand. May protect against anesthetic dysrhythmias. Use atropine for bradycardia, beta-agonist for severe hypotension.

Age
Can use with care of the elderly. Watch for increased side effects and pharmacokinetic changes.

General cautions

Non-cardioselective agents should be used with caution in patients with pulmonary, peripheral vascular disease, and CHF. Diabetic patients should be instructed that all beta-blocking agents can mask the signs and symptoms of hypoglycemia (e.g., tachycardia, jittery feelings).

General Side Effects

CV: bradycardia, AV block, hypotension, signs of peripheral vascular disease—intermittent claudication, cold extremities, Raynaud's phenomenon; **CNS:** dizziness, insomnia, fatigue, depression, vivid dreams or nightmares, insomnia; **GI:** nausea, vomiting, diarrhea; **Respiratory:** laryngospasm, bronchospasm, respiratory distress; **Other:** decreased libido, impotence, dry mouth, eyes, or skin.

General Nursing Considerations

Avoid abrupt withdrawal of beta-blockers, especially in patients being treated for angina, as sudden discontinuation can exacerbate anginal symptoms. AMI has been reported to occur after abrupt withdrawal of therapy. Instruct patient to avoid sudden position changes to prevent dizziness and not to stop taking drugs abruptly. If symptoms of dizziness, depression, fatigue, or dyspnea on exertion occur, instruct patient to notify physician.

NON-SELECTIVE BETA-BLOCKING AGENTS
Propranolol (Inderal)

Propranolol is a nonselective agent that causes a decrease in HR, preload, and afterload, which results in decrease in LVEDP and SVR.

Indications: HTN, angina, supraventricular dysrhythmias, and migraine.

Usual dosage: PO: starting 60-120 mg bid, qid; **Maintenance:** 80-320 mg bid, qid; **Maximum:** 320

mg q d; **IV:** push 1-5 mg slowly within 10 min (<1 mg/min).

Precautions/contraindications: Pregnancy and renal disease. See also Contraindications, page 290.

Side effects/adverse reactions: See General Side Effects, page 290.

Pharmacokinetics: Plasma half-life: 1-6 h; **Route of elimination:** liver; **Properties:** Cardioselective—no; ISA—no; Lipophilicity—strong; Bioavailability (Percentage of dose)—30%.

Interactions: Increases effects of barbituates, digitalis, and neuromuscular blocking agents.

Nursing considerations: High lipophilicity is reason for potential side effects of weakness, fatigue, vivid dreams, nightmares, and/or depression. Taking drugs with food increases bioavailability. See also General Nursing Considerations, page 290.

Nadolol (Corgard)

Nadolol is similar to propranolol but has the advantage that it has a long half-life and is not metabolized by the liver, which permits a once-per-day dose.

Indications: Moderate to severe HTN, chronic stable angina.

Usual dosage: PO starting: 40-80 mg/day, **Maintenance:** 8-160 mg/day; **Maximum:** 200 mg; **IV:** not available.

Precautions/contraindications: See Contraindications, page 290.

Side effects/adverse reactions: See General Side Effects, page 290.

Pharmacokinetics: Plasma half-life: 12-17 h; **Route of elimination:** renal; **Properties:** cardioselective—no; ISA—no; Lipophilicity—low; Bioavailability (percentage of dose)—30%.

Interactions: None.

Nursing considerations: Caution in patient with severe renal disease. Because of once-per-day dose, may be helpful in management of the noncompliant patient. See also General Nursing Considerations, page 290.

Pindolol (Visken)

Pindolol is a non-selective beta-adrenergic blocking agent with a strong ISA, demonstrated by its non-reduction of the resting heart rate.

Indications: HTN.

Usual dosage: PO starting: 7.5 mg tid; **Maintenance:** 10-15 mg tid; **Maximum:** 15-60 mg/day; **IV:** 0.4-2.0 mg.

Precautions/contraindications: See Contraindication, page 290.

Side effects/adverse reactions: Insomnia, sleep disturbance, nervousness, fatigue, and weakness are significant. See also General Side Effects, page 290.

Pharmacokinetics: Plasma half-life: 4 h; **Route of elimination:** liver, renal (40%); **Properties:** Cardioselective—no; ISA—strong; Lipophilicity—moderate; Bioavailability—90% of dose.

Interactions: None.

Nursing considerations: Obtain baselines in liver and renal function prior to initiating therapy. See also General Nursing Considerations, page 290.

Timolol (Blocarden)

Timolol is a non-cardioselective agent that has been shown to decrease mortality and reinfarction following MI. Is five to six times more potent than propranolol.

Indications: HTN.

Usual dosage: PO starting: 5-10 mg bid; **Maintenance:** 20-40 mg bid; **Maximum:** 60 mg/day; **IV:** 0.4 mg-1.0 mg.

Precautions/contraindications: See Contraindication, page 290.

Side effects/adverse reactions: See General Side Effects, page 290.

Pharmacokinetics: Plasma half-life: 4-5 h; **Route of elimination:** liver, renal; **Properties:** Cardioselective—no; ISA—no; Lipophilicity—moderate; Bioavailability—75% of dose.

Interactions: None.

Nursing considerations: Monitor BP if given with other alpha-adrenergic agonist, which may lead to systemic HTN. See also General Nursing Considerations, page 290.

Labetalol (Normodyne, Trandate)

Labetalol is presently the only beta blocker with both alpha- and beta-blocking properties, with beta blockade predominating. Blood pressure is lowered by a combination of beta-blockade, alpha-blockade, and direct vasodilation.

Indications: Mild to moderate HTN.

Usual dosage: PO starting: 100 mg bid; **Maintenance:** 200-400 mg bid; **Maximum:** 1200-1400 mg/day; **IV:** 0.5 mg bolus. Repeat every 10 min; **Maximum:** 300 mg.

Precautions/contraindications: See Contraindications, page 290.

Side effects/adverse reactions: Can cause significant postural hypotension 2-4 h after dose. May cause a lupus-like syndrome. See also General Side Effects, page 290.

Pharmacokinetics: Plasma half-life: 3-4 h; **Route of elimination:** liver; **Properties:** Cardioselective—no; Lipophilicity—moderate; Bioavailability—33% of dose.

Interactions: None.

Nursing considerations: See General Nursing Considerations, page 290.

CARDIOSELECTIVE BETA-BLOCKING AGENTS
Acebutolol (Sectral)

Acebutolol, a beta 1 adrenergic blocking agent, has an inhibitory effect on the heart muscle, which results in a decrease in HR and CO at rest and during exercise. At higher doses, however, it may inhibit and block beta 2 receptors.

Indications: HTN, PVCs, and angina.

Usual dosage: PO starting: 100-400 mg/day, **Maintenance:** 600-1200 mg/day; **Maximum:** 1200 mg/day; **IV:** 12.5-50 mg.

Precautions/contraindications: Caution in patients with liver and renal disease. See also Contraindications, page 290.

Side effects/adverse reactions: See General Side Effects, page 290.

Pharmacokinetics: Plasma half-life: 3 h; **Route of elimination:** 60% renal, 40% liver; **Properties:** Cardioselective—yes; ISA—yes; Lipophilicity—moderate to low; Bioavailability—40% of dose.

Interactions: None.

Nursing considerations: See General Nursing Considerations, page 290.

Atenolol (Tenormin)

Atenolol is a long-acting beta-blocking agent that may be given in single daily doses.

Indications: Mild to moderate HTN, angina pectoris.

Usual dosage: PO starting: 50 mg/day; **Maintenance:** 50-100 mg/day; **Maximum:** 100 mg/day.

Precautions/contraindications: Caution in patients with severe renal disease. Better tolerated in patients with diabetes, peripheral vascular disease, and pulmonary problems. See also Contraindications, page 290.

Side effects/adverse reactions: See General Side Effects, page 290.

Pharmacokinetics: Plasma half-life: 6-9 h; **Route of elimination:** renal; **Properties:** Cardioselective—yes; ISA—no; Lipophilicity—weak to mild; Bioavailability—50% of dose.

Interactions: None.

Nursing considerations: See General Nursing Considerations, page 290.

Metoprolol (Lopressor)

Metoprolol in higher-than-usual doses will block beta 2 receptors located in bronchial and vascular smooth muscle.

Indications: HTN, AMI.

Usual dosage: PO Starting: 50-100 mg bid; **Maintenance:** 100-300 mg bid; **Maximum:** 400 mg; **IV:** 15 mg.

Precautions/contraindications: See Contraindications, page 290.

Side effects/adverse reactions: See General Side Effects, page 290.

Pharmacokinetics: Plasma half-life: 3 h; **Route of elimination:** liver; **Properties:** Cardioselective—yes; ISA—no; Lipophilicity—moderate to strong; Bioavailability—50% of dose.

Interactions: None.

Nursing considerations: Monitor BP—may increase at end of dosing interval. See General Nursing Considerations, page 290.

Esmolol (Brevibloc)

Esmolol is a very short-acting IV beta-blocker. May block beta 2 receptors at higher doses.

Indications: Supraventricular tachycardia, in emergency setting in which short-term control of ventricular rate is desirable, such as in the perioperative or postoperative periods.

Usual dosage: PO: not available; **IV:** loading infusion: 500 μg/kg/min; maintenance: 50 μ/kg/min for 4 min. If insufficient response, can repeat loading dose and increase maintenance infusion to 100 μg/kg/min for 4 min. Dosages >200 μg/kg/min are not recommended.

Precautions/contraindications: See Contraindications, page 290.

Side effects/adverse reactions: See General Side Effects, page 290.

Pharmacokinetics: Plasma half-life: 9 min; **Route of elimination:** hydrolyzed in human blood by esterases found in RBCs; **Properties:** Cardioselective—yes; ISA—no; Lipophilicity—low; Bioavailability—100% of dose.

Interactions: None.

Nursing considerations: Well tolerated when given with digoxin, morphine, and warfarin sodium. Not for direct IV push. Must be diluted prior to infusion. See General Nursing Considerations, page 290.

CALCIUM-CHANNEL BLOCKERS

The calcium-channel blockers, or antagonists, are a group of agents with a broad range of clinical applications. Currently three agents are approved for use in the United States: verapamil, nifedipine, and diltiazem.

THE ROLE OF CALCIUM IN CARDIAC ELECTROPHYSIOLOGY

Calcium ions play a critical role in the conduction of electrical impulses from the atria to the ventricles. Re-examination of the action potential found in cardiac tissue is helpful in identifying the principal sites of action for the calcium-channel blockers.

The action potential of myocardial cells is initiated by a rapid influx of sodium ions, which move the cell-membrane potential in a positive direction (phase 0). Phase 1 involves the closing of sodium channels and opening of calcium channels. During phase 2 (plateau phase) there is a slow influx of calcium ions by way of "slow channels," which are more selective for calcium than for sodium. The inward movement of calcium initiates a complex series of events known as excitation-contraction coupling. The net effect of this process is depolarization of the cell membrane into muscular contraction of the cell, with calcium serving as the messenger.

Depolarization and conduction of the SA and AV nodal tissue are mediated by the slow influx of calcium ions. Thus, because nodal or pacer tissue is calcium-driven, it is anticipated that the effects of calcium-channel blockade will be more profound in these tissues.

MECHANISMS OF ACTION

Electrophysiology

Calcium-channel agents block the intracellular movement of calcium. Their primary electrical effects include (1) depression of automaticity by slowing the rate of SA-nodal firing, (2) slowing of conduction through the AV node, thereby slowing ventricular response, and (3) negative inotropic effect on myocardial contractility, attributable to less calcium available for excitation-contraction coupling.

Because the cardiac effects of calcium-channel blockade are primarily confined to atrial tissue, the clinical utility of these agents is in the treatment of supraventricular tachyarrhythmias, including paroxysmal supraventricular tachycardia (PSVT) and atrial flutter or atrial fibrillation with a fast ventricular response.

Effect on Vascular and Cardiac Smooth Muscle

Calcium's role in excitation-contraction coupling is not limited to cardiac tissue. The contraction-relaxation response of other cell types is also determined by calcium. The calcium-channel agents, therefore, affect contraction in other types of muscle; the extent of the effect and the type of muscle affected are largely determined by the structure and dose of the calcium-channel agent used.

Currently available compounds have their most pronounced effects on vascular smooth muscle, both in the coronary arteries and in arterial beds in the periphery. Administration of these agents causes a decrease in peripheral vascular resistance through preferential dilation of the arterioles. This action decreases BP, afterload, and myocardial oxygen demands. There is also a reflexive increase in HR, which may be controlled by administration of a beta-blocking agent.

Dilation of the coronary arteries contributes to the clinical utility of these agents in the management of ischemic heart disease, including classic and variant angina pectoris.

Distinct differences exist between the relative degree of activity of various calcium-channel blockers at sites of action in the atria and peripheral vascular beds and on myocardial contractility. Table 8-1 summarizes the effects of calcium channel blockers on conducting fibers and vascular and cardiac smooth muscle.

Verapamil (Calan, Isoptin)

Verapamil acts primarily at the AV node to slow calcium channels, decreasing conduction and prolonging the effective refractory period. Electrophysiologically it is classified as a class IC antiarrhythmic agent. Because of its effect on SA and AV node conduction, verapamil is very effective in treating supraventricular tachyarrhythmias and particularly effective in treating reentrance dysrhythmias. In addition, hemodynamically verapamil produces coronary artery and peripheral vasodilation. It also has the most potent negative inotropic agents of the calcium antagonists currently in use. Generally speaking, these negative effects on myocardial contractility are adequately compensated for by the

Table 8-1

EFFECTS OF CALCIUM-CHANNEL BLOCKERS ON SITES OF ACTION

Drug	HR	SA Nodal Automaticity	AV Nodal Conduction	Myocardial Contractility	Arteriolar Vasodilation
Nifedipine	↑	—	0/↓	↓	↑↑↑
Verapamil	↑↓	↓↓	↓↓↓	↓↓	↑↑
Diltiazem	0/↓	↓	↓↓	↓	↑

decrease in afterload and sympathetic nervous system stimulation that is associated with these agents.

Indications: Supraventricular dysrhythmias, angina.

Usual dosage: Initial: PO 80 mg q 6-8 h, **IV:** 5-10 mg bolus (0.15-0.75 mg/kg) IVP over 2-3 min. Repeat q 30 min if no response. **Maintenance:** 80-120 mg q 6-8 h; **Maximum:** 480 mg/day; **SR tab:** 240 mg/day.

Precautions/contraindications: Contraindicated in patients with sick sinus syndrome, second- or third-degree AV block, or systolic pressures <90 mm Hg; caution in patients with preexisting ventricular dysfunction or patients receiving concomitant therapy with other agents known to depress contractility, e.g. disopyramide. Not teratogenic in laboratory animals.

Side effects/adverse reactions: Bradycardia, hypotension, peripheral edema, dizziness, headache, constipation, nausea.

Pharmacokinetics: Plasma half-life: 3-7 h; **Route of elimination:** metabolized by liver, excreted in urine.

Interactions: Additive cardiac depression possible when given with beta-blockers; increases digoxin levels by 50%-70% during first week of therapy.

Nursing considerations: Caution when giving IV because of interaction with beta-blockers. Monitor for digoxin toxicity. Monitor ECG for AV block (can increase PR interval).

Nifedipine (Procardia, Adalat)

Nifedipine is a potent vasodilator of coronary arteries and arterioles. It causes peripheral dilation, decreasing peripheral vascular resistance. It may increase HR through reflexive sympathetic stimulation. Has no appreciable effect on the SA or AV node.

Indications: All types of angina (stable, variant, unstable), HTN, and possibly the early stages of AMI. Because it has no effect on the SA or AV node, may be used in patients with AV disease.

Usual dosage: PO/SL: 10-40 mg q 6-8 h; **Maximum:** 180 mg.

Precautions/contraindications: Caution in pregnancy (shown to be teratogenic in laboratory animals).

Side effects/adverse reactions: Peripheral edema, hypotension, reflex tachycardia, palpitations, dizziness, headache, light-headedness, weakness, nausea, diarrhea.

Pharmacokinetics: Plasma half-life: 3-5 h; **Route of elimination:** metabolized in liver, 75% excreted in urine.

Interactions: Cimetidine may increase concentration of nifedipine; increases digoxin levels by 45%-50%.

Nursing considerations: Monitor for symptoms of digitalis toxicity; no effect on PR interval.

Diltiazem (Cardizem)

Diltiazem has a greater affinity for the SA node. It is a Class IV antiarrhythmic agent. Physiologically it decreases conduction through SA and AV node, resulting in decreased HR. Causes vasodilation of coronary and peripheral arteries. Has little to no negative inotropic effect. Incidence of side effects associated with diltiazem is appreciably lower compared with verapamil and nifedipine.

Indications: Angina pectoris caused by coronary vasospasm, stable angina not relieved by nitrates or beta-blockers, mild to moderate HTN.

Usual dosage: PO: 30 mg qid initially, increasing gradually to 90 mg tid; **Maximum:** 240 mg/day.

Precautions/contraindications: Caution in pregnancy (shown to produce skeletal abnormalities in laboratory animals).

Side effects/adverse reactions: Slight peripheral edema, headache, nausea, dermatitis, rash, petechiae, photosensitivity.

Pharmacokinetics: Plasma half-life: 2-6 h; **Route of elimination:** metabolized in liver, excreted in urine (35%) and GI (65%).

Interactions: In combination with beta-blockers or digoxin, may prolong AV conduction; diltiazem may increase carbamazepine concentration. Cimetidine may increase concentration of diltiazem.

Nursing considerations: Monitor ECG for prolonged PR interval and potential for AV block.

VASODILATORS

Vasodilators improve cardiac performance through relaxation of blood vessels. These agents cause various degrees of arteriolar and/or venous dilation. Vasodilators are widely used in therapy for heart failure and reduction of HTN. General indications include systemic HTN, severe CHF, ischemic heart disease, cardiomyopathy, aortic or mitral insufficiency, and AMI with associated heart failure or shock. The principal adverse reactions associated with vasodilator therapy are hypotension, tachycardia, and CNS disturbances (e.g., dizziness, syncope, and headache).

Vasodilators can be classified into four groups by primary mechanism of action (see box on page 295).

Mechanism of Action

The goal of vasodilator therapy is primarily to reduce afterload, preload, or both (see box on page 295).

CLASSIFICATION OF VASODILATORS

Direct Smooth Muscle Relaxants
Sodium nitroprusside	B
Nitrates	P
Hydralazine	A
Diazoxide	A
Minoxidil	A

Calcium Antagonists
Nifedipine	A

Angiotensin converting enzyme (ACE) inhibitors
Captopril	B
Enalapril	B

Alpha-adrenergic receptor blockers
Prazosin	B
Labetalol	A
Phentolamine	A

Site of action: A-primarily afterloads; P-primarily preload; B-balanced.

Afterload

Reducing resistance to LV ejection and aortic impedance (afterload) may increase stroke volume and CO without increasing myocardial oxygen demand. Afterload reduction implies a decrease in the myocardial oxygen uptake. The work of the heart and the oxygen uptake can also be reduced by adding inotropic and diuretic agents.

Preload

LV filling pressure (preload) is elevated in left heart failure. The effect of administering preload-reducing agents is to increase venous capacitance, which will result in a reduction of both RV and LV filling pressures. Drugs such as nitrates dilate the systemic veins, causing a decrease in venous return to the heart and thus ventricular filling pressure. In addition to reduction of preload, the combination of inotropic and diuretic agents may be effective.

DIRECT SMOOTH-MUSCLE RELAXANTS
Sodium Nitroprusside (Nipride)

Sodium nitroprusside is a potent, rapid-acting IV agent that has a balanced effect in dilating both arterioles and veins and decreases venous return.

Indications: CHF, AMI, acute hypertensive crisis.

Usual dosage: IV: 0.5-10.0 μg/kg/min; **Infusion:** 200 μg/ml (50/250 D5W).

Precautions/contraindications: Caution in patients with hepatic dysfunction, renal failure, hypothyroidism.

Side effects/adverse reactions: Nausea, retching, headache, ataxia, blurred vision, delirium, dizziness, vomiting, tinnitus.

Pharmacokinetics: Plasma half-life: 2-5 min (effect stops within 10 min of stopping infusion); **Route of elimination:** metabolized by liver, excreted by kidney; **Hemodynamic effects:** decreases SVR, CO, LVEDP, PVR, BP; increases HR.

Interactions: Do not mix with any drug in syringe or solution.

Nursing considerations: Sodium nitroprusside is photosensitive; cover solution with opaque material and change every 4 h. Administer by infusion pump only.

Avoid infusion with other medications because of "bolus effect." Obtain baseline hemodynamic readings and parameters before administering sodium nitroprusside. Monitor BP closely, avoid in diastolic BP less than 60 mm Hg. Monitor thiocynate levels and assess for signs and symptoms of cyanide poisoning (absent reflexes, coma, hypotension, dilated pupils, metabolic acidosis [early sign] and shallow breathing). Amyl nitrite inhalations and IV sodium thiosulfate are used to treat acute cyanide poisoning. Assess for signs of extravasation.

Nitroglycerin (Nitrostat, Nitro-Bid, Nitro-Dur, Transderm-Nitro)

Nitroglycerin dilates vascular smooth muscle, which decreases peripheral vascular resistance and decreases venous return.

Indications: Angina, CHF with elevated PCWP.

Usual dosage: SL: gr 1/150 (0.4 mg)-gr 1/200 (0.6 mg); **IV:** 200 μg/ml (50 mg/250 D5W), 5 μg/min titrated in 5 μg increments; **Oint (2%):** 1-2 in; **Transdermal:** 2.5-15.0 mg over 24 h.

Precautions/contraindications: None.

Side effects/adverse reactions: Postural hypotension, tachycardia, dizziness, syncope, headache, cutaneous flushing, vomiting.

Pharmacokinetics: Plasma half-life: SL—7 min, oint (2%)—3-6 hr, **IV**—1-2 min; **Route of elimination:** metabolized by liver; **Hemodynamic effects:** decreases LVEDP, SVR, PCWP, BP; increases HR. Little or no increase in CO.

Interactions: None.

Nursing considerations: Establish baseline parameters and monitor hemodynamic status closely. Avoid giving with either a systolic or diastolic BP less than 90/60 mm Hg. Monitor for orthostatic hypotension. Oral analgesics may be helpful for headache. Remove cotton to prevent absorption of medication. **Sublingual route:** Instruct patient to keep NTG tablets in dark, light-protected bottles. (A burning sensation indicates fresh tablets.) Have patient lie down with sublingual administration. If given for angina, instruct patient that if pain is not relieved by 3 NTG tablets, contact physician immediately. **IV route:** Do not exceed 120 μg/min normally. Use infusion pump and recommended IV tubing (polyethylene) to prevent absorption of NTG. **Ointment/patches:** Remove residual ointment and rotate sites for patch. Cover applicator paper with plastic wrap and secure with tape to protect clothing and promote absorption.

Hydralazine (Apresoline)

Hydralazine is an arteriolar vasodilator used in the treatment of HTN, usually given in combination with other agents.

Indications: Moderate to severe HTN.

Usual dosage: PO: 10 mg qid initially, gradually increasing dose to 50 mg qid; **IV/IM:** 10-20 mg q 4-6 h, given slowly.

Precautions/contraindications: Dosage should be reduced in severe renal failure. Contraindicated in patients with ischemic heart disease, dissecting aneurysm, SLE syndrome.

Side effects/adverse reactions: Common side effects include headache, palpitations, anorexia, nausea, vomiting, diarrhea, sodium retention; infrequent side effects at higher doses include a lupus-like syndrome (muscle aching, rash, joint pain, fatigue).

Pharmacokinetics: Plasma half-life: 3-6 h; **Route of elimination:** metabolized by liver, excreted in urine; **Hemodynamic effects:** decreases SVR, BP; increases CO, HR; no change in LVEDP.

Interactions: Do not mix with any drug in syringe or solution.

Nursing considerations: Monitor BP frequently during and after PO or IV use. Instruct patient to take drug with food and to avoid sudden changes in posture. If dizziness occurs, patient should flex legs and arms before getting up from bed or from sitting position. The patient should avoid extremely hot showers or baths and alcohol.

Diazoxide (Hyperstat)

Diazoxide is a direct-acting arteriolar vasodilator used for therapy in a hypertensive crisis. The vasodilator effect is not sustained, so this agent is unsuitable for chronic HTN and afterload reduction.

Indications: Hypertensive crisis.

Usual dosage: IV: 1-3 mg/kg given rapidly every 5 to 15 min up to 150 mg until diastolic pressure <100 mm Hg.

Precautions/contraindications: Contraindicated in dissecting aortic aneurysm, coarctation of the aorta, intracerebral hemorrhage.

Side effects/adverse reactions: Transient hyperglycemia, edema, CHF, hypotension, nausea, vomiting, dizziness, weakness.

Pharmacokinetics: Plasma half-life: 4-12 min; **Route of elimination:** excreted by liver (⅓) and kidney (⅓); **Hemodynamic effects:** decreases BP, SVR and increases CO, HR.

Interactions: Do not mix with any drug in syringe or solution. May increase effects of warfarin.

Nursing considerations: Monitor BP closely. Keep patient supine. Diazoxide can cause hyperglycemia; monitor serum glucose. Monitor intake and output and assess for signs and symptoms of fluid retention (can precipitate heart failure). IM injections can produce inflammation, pain, and sometimes necrosis.

Minoxidil (Loniten)

Minoxidil is a direct-acting vasodilator of arteriolar smooth muscle (similar to diazoxide). Requires concomitant beta-blockade and diuretics to reduce tachycardia and avoid sodium and fluid retention, which are associated with its administration.

Indications: Severe HTN refractory to other antihypertensive agents.

Usual dosage: PO initial: 1-2 mg bid to tid; **Maintenance:** 3-10 mg/day; **Maximum:** 20 mg/day.

Precautions/contraindications: Contraindicated in MI, dissecting aortic aneurysm, pheochromocytoma.

Side effects/adverse reactions: Angina, rebound HTN, tachycardia, increased T-wave, pericardial effusion, sodium and fluid retention, CHF, dizziness, drowsiness, hirsutism, rash, gynecomastia.

Pharmacokinetics: Plasma half-life: 3 h; **Route of elimination:** metabolized by liver, excreted in feces; **Hemodynamic effects:** decreases SVR, LVEDP, BP; increases CO.

Interactions: None.

Nursing considerations: Monitor for signs and symptoms of fluid retention, ECG changes, tachycardia, rebound HTN, pericardial effusion. Instruct patient to report dizziness, difficulty breathing, orthopnea, signs of peripheral edema, rapid weight gain, angina.

CALCIUM ANTAGONISTS
Nifedipine (Procardia)

Nifedipine acts as a potent vasodilator by dilating peripheral arterioles, thus reducing the total peripheral resistance (afterload) against which the heart works. Also dilates the main coronary arteries and coronary arterioles, causing relaxation and prevention of coronary artery spasm.

ANGIOTENSIN CONVERTING ENZYME (ACE) INHIBITORS
Captopril (Capoten)
Enalapril (Vasotec)

Captopril and Enalapril act as competitive inhibitors of ACE; inhibition of ACE leads to decrease in plasma levels of angiotensin II, a potent vasoconstrictor. Captopril and enalapril act as both arteriolar and venous vasodilators. Major advantages are lack of fluid retention and reduction of plasma aldosterone level; major disadvantage, especially with captopril, is hypotension.

Indications: HTN, patients with CHF who are unresponsive to conventional therapy.

Usual dosage:
Captopril
PO: For HTN 25 mg tid; may increase up to 450 mg/day. For CHF 6.25-12.5 mg bid, tid.
Enalapril
PO: initial: 2.5-5.0 mg/day; **Maintenance:** 10-40 mg as single dose or 2 divided doses; **Maximum:** 40 mg/day.

Precautions/contraindications: Caution in patients with renal disease or renal failure.

Side effects/adverse reactions: *Captopril:* Dysrhythmias, dizziness, light-headedness, orthostatic hypotension, angioedema, fever, agranulocytosis, neutropenia or proteinuria, hyperkalemia, metallic taste.
Enalapril: Headache, dizziness, fatigue, angioedema, hypotension, abdominal pain, nausea, neutropenia, hyperkalemia.

Pharmacokinetics: Plasma half-life: 6-12 h (Captopril), 11 h (Enalapril), **Route of elimination:** excreted by kidney; **Hemodynamic effects:** decreases BP, SVR, LVEDP; increases CO.

Interactions: Do not use with vasodilators (hydralazine, prazosin).

Nursing considerations: *Captopril* Instruct patient to avoid sudden changes in body position. Monitor BP closely. Administer 1 h before meals. Monitor for proteinuria; obtain protein estimates (dipstick) before therapy at 9 month intervals. Monitor WBCs and observe for neutropenia. Instruct patient on signs and symptoms of infection. Monitor serum potassium levels; do not give potassium-sparing diuretics or potassium supplements.
Enalapril: Good for patient compliance because of once-a-day-dosing. OK to take with food. Patients receiving diuretic therapy should be closely monitored for hypotension. Monitor WBCs; instruct patient to report signs and symptoms of infection. Monitor serum potassium levels. Hct and Hgb levels can decrease with enalapril; monitor CBC and assess for anemia.

ALPHA-ADRENERGIC RECEPTOR BLOCKERS
Prazosin (Minipress)

Prazosin is an alpha-adrenergic blocker with both arteriolar and venous vasodilatory properties.

Indications: Mild to moderate HTN.

Usual dosage: Initial: 1-2 mg bid, tid; **Maintenance:** 3-10 mg/day; **Maximum:** 20 mg/day.

Precautions/contraindications: Caution in patients with liver disease.

Side effects/adverse reactions: Dizziness, headache, syncope, weakness, orthostatic hypotension, depression, palpitations, blurred vision, dry mouth, nausea, vomiting, abdominal cramps, constipation, priapism.

Pharmacokinetics: Plasma half-life: 2-3 h, longer if CHF present; **Route of elimination:** metabolized by liver, excreted primarily in feces; **Hemodynamic effects:** decreases BP, SVR, LVEDP; increases CO.

Interactions: May increase hypotensive effects with beta blocker, nitroglycerine.

Nursing considerations: Assess for fluid deficit; monitor intake and output daily. If patient is potentially hypovolemic because of sodium-restricted diet or diuretics, correct first before starting therapy. Syncope may occur with first dose, so administer first "low" dose at night and gradually increase dose depending on patient's clinical response. Patients usually receive a diuretic with prazosin to potentiate its effect as an antihypertensive agent. A small-dose beta-blocker may also be given if tachycardia is present.

Labetalol (Trandate, Normodyne)

Labetalol is a combined alpha- and beta-blocking agent. Useful as a vasodilator in treatment and management of HTN. See section on Beta-Adrenergic Blocking Agents on pages 288-292 for specific information.

Phentolamine (Regitine, Rogitine)

Phentolamine has mainly been used as an IV arteriolar vasodilator in low-output LV failure. Increases CO and decreases SVR. Small effect when using on LV filling pressure. Primarily an alpha-blocking agent, but may also release norepinephrine, which may account for the tachycardia and increased inotropic effect.

Indications: HTN, pheochromocytoma.

Usual dosage: PO: 50-100 mg q 4-6 h; **IV:** 10 μg/kg/min increased by 10 μg every 15 min, up to 120 mg/h.

Precautions/contraindications: Contraindicated in patients with MI, angina.

Side effects/adverse reactions: Tachycardia, dysrhythmias, angina, hypotension, weakness, dizziness, flushing, nausea, vomiting.

Pharmacokinetics: Plasma half-life: unknown; **Route of elimination:** unknown; **Hemodynamic effects:** decreases SVR,BP; increases CO, HR; no change in LVEDP.

Interactions: May increase effects of certain antihypertensives. Not to be mixed in solution or syringe with any drug except levarterenol.

Nursing considerations: Monitor BP and HR closely during administration. Prolonged hypotension may occur with parenteral use. May be used for prevention and treatment of skin necrosis follow extravasation of norepinephrine.

DRUGS USED IN TREATMENT OF HYPERLIPOPROTEINEMIAS

Hyperlipoproteinemias are conditions in which the concentration of cholesterol or triglyceride-carrying lipoproteins in plasma exceeds normal limits. This condition is of clinical concern because elevated concentrations of lipoproteins can lead to development of atherosclerosis, thrombosis, and possible MI. Drug therapy in this area is aimed at lowering concentrations of the lipoproteins in plasma, either by decreasing production of them or by removing them from the plasma. The decision to initiate drug therapy should be acted on when serum lipid protein levels do not respond adequately to dietary intervention. For treatment purposes, if patient's total cholesterol is greater than 240 mg/dl, drug therapy is started. Blood-cholesterol levels are usually drawn every 3-4 mo to evaluate efficacy of the drug.

DRUGS THAT LOWER PLASMA CONCENTRATIONS OF LIPOPROTEINS

Niacin

Niacin acts by decreasing the production of "very low-density lipoproteins" (VLDL) as a result of the drug's inhibition of lipolysis in adipose tissue.

Indications: Hyperlipoproteinemia.

Usual dosage: Niacin: 1.5-6.0 g/day, given in 2-4 divided dosages. Some patients may require up to 9 g/day. **Alternative** dose schedules: Initiate with 100 mg tid, increasing dose by 300 mg/day at 4-7 day interval. Others recommend initiating therapy at 500 mg tid and gradually increasing dosage until desired effect is achieved.

Precautions/contraindications: Caution in patients with jaundice or liver disease, gallbladder disease, diabetes mellitus, gout, peptic ulcer, and allergy. Contraindicated in patients with arterial hemorrhaging, severe hypotension, liver disease, active peptic-ulcer disease; women who are pregnant or may become pregnant; women who are breast-feeding, unless the possible benefits outweigh the potential risks because toxicologic studies have not been conducted with large doses of niacin.

Side effects/adverse reactions: The majority of side effects are dose-related and generally subside with dose reduction. Most common adverse effects are GI upset and intense cutaneous flushing of face, neck, and upper body (flushing usually occurs within 15-20 min of administration and lasts for about 30-60 min). Other adverse effects include pruritus, burning or tingling of skin, diarrhea, nausea, vomiting, hypotension, dizziness, tachycardia, palpitations, and dysrhythmia. Can cause significant hepatic dysfunction. Can exacerbate diabetes mellitus by elevating FBS. Can elevate uric acid, thereby precipitating gouty arthritis attacks.

Interactions: None.

Nursing considerations: Niacin must be started in small doses (50-100 mg) and increased gradually over several weeks to avoid side effects. Instruct patient not to take niacin on an empty stomach. Monitor blood-glucose concentration periodically, especially in the early course of therapy. (Insulin or oral hypoglycemia dosage requirements may change in diabetic patients.)

Clofibrate (Atromid-S)

Clofibrate's primary action is to increase the activity of the enzyme lipoprotein lipase, which in turn enhances the rate of intravascular catabolism of very low-density lipoproteins (VLDL) and intermediate-density lipoprotein (IDL) to low-density lipoprotein (LDL).

Indications: Hyperlipoproteinemia.

Usual dosage: 2 g/day, given in 2-4 divided doses.

Precautions/contraindications: Contraindicated in patients with clinically important renal or hepatic dysfunction or primary biliary cirrhosis. Patients with biliary cirrhosis may have increased serum cholesterol after clofibrate administration. The safe use of clofibrate during pregnancy has not been established, so the drug should not be used in pregnant women. The drug is contraindicated in breast-feeding women because it is not known if clofibrate is distributed into breast milk.

Side effects/adverse reactions: Generally well tolerated, but may cause an acute "flu-like" muscular syndrome with myalgia or myositis and symptoms of cramping, weakness, and arthralgia. Causes nausea, diarrhea, skin rash, alopecia, weakness, breast tenderness, impotence, decreased libido, cholelithiasis, cholecystitis, dysrhythmias, renal dysfunction, hepatic dysfunction, blood dyscrasias.

Interactions: May potentiate effects of warfarin. Dosage adjustment of the oral anticoagulant may be required to maintain desired prothrombin time.

Nursing considerations: Administer with food or milk to minimize gastric irritation. Frequent determinations of prothrombin time should be performed to determine if the dose of the anticoagulant should be adjusted. Routinely evaluate CBC, liver-function tests, and electrolytes throughout the course of therapy. May cause an increase in CPK levels and a decrease in plasma-fibrinogen levels.

Gemfibrozil (Lopid)

Gemfibrozil is similar to clofibrate in its mechanism of action in lowering plasma VLDL. Not known whether gemfibrozil influences production or removal—or both—of VLDL.

Indications: Hyperlipoproteinemia.

Usual dosage: 600 mg tid 30 min before morning and evening meals.

Precautions/contraindications: Contraindicated in patients with preexisting gallbladder disease and in those with hepatic or severe renal dysfunction. Should be avoided if possible in patients with past medical history of gallstones because it may promote cholelithiasis and cholecystitis. Safe use in pregnancy has not been established; not known if drug is distributed into breast milk.

Side effects/adverse reactions: GI pain or distress, eosinophilia, skin rash, musculoskeletal pain, blurred vision, mild anemia, leukopenia. May increase cholesterol excretion in bile; therefore, cholelithiasis and cholecystitis may occur.

Interactions: May potentiate effects of warfarin. Dosage adjustment of the oral anticoagulant may be required to maintain desired prothrombin time.

Nursing considerations: Make frequent determinations of prothrombin time to determine if the dose of the anticoagulant should be adjusted. Routinely evaluate CBC, liver-function tests, and electrolytes throughout the course of therapy. May cause an increase in CPK levels and a decrease in plasma-fibrinogen levels. Blood sugar should be monitored because it may increase. Administer with food or milk to minimize gastric irritation.

Probucol (Lorelco)

Probucol's mechanism of action in lowering serum cholesterol is uncertain. It is not known whether it acts to decrease the synthesis of LDL or to stimulate its catabolism. Drug also lowers plasma concentrations of HDL by suppression of protein synthesis.

Indications: Hyperlipoproteinemia.

Usual dosage: 500 mg tid with morning and evening meals.

Precautions/contraindications: Contraindicated in patients with evidence of recent or progressive myocardial damage or findings suggesting ventricular dysrhythmia; pregnant women (safe use has not been established); women who are breast-feeding (not known if drug is distributed in human milk; however, it is known that the drug is excreted into the milk of lactating animals).

Side effects/adverse reactions: Diarrhea, flatulence, abdominal pain, nausea; prolonged QT intervals can occur. Other adverse effects include headache, dizziness, elevation in liver and renal enzymes, increases in BUN and blood glucose.

Interactions: Should not be administered concomitantly with clofibrate because the reduction in total cholesterol is not additive and pronounced reduction in HDL-cholesterol may occur.

Nursing considerations: ECGs should be performed before intiating therapy and after 6 and 12 mos of therapy.

BILE ACID-BINDING RESINS

Cholestyramine Resin (Questran)
Colestipol (Colestid)

Cholestyramine resin and colestipol act to lower concentrations of plasma LDL-cholesterol by absorbing and binding bile acids in the intestine. This combination forms a new absorbable complex that is excreted along with unchanged resin in feces, thus resulting in partial removal of bile acids from enterohepatic circulation.

Indications: Hyperlipoproteinemia.

Usual dosage: 12-16 g (cholestyramine resin) or 15-30 g (colestipol) divided into 2-4 portions to be taken daily either before or during meals and at bedtime.

Precautions/contraindications: Contraindicated in patients with complete biliary obstruction in which no bile products reach the intestine. Cholestyramine resin should be used with caution in pregnant women; the resin is not absorbed systemically and therefore is not expected to cause fetal harm. Caution in women who are breast-feeding. Safe use of colestipol during pregnancy or lactation has not been established.

Side effects/adverse reactions: Constipation, nausea, abdominal discomfort, bloating, indigestion. High doses may cause steatorrhea and may impair absorption of fat-soluble vitamins. Other adverse effects include fecal impaction, hemorrhoidal bleeding, increased prothrombin time, negative dermatologic effects. Preparations have an unpleasant sandy or gritty taste.

Interactions: Since resins are of an even exchange type, they are capable of binding a number of drugs in the GI tract and delaying or reducing absorption. This effect has been documented with thiazide diuretics, thyroid hormones, anticoagulants, phenylbutazone, phenobarbital, various digitalis preparations.

Nursing considerations: Monitor bowel function. Encourage patient to increase fluid intake and milk in diet. Stool softeners and laxatives may be required to minimize constipating effects of medication. May cause an increase in SGOT, phosphate, chloride, and alkaline phosphatase and a decrease in serum calcium, sodium, and potassium levels. In doses of 24 g/day or higher, supplements of fat-soluble vitamins and folate may be required.

Lovastatin (Mevacor) (formally called mevinolin)
Lovastatin exerts its LDL cholesterol lowering effect by indirectly inhibiting HMG CoA reductase (3-hydroxy-3 methyl glutaryl coenzyme A reductase), the enzyme responsible for the rate-limiting conversion of acetyl CoA to mevalonate, a precursor of steroids, including cholesterol.

Indications: Hyperlipoproteinemia.

Usual dosage: 20 mg bid, with total dose ranging from 10-80 mg/day; usually initiate therapy with 20 mg in evening and add or increase doses in 20-mg increments by adding tablets in the morning or evening.

Precautions/contraindications: Contraindicated in patients with liver-enzyme elevations, active liver disease, renal failure with predisposition to rhabdomyositis. Contraindicated in pregnant or breast-feeding women because of teratogenic effects in animals.

Side effects/adverse reactions: Headache, GI problems, such as diarrhea, constipation, flatus, abdominal pain, cramping. Other adverse effects include liver dysfunction (increases in AST, ALT, CPK), lens opacities (cataract formation), myositis myalgias.

Interactions: Up to 5% of patients receiving lovastatin concomitantly with gemfibrozil developed myositis characterized by symptoms of myalgia and very high CPK levels.

Nursing considerations: Perform liver-function tests every 4 to 6 wks during the first 15 mos of therapy and periodically thereafter; therapy should be discontinued if aminotransferase levels rise above 3 times the upper normal limit and are persistent. Baseline and yearly slit-lamp optometry examinations should be conducted. Patients should be withdrawn from therapy if symptoms of muscle tenderness and pain and elevated CPK levels occur.

ANTIHYPERTENSIVE AGENTS

Phamacologic therapy for the management of hypertension is initiated once it is clear that nonpharmacologic treatment is ineffective in controlling blood pressure. Using a stepped approach, small doses of one drug from one class are given, increasing its dose and then adding another drug from another class in gradual increasing doses until the desired blood pressure is achieved with minimal side effects. (See page 134 for additional information regarding the stepped approach.)

Drugs used in the treatment of hypertension include diuretics, beta-adrenergic agents, alpha-adrenergic agents, angiotension-converting enzyme inhibitors, arteriolar vasodilators, central acting adrenergic inhibitors, and adrenergic neuronal blocking agents. Some of these drugs are listed below (see also other categories of drugs included in this chapter).

Diuretics
　Thiazides
　　Chlorothiazide (Diuril): 0.5-1 g/day
　　Hydrochlorothiazide (Esidrix, Hydrodiuril): 50-100 mg/day
　　Bendroflumethiazide (Naturetin): 2.5-10 mg/day
　Loop diuretics
　　Furosemide (Lasix): 40-80 mg bid or qid
　　Ethacrynic acid (Edecrin): initial dose 25-50 mg
　Potassium-sparing diuretics
　　Spironolactone (Aldactone): 100-400 mg bid or tid
　　Triamterene (Dyrenium): 100-300 mg bid
　　Amiloride (Midamor): 5-20 mg/day or bid
Beta-adrenergic blocking agents
　Propranolol (Inderal): 10-80 mg PO bid or qid
　Metoprolol tartrate (Lopressor): 50-200 mg PO qid or bid
　Pindolol (Visken): 15-60 mg/day
　Atenolol (Tenormin): 50-100 mg/day
　Timolol maleate (Blocadren): 20-40 mg/day
　Nadolol (Corgard): 80-320 mg/day
Antihypertensive agents
　Methyldopa (Aldomet): up to 2 g/day PO bid, tid, or qid
　Guanethidine (Ismelin): 5-200 mg/day PO
　Clonidine (Catapres): 0.1-1.2 mg PO bid
　Captopril (Capoten): 24-150 mg tid
　Hydrazaline (Apresoline): 10-50 mg PO qid
　Sodium nitroprusside (Nipride): 0.5-10 μg/kg/min IV
　Diazoxide (Hyperstat): 300 mg by rapid IV bolus
Alpha-adrenergic blocking agents
　Phentolamine (Regitine): 1-5 mg IV intermittently
　Prazosin (Minipress): initial dose 1 mg PO, slowly increased to 10-15 mg/day

References

1. Akhtar: Practical considerations in the treatment of ventricular arrhythmias with Mexiletine, Am Heart J, 107(5):1086.

2. American Heart Association: Heart Facts—1989, Dallas, Texas, 1980, National Center.

3. American Heart Association Standards and guidelines for cardiopulmonary resuscitation and emergency cardiac care, JAMA 225:2841, 1986.

4. Anastasiou-Nana MI, Anderson JL, Askins JC et al: Long-term experience with Sotalol in the treatment of complex ventricular arrhythmias, Am Heart J 114(2):288, Aug 1987.

5. Anderson CS: The pathophysiology of shock: an overview. In Guthrie MM, New York, 1982, Churchill Livingstone, Inc.

6. Andreoli KG et al: Comprehensive cardiac care, ed 6, St Louis, 1987, The CV Mosby Co.

7. Reference deleted in page proof.

8. Balwin JC and Shumway NE: The status of cardiac transplantation. In Rapaport E editor: Cardiology update: review for physician, New York, 1986, Elsevier-New York Inc.

9. Barry J and Dieter WG: Endocarditis: an overview, Heart Lung 11(2):138, March—April 1982.

10. Belloni FL: The local control of coronary blood flow. Cardiovasc Res, 13.63, 1979.

11. Blake S: The clinical diagnosis of constrictive pericarditis, Am Heart J 106(2):432, August 1983.

12. Bobak IM, Jensen MD, and Zalar MK: Maternity and gynecologic care, ed 4, St Louis, 1989, The CV Mosby Co.

13. Braunwald E, editor: Heart disease: a textbook of cardiovascular medicine, Philadelphia, 1988 WB Saunders Co.

14. Breu CS, Lindenmuth JE, and Tillisch JH: Treatment of patients with congestive and cardiomyopathy during hospitalization: a case study, Heart Lung, 11(5)229, May—June 1982.

15. Brown WJ: A classification of microorganisms frequently causing sepsis, Heart Lung, 5:397, 1976.

16. Bulkley B, Weisfeldt and Hutchins GM: Asymmetric septal hypertrophy and myocardial fiber disarray, Circulation 56(2): 292 Aug 1977.

17. Burke LH, O'Brien S, and Norris S: Nursing care of patient with recurrent ventricular dysrhythmias. In Kern L, editor: Cardiac critical care nursing, Rockville, MD, 1988, Aspen Publishers, Inc.

18. Cain R, Ferguson RM, and Tillisch J: Variant angina: a nursing approach, Heart Lung 8:1122, Nov—Dec 1979.

19. Cairns JA, Gent, M, Singer J et al: Aspirin, sulfinpyrazone, or both in unstable angina, N Engl J Med 313:1369, 1985.

20. Cannom DS and Winkle RA: Implantation of the automatic implantable cardioverter defibrillator (AICD): practical aspects, PACE 9:723, 1987.

21. Canobbio MM, editor: Congenital heart disease in adults, Nurs Clin North Am 19:469, 1984.

22. Canobbio MM: The Eisenmenger syndrome, Nurs Clin North Am 19:537, 1984.

23. Choong CY, Roubin GS, Harris PJ et al: A comparison of the effect of beta-blockers with and without ISA on hemodynamics and left ventricular function at rest and during exercise in patients with coronary artery disease, J Cardiovasc Pharmacol 8(3)441, May—June 1986.

24. Clark S: Ineffective coping: patient and family. In Kern LS, editor: Cardiac critical care, 1988.

25. Collen D et al: Coronary thrombolysis with recombinant human tissue type plasminogen activator: a prospective randomized, placebo trial, Circulation 70:1012, 1984.

26. Colucci WS: Usefulness of calcium antagonists for congestive heart failure, Am J Cardiol 59:52B, Jan 30, 1987.

27. Conolly ME, Kersting F, and Dollery CT: The clinical pharmacology of beta-adrenoceptor-blocking drugs, Prog Cardiovasc Dis 19:203, 1976.

28. Conover MB: Cardiac arrhythmias: exercises in pattern interpretation, ed 2, St Louis, 1978, The CV Mosby Co.

29. Conover MB: Exercises in diagnosing ECG tracings, ed 3, St. Louis, 1984, The CV Mosby Co.

30. Conover MB: Understanding electrocardiology: physiological and interpretive concepts, ed 5, St Louis, 1988 The CV Mosby Co.

31. Cooper DK, Valladares, and Futterman LG: Care of the patient with automatic

implantable cardioverter defibrillator: a guide for nurses, Heart Lung 16:640, 1987.

32. Craven RF and Curry TD: When the diagnosis is Raynaud's, AJNR, 8(5):1007, May 1981.

33. Danilo Jr P: Aprindine, Am Heart J, 97:119, 1979.

34. DeWood MA et al: Coronary arteriographic findings of acute transmural myocardial infarction, Circulation 58:139, 1983.

35. Dixon MB, and Nunnelee J: Arterial reconstruction for atherosclerotic occlusive disease, J Cardiovasc Nurs 1:36, 1987.

36. Dixon MB: Acute aortic dissection, J Cardiovasc Nurs, 1:24, 1987.

37. Doenges ME, Jeffries MF, and Moorhouse MF: Nursing care plans: nursing diagnosis in planning patient care, Philadelphia 1984, FA Davis Company.

38. Dole WP and O'Rourke RA: Pathophysiology and management of cardiogenic shock. In Harvey WP, editor: Current problems in cardiology, 8:1, 1983.

39. Doyle B: Nursing challenge: the patient with end stage heart failure. In Kern LS: Cardiac critical care, Rockville, MD, 1988, Aspen Publishers, Inc.

40. Doyle JE: Treatment modalities in peripheral vascular disease Nurs Clin North Am, 58:139, 1983.

41. Fergenbaum H: Echocardiography. In Braunwald E, editor: Heart disease: a textbook of cardiovascular medicine, Philadelphia, 1988, WB Saunders Co.

42. Ferlinz J: Nifedipine in myocardial ischemia, systemic hypertension, and other cardiovascular disorders, Ann Intern Med 105(5):714, Nov 1986.

43. Flaherty JT, Becker LC, Bulkley BH et al: A randomized prospective trial of intravenous nitroglycerin in patients with acute myocardial infarction, Circulation 68(3):576, Sept 1983.

44. Franciosa JA: Nitroglycerin and nitrates in congestive heart failure, Heart Lung 9(5):873, Sept—Oct 1980.

45. Frankl WS and Greenspan AJ: Electrophysiology testing: clinical applications, Cardiovasc Clin 13(3):301, 1982.

46. Funk M: Diagnosis of right ventricular infarction with right precordial ECG leads, Heart Lung 15:562, 1986.

47. Funk M: Heart transplantation: postoperative care during the acute period, Crit Care Med 6:27, 1988.

48. Gabriel Khan MI: Manual of cardiac drug therapy, London, 1984, Baulliere Tindall.

49. Gardner PE and Laurent-Bopp D: Continuous $S_V O_2$ monitoring: clinical application in critical care, Prog Cardiovasc Nurs 2:9, 1987.

50. Ginzton LE and Laks MM: Acute pericarditis: recognition by ECG, Prim Cardiol 10:73-84.

51. Girlando RM, Belew B, and Klara F: Coarctation of the aorta, Crit Care Nurs 8:38, 1988.

52. GISSI trial: Effectiveness of intravenous thrombolytic treatment in acute myocardial infarction, Lancet, 1:397, 1986.

53. Glagov S and Zairns C: Pathology of aneurysm formation. In Aneurysm, Baltimore, 1983, Williams & Wilkins, Inc.

54. Goldberger E: Textbook of clinical cardiology, St. Louis, 1982, The CV Mosby Co.

55. Goldstein JL and Brown MS: Genetics and cardiovascular disease. In Braunwald E: Heart disease: a textbook of cardiovascular medicine, Philadelphia, 1988, WB Saunders Co.

56. Goodwin JF: Hypertrophic cardiomyopathy: a disease in search of its own identity, Am J Cardiol 45:177, 1980.

57. Gregoratos G and Karlinger JS: Infective endocarditis: diagnosis and management, Med Clin North Am 63:173, 1979.

58. Groer MW and Shekleton ME: Basic pathophysiology: a conceptual approach, St Louis, 1983, The CV Mosby Co.

59. Guazzi M, Olivari MT, Polese A et al: Repetitive myocardial ischemia of Prinzmetal type with angina pectoris, Am J Cardiol 37:923, 1976.

60. Guthrie MM, editor: Shock, NY, 1982, Churchill Livingstone, Inc.

61. Guyton AC: Textbook of medical physiology, ed 8, Philadelphia, 1980, WB Saunders Co.

62. Guzzetta CE and Dossey BM: Cardiovascular nursing: body, mine, and tapestry, St Louis, 1984, The CV Mosby Co.

63. Hammill SC, Sorenson PB, Wood DL et al: Propafenone for the treatment of refractory complex ventricular ectopic activity, Mayo Clin Proc 61(2)98, Feb 1986.

64. Harris L et al: The cardiovascular effects of caffeine post-myocardial infarction, Circulation 72 (suppl III): 116, 1985.

65. Herling IM: Intravenous nitroglycerin: clinical pharmacology and therapeutic considerations, Am Heart J 108(1):141, July 1984.

66. Hess ML et al: The noninvasive diagnosis of acute and chronic cardiac allograft rejection, Heart Transplant 1.

67. Hirman JA: Nursing assessment and nursing diagnosis in patients with peripheral vascular disease, Nurs Clin North Am 21:219, 1986.

68. Hoffman BF and Cranefield PF: The physiological basis of cardiac arrhythmias, Am J Med 37:670, 1964.

69. Hoffman JE: Natural history of congenital heart disease: problems in its assessment with special reference to ventricular septal defects, Circulation 37:97, 1968.

70. Holmes DR, et al: Percutaneous transluminal coronary angioplasty alone or in combination with streptokinase therapy during MI, Mayo Clin Proc 60:449, 1985.

71. Hume M: Examination of the arterial system, Hosp Med, Oct 1970.

72. Irvin JD and Viau JM: Safety profiles of angiotensin converting enzyme inhibitors captopril and enalapril, Am J Med 81(suppl 4C), Oct 31, 1986.

73. Isner JM and Roberts WC: Right ventricular infarction complicating left ventricular infarction secondary to coronary heart disease, Am J Cardiol 42:885, 1978.

74. Jaffe AJ and Sobel BE: Thrombolysis with tissue type plasminogen activator in acute myocardial infarction: potentials and pitfalls, JAMA 1986.

75. Jamieson SW et al: Heart transplantation for end-stage ischemic heart disease: the Stanford experience, Heart Transplant 3:224, 1984.

76. Joint National Committee: The 1984 Report of the National Committee on Detection, Evaluation, and Treatment of High Blood Pressure, Arch Intern Med 144:1045, 1984.

77. Josephson M, Harken A, Horowitz L: Endocardial excision: a new surgical technique for the treatment of recurrent ventricular tachycardia, Circulation, 60:1430, 1979.

78. Josephson M and Horowitz L: Electrophysiologic approach to therapy of recurrent sustained ventricular tachycardia, Am J Cardiol 43:631, 1979.

79. Kannel WB, McGee D, and Gordon T: A general cardiovascular risk profile: the Framingham Study, Am J Cardiol 38:46, 1976.

80. Kasper W, Msinhertz T, Wollschlager M et al: Coronary thrombolysis during myocardial infarction by intravenous BRL-26921, a new anisoylated plasminogen-streptokinase activator complex, Am J Cardiol 68:418, 1986.

81. Kennedy JW et al: Western Washington randomized trial of intracoronary streptokinase in acute myocardial infarction, N Engl J Med 309:1477, 1983.

82. Kennedy JW et al: Acute myocardial in-

farction treated with intracoronary streptokinase: a report of the society for coronary angiography, Am J Cardiol 55:871, 1985.

83. Kenny J: Calcium channel-blocking agents and the heart, Br Med J (Clin Res), 26,291:1150, Oct 1985.

84. Kent KM: Percutaneous transluminal angioplasty: report from Registry of National Heart Lung and Blood Institute, Am J Cardiol 49:2011, 1982.

85. Kent KM: Transluminal coronary angioplasty. In Rackey CE, editor: Advances in critical care cardiology, Cardiovasc Clin 16:53, 1986.

86. Kern L: Mechanical support of failing heart in congestive heart failure. In Michaelson C editor: Congestive heart failure, St Louis, 1983, The CV Mosby Co.

87. Kim MJ et al: Pocket guide to nursing diagnoses, ed 2, St Louis, 1987, The CV Mosby Co.

88. King SL: Patient care in vascular surgery, AORNJ, 33(5)843, April 1981.

89. Kirchhoff KT: An examination of the physiologic basis for coronary precaution, Heart Lung 15:874, 1981.

90. Kistner RL, Ball JJ, Nordyke RA, and Freeman GC: Incidence of pulmonary embolism and thrombophlebitis of lower extremities, Am J Surg 124:169, 1972.

91. Kloner RA and Braunwald E: Effects of calcium antagonists on infarcting myocardium, Am J Cardiol 30:59(3):84B, Jan 1987.

92. Krikler DM: Calcium antagonists for chronic stable angina pectoris, Am J Cardiol 59:95B, Jan 30, 1987.

93. Laffel O and Braunwald E: Thrombolytic therapy: a new strategy for treatment of acute myocardial infarction, Part I, N Engl J Med 311:710, 1984.

94. Lai WT, Huycke EC, and Sung RJ: Supraventricular tachyarrhythmias: mechanisms, types and management, Postgrad Med J 83:209, 1988.

95. Lees RS and Lees AM: Lipid lowering drugs: renewed enthusiasm, Drug Therapy, pp. 57-74, May 1984.

96. LeFrock JL, Ellis CA et al: Transient bacteremia associated with sigmoidoscopy, N Engl J Med 289:469, 1973.

97. LeFrock JL, Klainer AS et al: Transient bacteremia associated with nasotracheal suctioning, JAMA 236:1610, 1977.

98. Levitt JM and Karp RB: Heart transplantation, Surg Clin North Am 65:613, 1985.

99. Lewis HD, Davis JW, Archibald DG et al: Protective effects of aspirin against acute myocardial infarction and death in men with unstable angina, N Engl J Med 309:396, 1983.

100. Lewis SM and Collier IC: Medical surgical nursing: assessment and management of clinical problems, New York, 1983, McGraw-Hill Book Co.

101. Lipid Research Clinics Program: The lipid research clinics coronary primary prevention trial results: I. reduction in incidence of coronary artery disease, JAMA, 251:351, 1984.

102. Lough ME: Quality of life issues following heart transplantation, Prog Cardiovasc Nurs 1:17, 1986.

103. Ludmer P and Goldschlager N: Cardiac pacing in the 1980's, N Engl J Med 311:1671, 1984.

104. Malasanos L, Barkauskas V, and Stoltenberg-Allen K: Health assessment, ed 4, St Louis, 1990, The CV Mosby Co.

105. Marcus FI, Fontaine GH, Frank R et al: Clinical pharmacology and therapeutic applications of the antiarrhythmic agent, Amiodarone, Am Heart J 101:480, 1981.

106. Marriott HJ and Conover MHB: Advanced concepts in arrhythmias, St Louis, 1983, The CV Mosby Co.

107. Massy JA: Diagnostic testing for peripheral vascular disease, Nurs Clin North Am 21.207, 1986.

107a. McCance K and Huether SE: Pathophysiology, ed 1, St Louis, 1990, The CV Mosby Co.

108. McFarland GK and McFarlane EA: Nursing diagnosis and intervention: planning for patient care, St Louis, 1989, The CV Mosby Co.

109. Mercer M: The electrophysiology study: a nursing concern, Crit Care Nurs 7:58, 1987.

110. Michaelson CR, editor: Congestive heart failure, St Louis, 1983, The CV Mosby Co.

111. Miller DC and Roon AJ: Diagnosis and management of peripheral vascular disease, Menlo Park, CA, Addison-Wesley Publishing Co, Inc.

112. Minowski N: The automatic implantable cardioverter-defibrillator: an overview, J Am Coll Cardiol 6:461, 1981.

113. Moore S: Pericarditis after acute myocardial infarction: manifestations and nursing implications, Heart Lung 8(3):551, May-June 1979.

114. Moore WS: What's new in peripheral vascular surgery, J Cardiovasc Surg 24:49, 1983.

115. Murdaugh C: Coronary heart disease in women, Prog Cardiovasc Nurs 1:9, Oct-Dec 1986.

116. Myerberg RJ and Castellanos: Cardiac arrest and sudden death. In Braunwald E, editor: Heart disease: a textbook of cardiovascular medicine, Philadelphia, 1988, WB Saunders Co.

117. Nathan A, Hellestrand K, Bexton R et al: The pro-arrhythmic effect of the new "antiarrhythmic" drug, Flecainide Acetate, (Abstract), J Am Coll Cardiol 1:709, 1983.

118. Neil CA: Etiology of congenital heart disease, Cardiovasc Clin 4:138, 1972.

119. Norwegian Multicenter Trial: Timolol-induced reduction in mortality and reinfarction in patients surviving acute myocardial infarction, N Engl J Med 304:801, 1981.

120. Reference deleted in page proof.

121. Opie LH, Sonnenblick EH, Kaplan NM et al, editors: Beta-blocking agents: drugs for the heart, Orlando, New York, 1984, Grune and Stratton, Inc.

122. O'Rourke MF: Cardiogenic shock following myocardial infarction, Heart Lung 3:353, 1974.

123. Ortho Multi Center Transplant Study Group: A randomized clinical trial of OFT3 monoclonal antibody for acute rejection of cadaveric neural transplants, N Engl J Med 313:337, 1985.

124. Painain GA et al: Cardiac transplantation: indications, procurement, operation and management, Heart Lung 14:484, 1985.

125. Parsonnet V et al: A revised code for pacemaker identification: pacemaker study group, Circulation 64:60A, 1981.

126. Patrick ML, Woods SL, Cravel RF et al: Medical-surgical nursing: pathophysiology concepts, Philadelphia, 1986, JB Lippincott Co.

127. Perez MM and Pintos Diaz G: Arteriosclerosis obliterans of the lower limbs, Cardiovasc Rev and Reports 4:1357, 1983.

128. Perloff JK: Clinical recognition of congenital heart disease, ed 3, Philadelphia, 1987, WB Saunders.

129. Perloff JK: Physical examination of the heart and circulation, Philadelphia, 1982, WB Saunders.

130. Perloff JK, Child JS, and Edwards JE: New guidelines for the clinical diagnosis of mitral valve prolapse,

131. Perry AG and Potter PA: Shock: comprehensive nursing management, St Louis, 1983, The CV Mosby Co.

132. Pottage A: Clinical profiles of new class I antiarrhythmic agents—Tocainide, Mexiletene, Encainide, Flecainide and Lorcainide, Am J Cardiol 52:24C, 1983.

133. Pratt CM and Roberts R: Chronic beta blockade therapy in patients after myocardial infarction, Am J Cardiol 52:661, 1983.

134. Rahimtoola SH: Surgery for infective endocarditis, Crit Care Q, 4:51, 1981.
135. Rahimtoola SH et al: Consensus statement of the conference on the state of the art of electrophysiologic testing in the diagnosis and treatments of patients with cardiac arrhythmias, Circulation (suppl III):3, 1987.
136. Rao AK and TIMI Investigators: Thrombolysis in myocardial infarction trial (phase I): effect of intravenous tissue plasminogen activator and streptokinase on plasma fibrinogen and the fibrinolytic system, Circulation 72(111): 416, 1985.
137. Reid CL et al: Infective endocarditis: improved diagnosis and treatment, Curr Probl Cardiol 10:6, 1985.
138. Rentrop KP et al: Effects of intracoronary streptokinase and intracoronary nitroglycerin infusion on coronary angiographic patterns and mortality in patients with acute myocardial infarction, N Engl J Med 311:1457, 1984.
139. Roberts B: Balloon angioplasty in the treatment of peripheral vascular disease, J Cardiovasc Surg 23:225-228, 1982.
140. Roden DM and Woosley RL: Pharmacology and clinical use of Encainide, Internal Med Spec, April 1987.
141. Rogu EF, Amuchastegui LM, Lopez Morillos MA et al: Beneficial effects of Timolol on infarct size and late ventricular tachycardia in patients with acute myocardial infarction, Circulation, 76(3):610, September 1987.
142. Rosenbaum MD et al: Clinical efficacy of amiodarone as an antiarrhythmic agent, Am J Cardiol 38:934, 1976.
143. Rosenberg L, Kaufman DW, and Helmrich SP: Myocardial infarction in women under 50 years of age, JAMA 253:2965, 1985.
144. Ryan W, Engler R, Lewinter M et al: Efficacy of a new oral agent (Tocainide) in the acute treatment of refractory ventricular arrhythmias, Am J Cardiol 43:285, 1979.
145. Saunderson RG and Kurth CL: The cardiac patient, ed 2, Philadelphia, 1983, WB Saunders Co.
146. Savage DD, Garrison RJ, and Devereux RB: Mitral valve prolapse in the general population: epidemiologic features—the Framingham Study, Am Heart J 106:571, 1983.
147. Sawaya J, Muyais S, and Armenian H: Early diagnosis of pericarditis in acute myocardial infarction, Am Heart J 100:144, 1980.
148. Schneider RE, Trolich ED, and Messerli FH: Pathophysiology of hypertension in the elderly, Cardiol Clin 4:235, 1986.
149. Schneider JR: Effects of caffeine ingestion on heart rate, blood pressure, and myocardial oxygen consumption, and cardiac rhythm in acute myocardial infarction patients, Heart Lung 16:167, 1987.
150. Scott AK, Rigby JW, Webster J et al: Atenolol and Metoprolol once daily in hypertension, Br Med J 284:1514, 1982.
151. Seidel HM, Ball JW, Dains JE et al: Mosby's guide to physical examination, St Louis, 1987, The CV Mosby Co.
152. Shabetai R: Cardiomyopathy: how far have we come in 25 years, how far yet to go? J Am Coll Cardiol 1:252-63, 1983.
153. Shah PK, Abdulla A, Pichler M et al: Effects of nitroprusside-induced reduction of elevated preload and afterload on global and regional ventricular function in acute myocardial infarction, Am Heart J 105(4):531, April 1983.
154. Sheehy SB and Barber JM: Emergency nursing: principles and practices, ed 2, St Louis, 1985, The CV Mosby Co.
155. Shellock FG and Reidinger MS: Reproducibility and accuracy of using room temperature vs ice temperature for thermodilution cardiac output determination, Heart Lung 12:175, 1983.
156. Silva J: Anaerobic infections, Heart Lung 5:406, 1976.
157. Silver D and Stubbs DH: Venous thrombosis, pulmonary embolism, and the post phlebitis syndrome. In Miller and Roon, editors: Diagnosis and management of peripheral vascular disease, Menlo Park, CA, 1982, Addison-Wesley Publishing Co, Inc.
158. Singh BN, Collett JT, and Chew C: New perspectives in the pharmacologic therapy of cardiac arrhythmias, Prog Cardiovasc Dis 22:243, 1980.
159. Singh BN and Hauswirth O: Comparative mechanisms of action of antiarrhythmic drugs, Am Heart J 87:367, 1974.
160. Singh S: Systemic hypertension. In Kaye D and Rose, editors: Fundamentals of internal medicine, St Louis, 1982, The CV Mosby Co.
161. Sleight P: Beta blockade early in acute myocardial infarction, Am J Cardiol 60:6A, July 1987.
162. Smith PK, Holman WL, and Cox JL: Surgical treatment of supraventricular tachyarrhythmias, Surg Clin North Am 65:553, 1985.
163. Sobel BE: Fibrinolysis and activators of plasminogen, Heart Lung 16:776, 1987.
164. Spittell JA: Office and bedside diagnosis of occlusive arterial disease, Curr Probl Cardiol 7:(2) May 1983.
165. Spodic DH: Acute pericardial disease, Heart Lung 14:599, 1985.
166. Stoddart JC: Gram-negative infections in the ICU, Crit Care Med 2:17, 1974.
167. Subcommittee on Definition and Prevalence of the 1984 Joint National Committee: Hypertension prevalence and status of awareness, treatment, and control in the United States, Hypertension 7:457, 1985.
168. Swearingen PL, Sommers MS, and Miller K: Manual of critical care: applying nursing diagnoses to adult critical illness, St Louis, 1988, The CV Mosby Co.
169. Thelan L, Urden L, and Davie J: Textbook of critical care nursing: diagnosis and management, St Louis, 1990, The CV Mosby Co.
169a. Thibodeau GA: Anatomy and physiology, ed 13, St Louis, 1990, The CV Mosby Co.
170. Thompson DA: Cardiovascular assessment: guide for nurses and other health professionals, St Louis, 1981, The CV Mosby Co.
171. Thompson JM, McFarland GK, Hirsch JE et al: Mosby's manual of clinical nursing, ed 2, St Louis, 1989, The CV Mosby Co.
172. Tilkian AG and Daily EK: Cardiovascular procedures: diagnostic techniques and therapeutic procedures, St Louis, 1986, The CV Mosby Co.
173. Tilkian SM, Conover MB, and Tilkian A: Clinical implications of laboratory tests, St Louis, 1983, The CV Mosby Co.
174. TIMI Study Groups: The thrombolysis in myocardial infarction (TIMI) trial: phase I findings, N Engl J Med 312:932, 1985.
175. Topol EJ: Clinical use of streptokinase and urokinase therapy for acute myocardial infarction, Heart Lung 16:760, 1987.
176. Tucker S and Canobbio M et al: Patient care standards, ed 4, St Louis, 1988, The CV Mosby Co.
177. Tyndall A: A nursing perspective of the invasive electrophysiologic approach to treatment of ventricular arrhythmias, Heart Lung 12:620, 1983.
178. Underhill S et al: Cardiac nursing, ed 2, Philadelphia, 1989, JB Lippincott Co.
179. Urban N: Integrating hemodynamic parameters with clinical decision making, Crit Care Nurs 6:48, 1986.
180. Vandebelt RJ et al: Cardiology: a clini-

cal approach, Chicago, 1979, Year Book Medical Publishers, Inc.

181. Verstraete M et al: Randomized trial of intravenous streptokinase tissue-type plasminogen activator versus intravenous streptokinase in acute myocardial infarction, Lancet, 1:842, 1985.

182. Reference deleted in page proof.

183. Wagner MM: Pathophysiology related to peripheral vascular disease, Nurs Clin North Am 21:195, 1986.

184. Warbinek E and Wyness MA: Designing nursing care for patients with peripheral arterial occlusive disease, Part I, Cardiovasc Nurs 22:1, 1986.

185. Warbinek E and Wyness MA: Peripheral arterial occlusive disease: Nursing assessment and standard care plans, Part II, Cardiovasc Nurs 22:6, March—April 1986.

186. Warth DC, King ME, Cohen JM et al: Prevalence of mitral valve prolapse in normal children, J Am Coll Cardiol 5:1173, 1985.

187. Watson JE: The National Cholesterol Education Program: the role of nursing, J Cardiovasc Nurs 24:13, May—June 1988.

188. Wetstein L, Landymore RW, and Herre JM: Current status of surgery for ventricular arrhythmias, Surg Clin North Am 65:571, 1985.

189. Whitman GR and Hicks LE: Major nursing diagnosis following cardiac transplantation, J Cardiovasc Nurs 2:1, 1988.

190. Wilson CM, Allen JD, and Adgey AA: Death and damage after multiple DC countershocks, Br Heart J 53:99, 1985.

191. Wilson RF and Wilson FA: Sepsis. In Kinney MR et al, editors: AACN's Clinical Reference for Critical Care Nurses, New York, 1981, McGraw-Hill Inc.

192. Winslow EH: Cardiovascular consequences of bedrest, Heart Lung 14:236, 1985.

193. Winston TR, Henly WS, and Geis RC: Surgery for peripheral vascular disease, AORN J 33:849, 1981.

194. Wirsing P, Andriopoulous A, and Botticher R: Arterial embolectomies in the upper extremity after acute occlusion, J Cardiovasc Surg 24:40, 1983.

195. Wit AL and Rosen MR: Pathophysiologic mechanisms of cardiac arrhythmias, Am Heart J 106:798, 1983.

196. Wynne J and Braunwald E: The cardiomyopathies and myocarditis. In Braunwald, editor: Heart disease: a textbook of cardiovascular medicine, WB Saunders Co.

197. Yasue H, Touyame M, Kato H et al: Prinzmetal's variant form of angina as a manifestation of alpha adrenergic receptor-mediated coronary artery spasm: documentation of coronary arteriography, Am Heart J 91:148, 1976.

Index

CARDIOVASCULAR YELLOW PAGES

ORGANIZATIONS AND AGENCIES

American Association of Critical Care Nurses (AACN)
One Civic Plaza, Suite 330
Newport Beach, CA 92660
714/644-9310

American Heart Association
National Center
7320 Greenville Ave.
Dallas, TX 75231
214/373-6300   (For general public)

The Coronary Club
Cleveland Clinic Education Foundation
9500 Euclid Ave., Ste. E4-15
Cleveland, OH 44195
216/444-3690   (For general public)

Council of Cardiovascular Nurses
American Heart Association
7320 Greenville Ave.
Dallas, TX 75231
214/373-6300

Medic Alert Foundation
P.O. Box 1009
Turlock, CA 95381-1009
209/668-3333   (For general public)

The Mended Hearts, Inc.
7320 Greenville Ave.
Dallas, TX 75231
214/373-6300   (For general public)

High Blood Pressure Information Center
4733 Bethesda Ave., Ste. 530
Bethesda, MD 20814
301/951-3260   (For general public)

National Heart, Lung, and Blood Institute
National Institutes of Health
9000 Rockville Pike
Building 31, Room 4A21
Bethesda, MD 20892
301/496-4236   (For general public)

ORGAN DONATIONS

The Living Bank
4545 Post Oak Place, Ste. 315
Houston, TX 77027
713/528-2971   800/528-2971
(For physicians and medical personnel only)

North American Transplant Coordinators Organization (NATCO)
P.O. Box 15384
Lenexa, KS 66215
913/492-3600   (For health professionals)

United Network for Organ Sharing
National Organ Procurement and Transplantation Network
1100 Boulders Pkwy., Ste. 500
P.O. Box 13770
Richmond, VA 23225
800/24-DONOR (For public education, media, and health professionals)

FREE MATERIALS AVAILABLE ABOUT CARDIOVASCULAR DISORDERS

American Heart Association
Box DIR
7320 Greenville Ave.
Dallas, TX 75231
214/373-6300

After a heart attack, 20 pages
E is for exercise, 8 pages
Facts about stroke, 4 pages
High blood pressure, 4 pages
Nutrition labeling, 8 pages

High Blood Pressure Information Center
4733 Bethesda Ave., Ste. 530
Bethesda, MD 20814
301/951-3260

Blacks and high blood pressure, 8 pages
High blood pressure and what you can do about it, 32 pages
High blood pressure: things you and your family should know, Brochure, English and Spanish
Questions about weight, salt, and high blood pressure, 8 pages

National Heart, Lung and Blood Institute
National Institutes of Health
9000 Rockville Pike
Building 31, Room 4A21
Bethesda, MD 20892
301/496-4236

Heart attacks, 20 pages
Facts about exercise: how to get started, fact sheet
Facts about exercise: what is fact and what is fiction, fact sheet
Facts about exercise: sample exercise program, fact sheet
Healthy heart handbook for women, 31 pages